TALES FROM AN ANCIENT MARATHONER

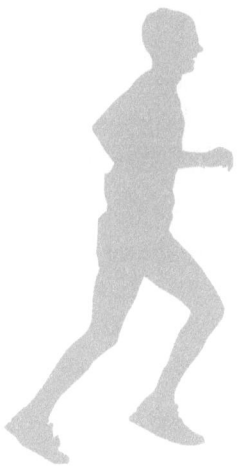

GREG WILSON

Published in Australia by Sid Harta Books & Print Pty Ltd,
ABN: 34632585293
23 Stirling Crescent, Glen Waverley, Victoria 3150 Australia
Telephone: +61 3 9560 9920, Facsimile: +61 3 9545 1742
E-mail: author@sidharta.com.au

First published in Australia 2024
This edition published 2024
Copyright © Greg Wilson 2024
Cover design, typesetting: WorkingType (www.workingtype.com.au)

The right of Greg Wilson to be identified as the
Author of the Work has been asserted in accordance with the
Copyright, Designs and Patents Act 1988.

All rights reserved. No part of this publication may be reproduced, stored in a retrieval system, or transmitted, in any form or by any means without the prior written permission of the publisher, nor be otherwise circulated in any form of binding or cover other than that in which it is published and without a similar condition being imposed on the subsequent purchaser.

ISBN: 978-1-7638601-7-9

ABOUT THE AUTHOR

Greg Wilson is a first time author aged 71, who resides in the beautiful Macedon Ranges region of central Victoria, Australia. Leaving school early, soon led to a 20 year career in the Australian Army, spent serving throughout Eastern Australia, with Active Service in Vietnam. Much more knowledge was acquired during his service and as this was the pre-computer era, prolific reading and regular diary keeping, laid the basis for his autobiography.

He is an accomplished distance runner with a marathon career which has spanned fifty years. Most recent has been the pursuit of Australian Age Group Records including those held by "folk legend" Cliff Young.

IF, BY RUDYARD KIPLING

If you can keep your head when all about you
    Are losing theirs and blaming it on you,
If you can trust yourself when all men doubt you,
    But make allowance for their doubting too;
If you can wait and not be tired by waiting,
    Or being lied about, don't deal in lies,
Or being hated, don't give way to hating,
    And yet don't look too good, nor talk too wise:

If you can dream—and not make dreams your master;
    If you can think—and not make thoughts your aim;
If you can meet with Triumph and Disaster
    And treat those two impostors just the same;
If you can bear to hear the truth you've spoken
    Twisted by knaves to make a trap for fools,
Or watch the things you gave your life to, broken,
    And stoop and build 'em up with worn-out tools:

If you can make one heap of all your winnings
    And risk it on one turn of pitch-and-toss,
And lose, and start again at your beginnings
    And never breathe a word about your loss;
If you can force your heart and nerve and sinew
    To serve your turn long after they are gone,
And so hold on when there is nothing in you
    Except the Will which says to them: 'Hold on!'

If you can talk with crowds and keep your virtue,
    Or walk with Kings—nor lose the common touch,
If neither foes nor loving friends can hurt you,
    If all men count with you, but none too much;
If you can fill the unforgiving minute
    With sixty seconds' worth of distance run,
Yours is the Earth and everything that's in it,
    And—which is more—you'll be a Man, my son!

DEDICATION

As the years roll on, many of the people who have enriched my life are no longer with us, but it is fitting to mention them here along with those thankfully still enjoying life.

There were runners and cyclists who brightened my early days with their world-class performances.

Names such as Herb Elliot, John Landy, Abebe Bikila, Ron Clarke and Derek Clayton, Bill Emmerton, George Purdon, Barry Waddell and Sid Patterson. No doubt their deeds shaped the path of my future sporting life.

The Army ensured that I grew up fast, as did serving with the legendary veterans of the Australian Army Training Team – Vietnam. John Nolan, Bruno Cabone, Roy Chamberlain and Don Targett with whom I shared youth and sport.

Two Army members influenced me the most, being Graham Moon, a champion orienteer, and Alan Batchelor, Army athletics veteran star and leader of the XXXX Army Around Australia Relay.

Townsville (Nth Qld) was where I commenced and grew as a runner and a person. Many of the friends I made there still remain in my life today. Foremost was local running legend Peter Lahiff who was both a close friend and a fine example of how to live your life.

Thanks also to Sandy with whom I shared thirty years of love and companionship and our children Daniel and Kimberley.

My post-Army years at Toolangi where great training mates Wally Butler and Brian Simmons and their wives provided solid competition and warm companionship. To enter the world of ultra running and team up with the world's greatest in Yiannis Kouros was an experience to treasure.

It was remarkable with my niece Rae Harvey's help to discover and enjoy an extended paternal family of Dennis and Margaret Tonks and Jack Chivers and their descendants.

In my latest 'running reincarnation' I have reunited with Townsville friends including foundation TRR members Peter Lahiff, David Wharton and Bob Down. Meeting local Macedon Ranges trail and road runners was vital to me continuing in the sport as was competition with Victorian Masters Athletics.

My amigos, Yassine Belaabed and Les Williams, continue to inspire with performances up to and into their seventies. With Yassine, I had the pleasure of meeting a Veteran running legend in John Gilmour, who was so inspirational in proceeding from a WWII Prisoner of War to be the greatest Masters runner in the world.

Finally to my Townsville mates, Peter Lahiff and John Nuttall. The knowledge that they held AURA Australian Age Group Records for ultra running, set me on the path to achieving similar goals. This in turn has extended my healthy and interactive lifestyle for more years than I could have imagined possible.

CONTENTS

About the Author		iii
If, by Rudyard Kipling		iv
Dedication		vii
Contents		x
Preface	Mt Macedon, November 2022	1
Chapter 1	My background	3
Chapter 2	Cycling in Kyneton	19
Chapter 3	Army training	32
Chapter 4	Townsville	43
Chapter 5	Townsville to Vietnam, 1972	67
Chapter 6	Marathoner and marriage	97
Chapter 7	Townsville champ	107
Chapter 8	Civilian life	113
Chapter 9	Back in the Army	131
Chapter 10	Retiring from running	144
Chapter 11	My comeback	151
Chapter 12	The Great Otway Classic	160
Chapter 13	To Sydney	175

Chapter 14	The XXXX Army Around Australia Relay Marathon	188
Chapter 15	Orienteering in Norway	244
Chapter 16	Ultramarathons	267
Chapter 17	Easing into the next millennium	293
Chapter 18	Paradise lost	305
Chapter 19	Back to Kyneton and family	321
Chapter 20	Running as a Master	337
Chapter 21	Trail to ultra	352
Chapter 22	Running through the Covid years	370
Chapter 23	On trail and track with Christy	383
Chapter 24	Chasing the records	394
Chapter 25	Record-breaking ultramarathoner	406
Chapter 26	My reasons for running	419
Chapter 27	Pie in the sky	424
Chapter 28	A marathoner again	433
Chapter 29	Male Ultra Runner of the Year — 2023	447

PREFACE
Mt Macedon, November 2022

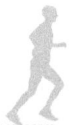

Our long Sunday run on a pleasant spring morning was the unusual genesis of this autobiography.

Although short of breath from the effort of keeping up with my younger running partner along sixteen hilly kilometres of Mt Macedon, I informed Christy that today was the eightieth birthday of Derek Clayton, Australia's former longtime holder of the world marathon record. I added that I had competed in a Victorian Country Marathon Championship that Derek won back in 1973, when I was running my second marathon aged twenty-one. Derek was at the fourteen-mile mark when he passed me, still heading out at twelve miles. Derek cruised to victory in 2 hours and 17 minutes while I was half an hour in arrears, recording 2 hours and 48 minutes.

'So, how many sub-three-hour marathons did you do? Was it five?'

'I had done thirty marathons in under three hours by the age of thirty.'

Almost accurate, and it rolls off the tongue well!

Christy replied, 'You ought to write a book.'

So, as it is the:

- sixtieth anniversary of the first Australian Army Training Team Vietnam (AATTV) members commencing Australia's involvement in the Vietnam War

- fiftieth anniversary of my posting to the AATTV

- fiftieth anniversary of the Townsville Road Runners

- fiftieth anniversary of the Victorian Masters Athletics

– it's an appropriate time for a memoir!

CHAPTER 1
My background

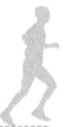

My earliest memories are of living in a very basic timber house beside the Calder Highway a few miles north of Woodend, a small town in central Victoria, Australia. The house was cold and draughty with no insulation and an earthen floor in places. The cooking stove was the only source of heating, icy tank water came from the tap and hurricane lamps provided illumination at night. There was no electricity.

The only neighbours within shouting distance were a farming family, the Boldistons, and on the Woodend side a large group of Mackaways. We had very little interaction.

In 1955, I was aged three, sharing the house with my mother Gwen, older brother Bryan and baby Lauren. My constant reminder of that time is my left hand, which has the tip of its index finger missing. The backyard contained an outside laundry copper, toilet and a chaff cutter. For some reason, Bryan decided we should play doctors. As the patient, I trustingly placed my finger on the chaff cutter while he performed surgery. A swish of the sharp blade and my fingertip was gone forever!

However, I was not deposited at Woodend North by aliens. It is only in recent years that I learned of my family background. I had no father that I was aware of and my mother never spoke of her past, so a further trip back in time is necessary to provide background to my earliest scant memory.

*

Richard Tonks was born in Wolverhampton, England on Christmas Day in 1799. While still a teenager, he was apprehended following an act of larceny and sentenced to seven years' imprisonment in the British penal colony of Tasmania. He was married and his wife Elizabeth remained in England, passing away in 1854. In 1820, Richard survived a voyage on the sailing ship *Coromandel* and then served out his prison sentence at Port Arthur.

Upon being released, he turned his hand, rather successfully, to running various grog shops. In 1855 Richard married Mary Russell. By 1870 he was licensee of the Jordan Inn on the Jordan River at Black Bush near New Norfolk. On the final day of 1870, his son Jeremiah was born at this location. Later his grandson Oscar lived at Prospect House which is now a bed-and-breakfast and a historic tourist attraction in Richmond. Oscar was on the local council, as his father had been in Black Bush. Unfortunately, Oscar seemed to be less than nice. It appears he owed his father a large sum of money and therefore Jeremiah left him nothing in his will.

My paternal grandfather, Gordon (Noel), born in 1900, was a son of Oscar who also resided at Prospect House. In 1922 he married Della Tilliack from Zeehan, who came from a large family, with its own colourful history. Della's father, William, was one of five children who travelled to Tasmania in the mid 1800s. William's father had been killed during the Prussian War and his wife fled to Tasmania to ensure her children did not suffer the same fate. Gordon and Della had four children, with my father Lloyd being born at Ulverstone, Tasmania in October 1924. Sometime later, the family relocated to Stanhope in northern Victoria where Gordon built a mudbrick house and worked at share farming. The oldest boys, Lloyd and Jack, worked very hard in helping with construction of the house and were not treated kindly by their father.

In 1939, World War II broke out and Lloyd joined the Royal Australian Air Force. After training he was employed in ground defence at airfields, including at Townsville in North Queensland. He also had active service on the island of Morotai.

When the war ended in 1945, Lloyd returned to

Stanhope and joined his brother Jack in employment, including carpentry, cartage and the timber industry. When he came south, he was accompanied by a young lady whom he had met while in Townsville. Winifred Williams had family in Ayr, a sugar town an hour south of Townsville. Winifred got a job working behind the bar at the Stanhope Hotel and got together with Lloyd whenever he returned from various jobs. On one such return, he was greeted by the news that young Wini was pregnant. Apparently, he had some misgivings regarding whether he was the father and so was not keen on marriage.

Della, his formidable mother, was having none of it. She forced the 'happy' couple into marriage, which occurred at Mooroopna in Victoria in June 1946. Unbelievably, the next day she put Winifred on the train and the new bride was returned to her family at Ayr, without a husband, but at least the new baby would have a father's name. Sometime after his brief encounter with marital bliss, Lloyd travelled to New Zealand. While in Auckland, he developed a romance with a young local girl named Gwen Harvey. As a youngster, Gwen had had ambitions to be a scientist and worked as a laboratory assistant at an ice cream factory. She enjoyed cycling around the hills of New Zealand's North Island and had climbed to the top of a nearby volcano.

One thing led to another, and sixteen-year-old Gwen

also became pregnant. Permission was granted by Gwen's divorced parents for her under-age marriage to Lloyd. The pertinent information that Lloyd was already married to Winifred does not seem to have been raised.

The young, engaged couple moved in together, living in the Auckland suburb of Inglewood. On 6 August 1949, my older brother was born in Auckland and named Bryan Alan Tudor Harvey.

There was no mention of a father on the birth certificate. Around this time, Gwen's mother, Dorothy, burned the family home down and committed suicide by walking out into the icy waters of Auckland harbour.

My mother's early life and background were a closed book. All I know is that her mother, Dorothy Grose, married Reginald Sethbridge Harvey. Gwen had a younger sister, Nola, and an aunt in Rhodesia, Africa, her mother's former homeland.

Lloyd and Gwen moved back to Australia and lived for a while in Edinburgh Rd, Mt Evelyn, a suburb to the east of Melbourne. Lloyd resumed working and playing with his brother Jack and the two were as 'thick as thieves'. A family anecdote has the young men leaving a pub after six o'clock closing and trying to work out how to get home. A nearby motorbike was borrowed and ridden to their block in Mt Evelyn. In their inebriated state, they decided to bury their 'borrowed' transport on the block!

In the early 1950s, Lloyd was working as a carpenter and

travelling to various jobs. He would take Gwen and baby Bryan along and if there was no onsite accommodation, they would live in his big, black Oldsmobile.

One such job was the renovation of the hospital in the small, south-western New South Wales town of Lockhart. A complication was that Gwen was heavily pregnant, but the bonus was the nearby hospital. On 9 June 1952, I arrived in the world as a New South Welshman, born in the Lockhart Hospital. I arrived in the world the same year as Queen Elizabeth was crowned.

I know little else of my father's brief life, except that he was involved in the construction of Dookie Agricultural College in central Victoria. He and Jack also worked driving trucks and felling trees in the forests around Orbost in far eastern Victoria. The earliest photo of me is in the backyard at the Mt Evelyn block.

My young sister Lauren was born on 3 March 1954. Sometime before or after her birth, Lloyd and Gwen separated. Lloyd was living in the Melbourne suburb of Blackburn and Gwen moved with two young boys and a newborn, to Woodend North, more than an hour up the Calder Highway, north-west of Melbourne.

What life was like can only be imagined. In the days before pensions, the only income would have been child endowment. No vehicle, no support and miles from the nearest shop. Somehow the young family survived, with the unfortunate exception of baby Lauren who passed away early in 1956, having lived less than two years. The cause of death was bronchopneumonia, no doubt due to the family's dire living conditions. Lauren's death certificate continued the tradition of 'convenient rewriting of history'. Lauren's father was listed as Lloyd Harvey and her mother as Gwen Bridge; the latter seems to be borrowed from Gwen's father's middle name of Sethbridge.

Six months later in another world, Lloyd Tonks had decided not to attend a Collingwood football match. Instead, he spent the Saturday afternoon in the pub at Box Hill. Upon leaving, he attempted to cross busy Whitehorse Road and was struck by a passing vehicle and passed away at age thirty-one.

*

There are many gaps in my childhood memories of Woodend, but I hope they suffice to give insight into that period of my life.

It seems that Gwen found a way out of her accommodation and financial dilemma. She placed or responded to a 'lonely hearts' advertisement in the rural newspaper, *The Weekly Times*. The result was that Gwen, Bryan and I moved into Woodend and resided there with a widower who had relocated from distant Warrnambool. Don Wilson was accompanied by his three boys, Brian,

Glen and Wayne, the latter two being of a similar age to my brother and me.

We rented the caretaker's cottage located just inside the main gate of the Woodend Cemetery, in Buckland Street. It was another old wooden building, dark and draughty, but a step up from the Woodend North house. The major improvement was a supply of electricity and linoleum that covered the floorboards.

A couple of name changes were considered necessary. Bryan had a name change to Garth, and we both adopted the surname Wilson in place of Harvey, our mother's maiden name. Don had a job working at nearby Shirley Park Stud Farm where racehorses were bred. It was owned by Hilton Nicholas, the son of the man who invented the pain medication, Aspro.

We had a large backyard which included a vegetable patch, a woodshed, an outside laundry and a 'long-drop' toilet. There were no internal fences, so the games played by four boys soon overflowed into the rows of gravestones. An old cow named Brindle was obtained to provide a regular supply of milk. Sometimes the cow escaped her chain and made a meal of floral arrangements on nearby graves.

It snowed regularly during winter in Woodend, as it is located near Mt Macedon, a high peak of the Great Dividing Range. Gwen and Don obviously found a way to keep warm, as over the next few years, we five boys were joined by a young sister, Donne, born on 15 May 1957, and brother Warrick, born on 23 February 1959.

As the family now had a breadwinner, living conditions should have been improved, but they were still very basic. Working for the minimum wage and supporting seven children didn't allow for much in the way of luxuries. This was in no way helped by Don's inclination to drink heavily, smoke cigarettes and gamble on racehorses. I was not aware of Gwen having these habits before her 1956 marriage to Don, but she had no problem joining in.

Gwen didn't seem to have a broad range of culinary skills but did enough to keep the large horde alive. Chops, stew, black pudding, liver, brains and tripe, along with boiled cabbage and squash, are foods that still turn my stomach. Fish and chips, various sandwiches and cups of tea were a bit more palatable. Entertainment was listening to the ABC on an old wireless and spending time outside playing various games. There was probably no time for love and affection from parents, and perhaps no inclination either. If the inhabitants became unruly, order was restored with a belt or electric jug cord freely applied to limbs.

There were various pets over the years. Storm was a Lavender Mere Scotch Collie who spent his days chasing cars through the fence; the postman was fortunate to have a gate in between. Cats, budgies, canaries, parrots, guinea pigs and rabbits added to the menagerie.

Ours was the residence nearest to the historic brick

and bluestone building of Woodend State School, as it was just across from our backyard. The school is on a hillside above a park and the Five Mile Creek. In 1956 the school population had a boost as three Wilson boys commenced their local schooling. A year later, Wayne and I began our formal education as 'preps'. At the start of each day, we would assemble and listen to the strains of *God Save The Queen* before trooping up the steps and into our compact classrooms, with well-worn desks, fountain pens, inkwells, lessons up on the blackboard and teachers imparting knowledge. It must have appealed to me, as I managed to win a book prize every year as the top student in my class. In these frugal post-World War II years, crates of small milk bottles were provided for students as an important supplement to their home nutrition. All too often, the bottles had been sitting in the sun all morning – the congealed milk was nauseating.

At the lowest point where the school grounds met the Calder Highway, a graded gravel rectangle served a variety of sports. Perhaps not the best surface for football and cricket, but I cannot use that as an excuse for not excelling. I was the smallest boy in the school and not keen on being upended onto the gravel surface.

Attending school allowed us to make some friends, and the occasional visit to their homes was a pleasant change from life in the Wilson household. Our usual playmates were members of the Gladman family who lived in nearby Dickens Street. They were a similarly large family of limited means.

Once I learned to read, I was a frequent visitor to the local library. This was my major recreational activity. There was no money for such luxuries as bicycles or tennis racquets. I went everywhere by foot and that included many hours roaming the Woodend Golf Course. Finding lost golf balls and reselling them to passing golfers was a handy supplement to rarely seen pocket money. I would also find soft drink bottles and return them to the milk bar for the refundable deposit.

Memories from my later primary school years include my first athletics competition. One afternoon students were herded down to the nearby Five Mile Creek Park. There we participated in a very short sprint where I finished second to a big red-headed kid named John Griffin. Most of the Wilson boys joined the Woodend Scouts, who gathered at a log cabin hall one evening a week. We played games and were taught some useful skills, like camping and living in the bush.

Nearby Mt Macedon had a firebreak running straight down its flank, below which Woodend was located. One evening we Scouts were taken to the top of the firebreak and let out, with instructions to proceed by foot back to the Scout Hall as fast as we could. I had never been on the mountain before and all I knew was that Woodend was down there somewhere! Anyway, I must have done something right as I arrived in solitary splendour well before the sun set.

During our years at Woodend Primary, my stepfather changed his employment. His new job was working at a Kyneton foundry called Ajax Pumps, the commute to work being nine miles. He purchased an old car, which was big and black. One weekend we all piled in and were taken for an outing in the Cobaw Range to the east of Kyneton. That was my first remembered outing by motor vehicle. Other trips were not so memorable. On weekends he would take us to supposedly closed hotels where he would get drunk, while his young passengers waited in the car.

Another trip was my first by train, when Gwen took some of us to Melbourne for a shopping trip and we had lunch at the Coles Cafeteria. A couple of times a year I would attend race meetings at Hanging Rock and Woodend and sell newspapers to the racegoers. Perhaps this was the catalyst for my lifelong interest in horse racing. I recall the Melbourne Cup being broadcast over the speakers at school and a New Zealand raider named Hi Jinks winning at long odds. I also listened as our old radio at home described the action of the trotters competing in the annual Inter Dominion series.

It was in Woodend that I remember attending my first visit to the picture theatre in High Street. It was a Walt Disney production called *Old Yeller*. A wholesome family movie was followed by a cold, dark walk past the pitch-black of the cypress trees near school. Heading for our cemetery house, it was rather scary hearing the possum calls as we scurried past.

Television had been invented, but it took some time to arrive in Australia. At first, curious residents would go to stand outside a shop window and enjoy the novelty of this new form of entertainment. After a period and due to the wonders of hire purchase, we spent evenings crowded around the set. Viewing was in black and white and generally cowboys and Indians or Robin Hood. The *Tarax Show* with Happy Hammond and regular Walt Disney shows increased our knowledge of the broader world around us.

In the early 1960s, our heads were spinning with the news that Russia had sent a Sputnik satellite into orbit around the Earth. The era of space travel was launched. Meanwhile in Woodend life was about to take a turn for the worse.

I guess the call went up: 'Where's Mum?' The house was searched and it was discovered that Garth's room, entered off the front verandah, was locked. With a bunch of family grouped around, the door was forced open. There on the bed was Gwen, and there was blood everywhere. Life must have gotten too much for her and she'd slashed her wrists. An ambulance arrived and took her away.

I have no idea who worked out the next few weeks of living arrangements for the family. I was taken in by a Mrs Killeen who lived on the Calder Highway on the south side of Woodend. She was very kind, and I received the best care in my life to date. I just enjoyed my time there and had no idea what the others were up to.

All too soon, it was back to the cemetery house. Gwen was back, pale, uncommunicative and with large bandages on her wrists. Life continued, but I doubt it was 'happy families'. I presume my home life was affecting my school studies and social interaction. I recall my Grade Five teacher grabbing me and attempting to 'shake me out of it'. Miss Milne was lovely, but I was sure she hadn't had a childhood like mine and just didn't understand. Another vivid memory was a group of us boys being chased out of the house and around the yard by Don, who was wielding an axe.

In 1964, I commenced secondary schooling at Kyneton High School. Kyneton was a larger town and the school catered for students from all around the district. We had to catch a bus for the return journey. Dick Lee was our bus driver, and he owned the slowest bus ever seen. It was so clapped out that it had trouble ascending the dual hills between the Campaspe River and Kyneton. We were envious of other student commuters who enjoyed big, modern, Organ's buses.

One enjoyable aspect of the bus commute was listening to music over the bus's speakers. During my brief stay at Mrs Killeen's, I had begun corresponding with a penpal in America. He was from California and mentioned that nearby Berkeley University had a great new singing duo called Tom and Jerry. Imagine my surprise when they changed their name to Simon and Garfunkel and their hit *Sounds of Silence* was played on my school bus.

As I was barely a teenager, I was not too involved with the 'pop culture' of the swinging sixties. However, with older brothers I soon became aware of such groups as The Beatles, The Rolling Stones and our own Easybeats. I spent Saturday mornings listening to the playing of the Top 40 hits as they counted down to number one.

Kyneton High is an historic building with a front verandah supported by imposing columns. The administrative and teachers' areas were across the front, with classrooms in wings along each side. In the centre of the U-shape was an assembly hall. A few demountable classrooms were added further down the hill as the number of students grew. There were basketball courts and down near the saleyards some sports grounds.

I did not flourish at Kyneton High School. It was perhaps my difficult home life, or leaving my safe little group of familiar faces at Woodend. I recall a science teacher who excelled in keeping control and terrifying his students. Imparting knowledge seemed a secondary consideration. As for mathematics, that was a total world of mystery. I could not see any use for these equations, and it was never explained well enough for me to grasp.

My eldest stepbrother Brian had left school and the

family home earlier. Garth had been a prefect during my early secondary years, but he soon left to begin his working career at Kyneton Drycleaners. He moved into a flat at the rear of the High St business. Glen and Wayne were in other classes, and I didn't have much in common with them anyway.

I was interested in various sports and an early trip to Gisborne to meet players from the top Victorian Football League club, Essendon, saw me become a lifelong supporter. In athletics it seemed that Australians were world-class. John Landy's battles with Roger Bannister and the four-minute-mile race were enthralling. He was soon followed by a young Western Australian named Herb Elliot, who was unbeatable at his chosen distance of the mile and 1500 metres. Newspaper headlines one day had an Australian called Bill Emmerton running the length of Death Valley (125 miles) in the USA and surviving. I thought it remarkable, apart from, 'Why the hell would you want to do that!'

CHAPTER 2
Cycling in Kyneton

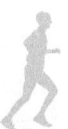

About 1965, Gwen left the cemetery house and moved with Donne, Warrick and me into the small flat that was Garth's accommodation behind Kyneton Drycleaners in High St. I don't know why the split occurred, but factors including Don's alcoholism and Gwen's mental illness no doubt contributed. No explanation was ever given.

The flat was solid bluestone and very dark, as the northern wall had no windows, being the back wall of the dry-cleaning shop. It also had two-storey buildings on each side and so felt very enclosed. My first experience of urban living was quite a change from the wide, open spaces of Woodend. My school commute was now a five-minute walk up High St.

Much of my leisure time was spent at the local swimming pool, diving, swimming or working on a suntan. I was not selected for team sports at high school, but when I reached Form 3, I found a sport that I was competitive in. Unfortunately, my career as a cross-country athlete lasted for only two events – a five-mile course from the school down to the Campaspe River, following it around the town on a muddy track to the racecourse and Barkly Square, and completing a loop through the back streets and back to the school. I was second to Glen Jacobs, with the top ten qualifying to represent Kyneton High at an inter-school cross-country event held in Castlemaine. I had the flu when it came time to compete at Castlemaine and the only Kyneton teammate I beat home was Glen Jacobs! I never had a chance to redeem myself as I had left school before the next year's event was held.

In these postwar years, many children were expected to leave school and enter the workforce as soon as they were legally allowed at age fifteen. This was certainly the case in the Wilson family, as no emphasis was put on the value of an education beyond the basics. The only way I could have continued through to a tertiary education was if I had earned a scholarship. In any case, my grades had slipped in arithmetic and mathematics, so I was no longer an 'egghead!'

I was still at school in 1966 when decimal currency was introduced into Australia in February. By June, after my birthday, I was off to join the workforce. It happened that one of Kyneton's major employers, the John Brown Knitwear sock factory, was right across the road from home. I soon had a position there as a knitting machinist. What can I say? It was routine and boring, but I was bringing home a pay packet.

Geoff Cordy was a workmate and a member of the Kyneton Amateur Cycling Club (now Macedon Ranges Cycling Club). He soon had me convinced to come along and try cycling as a sport. Now that I could afford it, I acquired a racing bike and soon joined in training rides and competition with a dozen local enthusiasts. Most of the cycle events were handicaps, which allowed all competitors the opportunity to have a win. No doubt the handicapper would also give a liberal start to young newcomers to encourage them. An advantage of being a beginner is having more scope for improvement than more experienced riders.

Taking the previous paragraph into account, I had never ridden a bike during my childhood. I joined in midwinter when the club was conducting its road race program. No doubt I had a few training rides before entering a race.

My second race was from Kyneton to Tylden return and provided my first ever victory in a sporting event. At fifteen years, I was a Juvenile cyclist and in open events would have raced against my own age group. In club races, we were often all in together, as numbers were small and it made conducting events simpler. Age and ability disparities were offset by having handicap races.

Another youngster, Jim Martin, was also having his

second ride and had a decent limit mark of six minutes in front of scratch (the back mark). I gave him two minutes start but nearing the finish, I had gathered him in as we rode away from the other outmarkers. Jim then had a mechanical issue and retired, leaving me to ride in alone. As I crossed the line, I was totally unaware that a mob of sheep on the loose had caused the finish line to be moved a mile closer. I wasn't even off my bike when the peloton of back markers crossed the line only eleven seconds behind. A very lucky victory!

A few weeks later the event was a fourteen-mile loop of Black Hill and Green Hill on the northern outskirts of Kyneton. With a generous start of 4 mins 30 secs from scratchman Ron Frazer, I overcame a strong crosswind and again tasted victory in front of my co-marker, Andrew Grady. I rode it in thirty-six minutes and so had 2 mins 30 secs to spare on third-placed Ron Frazer (34 minutes). I was quite enjoying my new sporting career but thought that the handicapper would not be so generous in future.

Meanwhile back in the real world, it seems that Don Wilson and Gwen had reconciled and for a brief time, our large family was crammed into Garth's rented flat. That situation was untenable and Garth, no doubt with a sigh of relief, saw us all move out to a rented miner's cottage in Hutton Street, on the western edge of Kyneton, where the end of the street became a gravel cul-de-sac as it met the bank of the Campaspe River.

With the coming of spring, it was time for the track cycling season, which in Kyneton was conducted at the local showgrounds in Mollison Street. The track had a gravel surface with no banking and circumnavigated the local football oval. I had enjoyed competing in road races, but this was a whole new ball game. Races were short, sharp and dangerous!

On the rare occasion that a junior race was held, I noticed that the handicapper had been watching. In a one-mile race, I was on scratch and gave away starts of up to 400 yards. John Robinson, who became Kyneton's top local junior when I later rode with the seniors, had 260 yards start on me.

Sometimes there was the opportunity to compete against riders of the same age from other Victorian country clubs. These events were often held in nearby towns in conjunction with professional athletics events. The surface was invariably the local football oval where the grass tracks were flat and slippery. Go too fast around the corner and you were off your bike and nursing abrasions, mulling over what could have been.

One such meeting was held in 1968 at nearby Lancefield. With riders from half a dozen central Victorian clubs attending, it was a good chance to discover what level we Kyneton riders were at. In my heat, I was handicapped on 10 yards and giving away 150 yards over two laps to the limit rider. I would have to ride really fast to make up that leeway. I did just that – until my wheel slid sideways and down I went.

The only rider with a tougher mark than mine was Neville Dellar from Maryborough. In the other heat, he gave 160 yards away to the winner, Kyneton's John Robinson. Surely the six-lap scratch race would be easier, as we all competed from the same mark. My fellow back markers, John Linaker (from Ballarat) and Neville, filled the first placings. I have no idea where I fitted in against these boys, as I fell off again!

There was a similar event held over three laps of the Sebastopol velodrome in Ballarat, a proper cycling track with banked corners. I was handicapped on ten yards along with Shane Landy (from Bendigo) who in future years became a top professional cyclist. I am not aware of being competitive, but at least the banking allowed me to stay on my bike.

Our senior riders, in particular cousins Ron and Kevin Frazer and Jeff Brown, did a great job of organising and carting us youngsters to events all over Victoria. The colour and atmosphere of these professional athletics carnivals provided a whole new level of excitement and sporting interest. Without their help, we would have been in own little world of events at the Kyneton showgrounds.

Kyneton had one fine professional athletics sprinter, Lloyd Stringer. As we rode training laps around the local track, Lloyd would often be practising his sprint technique on a track he mowed along the football field. I am not sure how successful Lloyd was, but he is renowned for placing second in the 120-yard Bendigo Gift on four occasions.

Employment at the sock factory wasn't fulfilling and after a year I left and decided to see what life was like in the big city. I took my racing bike on the train to suburban Brunswick and rented a room with some of the Mackaway family, who had been our neighbours in my early days at Woodend North. I obtained a job as a laboratory assistant at the Victorian College of Pharmacy in nearby Royal Parade, Parkville. I commuted on my bike and was enjoying the change of employment, but it ended all too soon. I soon worked out that my hosts were not the type of people I wanted to share a house with; they must have been bad to have me heading back to Hutton Street. After a couple of weeks, I gathered there was criminal activity going on and so I headed back to Kyneton with my tail between my legs.

I got a job alongside Garth as a presser at Kyneton Drycleaners. I quite enjoyed learning some new skills and putting them into practice. Still, for me a job was just a method of getting a wage to pay my board and continue my sporting interests.

The Kyneton cyclists also formed a basketball team called the Cyclones. I joined them in a district competition which took place on weeknights at the old drill hall in Market Street. At five feet seven inches tall, basketball was an unlikely sport for me to participate in successfully; I think it was very much a second sport for the other cyclists too, However, we had a secret weapon.

The local police sergeant's son, Brian Meehan, was not a cyclist, but he was the star of our team. All we had to do was make up the numbers and get the ball to Brian. He would regularly amass seventy per cent of our score and is the only reason a bunch of bike riders won a basketball premiership.

The cycling club conducted a points aggregate during the track season, to encourage riders to turn up often and race hard. In my first year as a fifteen-year-old Juvenile, I won the senior track aggregate. No doubt my encouraging handicap mark assisted, but I was pleased with the achievement in my first season of riding.

My second season was during the summer of 1968. One local meeting was held in temperatures of over one hundred degrees. During the afternoon I contested three events. I won the half-mile handicap and then came second to Kevin Frazer in the one-mile handicap. In the scratch race, with no handicap start, I came second to our track champion Ron Frazer.

In that year's club championships, the title was taken by Woodend's Russell Poletti, as Ron Frazer had the misfortune to fall during the second of three deciding events. I was now a sixteen-year-old Junior and managed two seconds and a third for an overall second in the championship.

A twenty-lap point score race was held and I swapped turns with Jeff Brown as we lapped all the other riders. He was a clear winner and I was happy to ride his coat-tails for second place. I was still a novice but was pleased to be able to compete with my older clubmates.

I must have missed a few races along the way, due to my ambition to go fast outweighing my ability to keep my bike upright on the treacherous Kyneton gravel track. In one fall, my elbow guard was torn off and I received a deep laceration to the right elbow. As soon as it was better, I was back on the track. Unbelievably, a spectator walked out onto the track and, crash, down I went again. My recently repaired elbow was torn to ribbons again. Off to the doctor to receive the news that there was nothing left to sew up. I had a course of antibiotics to subdue the infection caused by all the chunks of embedded gravel. I then had a period of recuperation while my flesh 'granulated' back into a functioning elbow.

As Juveniles, there were Shane Landy, Neville Dellar, John Linaker and I with a gap of 100-metres handicap out to the other country riders. No doubt there were as many fine riders in the city, but we seldom competed down there. I was about to find life a bit tougher as a Junior, riding in open events against more senior riders.

One memorable trip was to the Warragul Velodrome for the Country Victorian Championships. I had been entered in the sprint; however, my mentors neglected to explain the tactics that were involved. In all my races, I rode as fast as I could and that suited my opponents just fine. They sat on my pace-making and surged past me in the finishing straight. Later we trekked down to Geelong where I was in the time trial at my first Victorian Championships. This was more my go – ride solo as fast as you can for a number of laps. Flopped again! Not near fast enough. I began to think I was better suited to road races where endurance and determination were more important than raw speed. All the same, in my second and final year as a Kyneton track cyclist, I narrowly defeated Geoff Cordy to again win the club's senior track aggregate.

On New Year's Day, we had races at the annual Maryborough Highland Gathering. Again, I was taken with the atmosphere as pipes and drums played and top professional runners competed. In the C Grade scratch race, I managed third place behind Lance Dixon, a friend of mine from the city. Lance possessed similar ability to me, but he was bred to be a champion. Both his parents had been Australian cycling champions.

In 1969 as a sixteen-year-old, I joined my Kyneton clubmates in riding some of Victoria's open road races. First, there were a couple of combine races which featured our top Central Victorian riders. In a forty-eight-mile loop from Maryborough, from my liberal handicap and riding solo, I was first over the line at the Newstead and Maldon intermediate sprints before my race ended with a flat tyre.

Chapter 2 Cycling in Kyneton

Our local combine was a Tylden loop, consisting of four laps that totalled forty miles. I won the first three lap prizes before, this time, succumbing to cramp in the final lap. I also rode in the classic Bendigo to Charlton over sixty-five miles. I completed the course and the next day, back in Kyneton, came third in our thirty-mile scratch race.

(As a child of the 'pre-decimal era', it will become obvious that I continue to refer to the Imperial measurement of miles for my training right into the 1980s. It was maintained in order to compare the progression of my workload over the years, and I hope it does not cause confusion now, as most of my races were over metric distances.)

Considering that I had very little training and zero knowledge of cycling tactics and essential nutrition, my next event was a memorable step into the unknown. In midwinter, I rode off second limit in the open road race from Dandenong to Wonthaggi. The event covered a hilly eighty-nine miles and the field contained many of Victoria's elite senior road riders. I rode away from my co-markers after just a few kilometres as I felt they were riding too slowly. Pretty soon I caught the limit markers and went straight on by. I was now solo, in front of 160 mainly superior riders who were intent on chasing me down. I continued to do what I had learned back at Kyneton and rode as fast as I could, as far as I could.

The remainder of the race is just a blur. I had no idea

how many opponents caught and passed me, or when it happened. I remember it was snowing as I rode through Leongatha, and I was exhausted, as I had taken no food and very little fluids to sustain myself. It was freezing and hypothermia was a real danger, not that I knew anything about that.

Still I rode on, no doubt very slowly, and eventually crossed the finish line in Wonthaggi. On completion I was in a daze and had to be lifted off my bike. Later I found that I had finished last of forty riders who managed to survive the course. I was out there for three hours longer than the winner, an Olympian named Greg Minne. Though I finished last, I consoled myself with the fact that I had defeated 120 much more experienced riders who had pulled out.

That last placing remains as perhaps my finest cycling achievement. It was a lesson in how to not tackle an endurance cycling event, but also a demonstration that if you have enough determination, you can get there. My final race before the next phase of my life was a club race at Spring Hill, which I managed to win.

I was not happy with the junior wages I was receiving for working hard at Kyneton Drycleaners. Living with my dysfunctional blended family down in Hutton Street also weighed on my mind. Having seen advertisements for Army enlistment which spruiked 'full adult wages at seventeen', I approached my boss, Lionel Trickey, for a wage increase. I pointed out that I could get full adult wages elsewhere. The response was negative, so I began the process of applying to join the Australian Army. Later when I was due to leave, Lionel came back with a pay offer. My response was, 'No, thanks, you are too late.'

CHAPTER 3
Army training

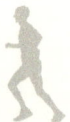

My decision to become a member of the Australian Army was multi-faceted. Compared to living with my family, there was the attraction of full adult wages at age seventeen, the lever of my current workplace wages being improving upon and a perceived improved lifestyle, but there was also the likelihood of being 'called up' for national service in the near future.

The Vietnam War was on the news most nights and there were many protests regarding Australia's involvement and the national service scheme. The thought of being trained to kill people and facing an enemy who wanted to kill me never crossed my mind; as a young civilian, I had no idea of what my chosen career would involve.

As soon as I turned seventeen in June 1969, I attended a defence recruiting centre in Bourke Street, Melbourne. I completed application forms and was given further appointments to complete medical, psychological and academic testing. With my family background and limited secondary schooling, I was barely hopeful of passing the tests.

In July I was informed that I had been successful in my application for enlistment. I again travelled to Melbourne where I joined a group of young men in signing my enlistment papers and taking an oath of allegiance. In for a penny, in for a pound – I signed up for six years instead of three.

All the Army members I met during the recruitment process were positive, helpful and friendly. If required to stay in the city overnight, there was a pleasant hotel at nearby St Kilda Junction. Good food, clean sheets, a warm fire and a television had me wishing I could stay longer.

In August, two months after my seventeenth birthday, I again travelled to Bourke Street, but this time it was a one-way trip. I joined a group of fellow recruits, and we boarded a bus for the long trip to Kapooka in southern New South Wales.

After four hours travelling north on the Hume Highway and the Olympic Way (now the Olympic Highway), we turned up a side road and passed through a set of imposing stone columns on which we read 'Blamey Barracks Kapooka'. They were set in the rolling plains of the Australian bush. The buildings we saw were spread over quite a distance. There were barrack blocks, large mess and administration buildings, parade grounds and flag poles.

The bus rolled to a halt and our whole world changed in an instant. We were yelled at, formed into lines, and pushed and pulled in all directions. No doubt the staff of the 1st Recruit Training Battalion had a system and a plan for us; to me it was a bewildering rush of harassment and bullying. It was best to just shut up and do as they commanded. Anyone who asked questions or queried orders was confronted by a very loud and angry non-commissioned officer (NCO).

All our new uniforms and equipment were carried to the upper floor of a barrack block that was to be our home for the next twelve weeks. The rooms had a partition with two beds on each side. Suddenly you had a new family numbering about thirty, four of them in your bedroom, and one you had no privacy from. Too bad if you were incompatible! My new family was titled 18 Platoon, C Company.

As it commenced, so it continued. As new recruits in the Australian Army, we formed lines, marched around as best we could and were equipped with the necessities of life. We received haircuts; the rule seemed to be that the longer your hair was when you sat down, the shorter it was upon standing again. Orders were constantly given on where to go and what to do. There was always an aggressive NCO around to see they were obeyed promptly.

Chapter 3 Army training

I could truncate this segment by just stating what I still feel today: recruit training at 1RTB was the most mentally and physically exhausting experience of my life. I found it horrendous and, indeed, it was designed to have exactly that effect. The system was devised to test your limits of endurance and see if you would crack. We would be loudly awoken before dawn and made to line up on the freezing parade ground, with only our bed sheet for a covering. What followed was intense activity all day and most evenings, and by the time you prepared for the next morning, it was 10 pm.

Meals were partaken by marching as a group to an enormous mess hall and joining a long line. Usually there was barely enough time to eat before we had to march off to our next lesson. For the first six weeks, we were confined to the base and the only day off was Sunday.

One of the important skills we had to perfect was drill. Learning how to follow commands, keeping in step and working as a team during increasingly complicated manoeuvres was deemed essential. If you stuffed up, you were embarrassed before your platoon mates and made to do remedial training. I could see little sense in it and the lessons were just endured.

We were all issued with self-loading rifles (SLRs) complete with magazines, drill rounds (bullets) and bayonets. They were big and heavy, and as I weighed fifty-seven kilograms, they were no fun to lug around.

Once we had a bit of proficiency at drill, then we were introduced to rifle drill. I found that even worse!

Rifles had to be kept secure, and it was just about the end of your career if you forgot. We endlessly practised stripping and assembling our SLRs and laying out the components so you could even reassemble them in the dark. Fingers would be red raw from constant loading and unloading of drill rounds (bullets) into the magazines as rapidly as possible.

Then came long days on the rifle range where it was essential to shoot straight. This was difficult for me; I was so 'weedy' that after a few seconds of raising and aiming the SLR, it began waving all over the place. They decided that I couldn't see well enough to hit the distant targets and I had a morning of 'freedom' visiting the optometrist at nearby Wagga Wagga. Soon after, I had my first set of spectacles to cure my short-sightedness. They sure did that; however, my scores on the rifle range did not magically improve.

There were many other subjects and lessons we had to absorb and retain while under mental and physical duress. There was always the threat of being 'back-squadded' should you not achieve a satisfactory standard. The unbearable thought of spending an extra period here, with one of the more recent intakes, was a huge incentive.

There were breakdowns, both physical and mental, a quiet removal and a gap in the ranks while the remainder just got on with it. Some recruits slept with a bayonet under their pillows for protection against perceived threats. If I suffer from any post-traumatic stress, it would stem from this introduction to life as a soldier and not from active service.

Physical training (PT) was another important aspect of the training. Most days saw us learning new skills and developing our fitness. How difficult this was depended a lot on your condition on arrival. As a cyclist, my heart and lung capacity and perhaps my leg muscles had a head start, but gymnastic and upper body strength were a work in progress.

Every now and then, we were required to race each other down to the front gate of Blamey Barracks and return. This run of a few kilometres was the one area in which I stood out from the crowd. I consistently finished well clear of my platoon mates, and it was a small ray of light to be above average in one element of the program.

Towards the end of our twelve weeks of training, we had a period learning how to conduct ourselves while living in the bush. Accommodation was an inflatable air mattress protected from the elements by a 'hutchie' (small tarpaulin) suspended from branches or sticks. This was followed by a twenty-mile route march while carrying a full pack, webbing and rifle. During this activity, my fitness advantage was offset by the testing weight we had to carry. I found it difficult just to lift the load, let alone carry it for that distance. I endured the march in the same manner as I endured all of recruit training – one foot in front of the other – and eventually I reached the finish.

That finish being our March Out Parade. I should have had a sense of satisfaction, but all I can recall is relief that it was finally over. During our training we had had the opportunity to request which Corps of the Army we preferred to serve in. After what I had experienced, I was certain that I preferred to join a service corps instead of one of the fighting arms. My rationale was that an 'arm' would involve more of the same and I couldn't stand that. I preferred to work in an area that served a useful purpose and achieved an aim. For no particular reason, I chose the Royal Australian Army Medical Corps (RAAMC), and training in that area was my next challenge.

With a few others bound for RAAMC, I had a long train journey from tiny Kapooka railway station to Melbourne, then out to the furthest north-eastern suburb of Lilydale. Darkness was settling in as we boarded a tiny diesel rail motor and travelled through the Yarra Valley to our terminus at the small town of Healesville.

We were met by the Duty Driver for a five-minute drive out of town to the School of Army Health (SOAH). A few minutes' march downhill and we arrived at some rows of tents. The tents were partitioned down the middle using wardrobes and contained only a bed and desk. Arriving in the dark, it was only over the following days we began to learn about our new training camp.

What a contrast to Kapooka! The SOAH was spread over a few acres, running down an isolated ridgeline. It was separated from Healesville by farmland, and on the eastern flank it bordered the Sir Colin Mackenzie Fauna Sanctuary.

At the high northern end of the ridge were the married staff quarters, a transport compound and many wooden outbuildings, serving as accommodation, work and storage spaces. In the centre, accessed through sandstone gates and a winding, tree-lined driveway was Summerleigh Lodge. This grand sprawling wooden building had a former life as a tourist destination, and I had never seen anything like it. A covered front verandah led to a large ballroom, which now served as the Officers' Mess. The NCOs and other ranks had a mess in other parts of the building. A rabbit-warren of rooms set over two storeys served as staff accommodation. The Sergeants' Mess was across a narrow road and clung to the ridge where it fell away steeply to where the Sanctuary was located. The building and surrounds were maintained to a very high standard as befitted a grand old lady. A swimming pool and gardens led down to tennis courts and then classrooms and a parade ground. Finally, past the quartermaster store and well apart from any grandeur, were our two rows of tented accommodation for trainees. The ablutions (toilet, shower and laundry) were a walk through the cold night air and were quite spartan.

There was still marching, inspections and saluting, but it was down a few levels from recruit training and not difficult now that we were trained. We were there for a three-week course designed to turn us into medical orderlies. A medical orderly is the bottom of the rank and skills pyramid in RAAMC. We numbered about twenty and had a few course staff to direct our every move. There were also other instructors charged with keeping our military skills fresh while imparting medical knowledge important for our future employment. The course involved gaining an understanding of how the human body functioned. Then there were a few first aid skills designed to enable us to keep it functioning. I had no idea of the background of my fellow trainees, only that they were generally older and most had more education than I had been able to achieve. It was a whole new world to me as I had no medical knowledge. I just put my head down and quietly tried to learn the lessons.

Ironically, one of my memories of that course was a joke told by one of the instructors, Sergeant Peter Hulsing. He had a broad Dutch accent and at times it was difficult to understand. He was enlightening us on the subject of shock and how this medical condition could kill people. We were informed that one person was bitten by a horse and died of shock. I am not sure if he expected a bunch of confused looks and mutters of 'What the hell?' Anyway, it was sometime later that we discovered he had actually said 'bitten by a hose', and thinking it was a snake, the individual died of shock. Makes a bit more sense, but the joke lost a little impact during translation.

We had weekends off, so I decided to take a train back to Kyneton to collect my racing bike; for some reason I decided it would be a good idea to ride back to Healesville. It was some 120 kilometres across an undulating Great Dividing Range in hot weather, and it turned out an epic undertaking, considering I hadn't seen my bike for four months. I was just over halfway, climbing back up the range from Whittlesea to Kinglake West when I realised how difficult a task I had set myself. I made it before dark, but it's a journey I have not tried to repeat.

When we marched out of the SOAH, I did so having attained top student marks, so I guess I absorbed more than just the snake joke. Again, we had been asked to nominate our preferred trades within the Corps and the location we would prefer to be posted to upon completion of training. I had no keen desire or knowledge of employment in the medical field and nominated for posting as a storeman. As for location, I requested my home state and those nearby.

One out of two had to do. I was to become a storeman but in a place called Townsville in north Queensland.

Following a leave break at Kyneton, I took the train to Melbourne and changed at Spencer Street Station for an epic train trip to my new home.

It took all of five days, which included overnight stops in Melbourne, Sydney and Brisbane. By the time I reached Brisbane, I was only halfway and the *Sunlander* train seemed to crawl up the endless east coast of Queensland with many stops in the middle of nowhere.

CHAPTER 4
Townsville

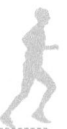

The *Sunlander* finally arrived at Townsville railway station and with equal measures of relief and anticipation, I stepped out into a blast of tropical heat and humidity. All my possessions were in a canvas Army bag and I was wheeling my racing bike. I located a movement control officer (MCO) who arranged for a vehicle to transport me to my new home, a place called 4 Camp Hospital.

The railway station was located at the inland end of Flinders Street, the main street of Townsville, between Ross Creek and Castle Hill. Through the shopping strip and then over a ridgeline, we dropped into a pleasant beachside suburb called North Ward. It seemed a most attractive place, with the towering red cliff of Castle Hill on one side and Cleveland Bay, stretching out to nearby Magnetic Island, on the other.

After half a lap of the hill, we turned north along Rowes

Bay and left the suburbs, proceeding five miles along the foreshore. Now the countryside was uninhabited flat scrubland on the left and miles of sandy beach, blue ocean and Magnetic Island on the right. After ten minutes we entered a small suburb called Pallarenda and where the road ended, there was a gate and signage, indicating a quarantine station and 4 Camp Hospital. I am not sure of what I expected my first Army posting to look like, but certainly this was not it. The Many Peaks Range follows the northern coastline for some miles before terminating at Cape Pallarenda. There is just room for an access road, which winds through the coastal scrub of a compact basin, surrounded by hills on three sides. To the east is a deserted beach with a jetty and not far across the water, a remote area of Magnetic Island.

On arrival, I was welcomed and given a familiarisation tour of the unit. The entry road passed a few outbuildings and the quarantine caretaker's residence, before completing a semicircle and ending just below a few long, spartan buildings, comprised of steel and entire walls of glass louvres. These were the quartermaster store (Q store), administration and, above them, a hospital ward. A compact parade ground and flag poles indicated the presence of a military establishment.

The other nearby buildings were half a dozen historic 'Queenslanders' of light timber construction, and some were high set. All had wraparound verandahs that were enclosed by insect screens. Covered walkways and ramps joined all these buildings, which allowed movement around the camp without getting soaked by the regular wet season downpours.

With my head spinning, I was guided to one of the Queenslanders and into a large room containing six bed spaces. I got myself settled in and with a smile on my face, prepared to enjoy the next phase of my life.

I soon discovered the next building was a vital hub, as it contained the Officers' and Sergeants' Mess, and the Other Ranks' Mess, as well as dining rooms for all staff. An ascending ramp led to a kitchen building from where we collected our food before proceeding back to the dining room. Other walkways led to the nurses' quarters and transport, and a final Queenslander served as a treatment room, doctor's office and isolation ward.

Nursing staff worked on a rotating twenty-four-hour roster to ensure optimum patient care. Most of the administration and service staff completed an eight-hour day and then after hours the camp was left as the responsibility of the duty officer and NCO. The unit was run by an Officer Commanding (OC), Captain Dave Schaper, and the Company Sergeant Major (CSM), Robert Allen.

My initial employment was in the Q store where I worked as a storeman under the regimental quartermaster sergeant (RQMS), Staff Sergeant Joe Christensen, and Corporal Terry Betterman. I arrived wearing summer dress and was soon issued the tropical adaption of this uniform, some pairs of polyester dress shorts. Our job was to order in supplies and to issue them out as requested. I only worked for a brief period in the Q store at 4 Camp Hospital when I realised that I didn't find it fulfilling. For reasons that escape me, I requested that I be allowed to work in the ward as a medical orderly, with a view to changing my employment from storeman to medical assistant.

For recreation, I soon located the nearest local cycling club and commenced track racing at the Garbutt velodrome in suburban Garbutt with the Rising Sun Amateur Wheelers. I would ride from Pallarenda to the track and then compete, before riding home again. I also competed with Royals at their velodrome, which was a further five miles across Ross River, near the abattoir.

Having come from a cycling club in a small Victorian town, I had no idea how competitive I would be riding on a proper track with a completely new group of senior and junior riders. I needn't have worried, as I was regularly in the results during my brief career. At Rising Sun, I was soon placed second in a five-mile motor-paced race and later combined with young local talent Lloyd Nowland to set a junior tandem record at our only attempt.

One meeting at Royals, I tasted victory in both events I contested, and was considered a most promising junior. However, after a few meetings, my career as a cyclist in

Townsville ground to a halt, although with no conscious decision on my part.

There were plenty of sporting events down south that I would read about and I absorbed both cycling and athletic results with great interest. I was not involved in running, but during the previous couple of years, a great Melbourne runner named Derek Clayton had set an incredible world record for the marathon, breaking 2 hrs 10 mins for the distance. The only person who could challenge it was Derek himself, who in 1969 at Fukuoka in Japan broke 2 hrs 9 mins and set a world record that would stand for a dozen years.

At the same time, the brother of the Essendon Football Club captain was making a name for himself at shorter distances. Ron Clarke went on to set numerous world records over a variety of long distances. This world domination of distance running followed on from those Australian middle-distance runners such as John Landy and Herb Elliot during my childhood. I am certain these well-publicised exploits influenced my future sporting choices.

Meanwhile, though I had left school two years ago and was now in the Army, my peer group of sports achievers were still completing secondary schooling. At Kyneton High School, the 800 yards and one mile were won in record time by Robert Falloon, who defeated Andrew Grady, my former cycling co-marker from Kyneton.

I occasionally wonder how I would have measured up

in the Australian Schoolboys' Cycling Championship, had I been able to complete my full education. It would have been pretty competitive. The winner was a youngster from northern Tasmania called Danny Clark. He later travelled to Europe as a professional cyclist and over many years won more six-day cycling races than anyone in history.

In Townsville, I joined some of my new workmates in playing Australian Rules football with Hermit Park Football Club and basketball with a team called the Whirlwinds. My ability at these ball sports was quite limited, but they were fun group sports activities. There were many national servicemen serving in Townsville and they included some fine sportsmen. Hermit Park must have had a great recruiter, as they were redolent with Army sporting talent and won every match during the 1970 season. One of the lesser lights, battling away with me in the reserve team, was a driver from my unit called Doug Boldiston. He went to Kyneton High School with my older brother and was my next-door neighbour when I was a toddler living at Woodend North. What a small world!

At some stage, I must have told the OC that I could run a bit. The unit nominated me to run in the annual 3 Task Force Inter-Unit Athletics Championships, to be held in April at Lavarack Barracks. I had been in Townsville for three months, yet this was my first visit to the huge

Army base that stretched along the base of Mt Stuart, on the south-western outskirts of the city.

My first ever event of athletics competition was held over five kilometres on a rough grass track in the heat of a tropical afternoon. I knew nothing about training and just turned up and ran. For most of the distance, I stayed on the leader's shoulder until the later stages where I dropped off the pace. The five-kilometre race was won by forty-two-year-old Officer Commanding (OC) of the District Support Unit at Lavarack, Major Jim Goodwin, with a time of 18 mins 45 secs, with me at age seventeen some hundred yards behind. I also placed second in the 1500 metres, beaten by three yards in 4 mins 48 secs.

Two weeks later, the qualified placegetters represented 3 Task Force against the visiting Brisbane team in the Queensland Inter-Area Championships, again held at Lavarack Barracks. Once again, I clung on behind Jim Goodwin as we left the opposition in the rear. With a couple of laps to go, I was still feeling okay, so I went past, and by the time we finished, I was a hundred yards clear of Jim. I improved my time to 18 mins 30 secs. I also won the 1500 metres by a hundred yards, in an improved time of 4 mins 30 secs.

To cap a remarkable upward spiral, before April was over, I travelled all the way to the RAAF Base at Amberly in south-western Queensland and represented the Army in the Queensland Inter-Service Championships. I won both distance running events, completing the one-mile race in 5 mins 2 secs. I then followed up with victory in the three-mile in a record 17 mins 21 secs.

Fair to say that I was pleasantly surprised, to progress from being a cyclist to being the best distance runner of the Australian Defence Force in Queensland in just one month. Even so, I was not awarded the accolade of Best Athlete at the meeting. It seems that Graham Taylor, the Queensland decathlon champion, was completing his national service and won almost every other event on the program! He also won five events at the Queensland Athletics Championships in 1970.

Back in the obscurity of being an untrained medic and working in the ward as a nurse, I picked up the skills necessary to do my job. After a few months of this, I was about to be sent to 1 Military Hospital in Brisbane to belatedly complete my Medical Assistant course. My brief career as a storeman ended with a whimper when I attended a trade test at the Ordnance Unit at Lavarack. I had received no training or information on how to pass this test, and so of course I failed it.

Before leaving for three months at Yeronga in suburban Brisbane, I had become a registered athlete with Townsville Amateur Athletic Club. They had competition on a Friday evening on a 330-yard track at Corcoran Park in the suburb of Hermit Park. As I was no longer cycling everywhere, I purchased my first motor vehicle, a 50cc Suzuki motor scooter. I obtained my licence by riding into the Motor Registration Office and riding for a city block without falling off in sight of the testing officer. In true North Queensland style, I rode with no helmet and wearing thongs on my feet.

In the latter part of the year, I was again on the *Sunlander* for the thousand-mile journey down the coast to Brisbane and 1 Military Hospital. The hospital grounds are enclosed within a bend of the winding Brisbane River. For some reason, I decided to seek accommodation off the base and for the duration of my Medical Assistant course, I resided at nearby Rocklea.

No doubt many of my fellow trainees had some medical knowledge; however, for me it was a sharp learning curve. There were lessons on anatomy and physiology, and once we knew how the human body worked, there were myriad diseases and conditions to be diagnosed and treated. Apart from copious theory, we had regular shifts of working at nursing on the wards and gaining practical skills. In the intense limited duration of the course, we received a range of medical and nursing knowledge across a broad sphere. We absorbed first aid, ambulance work, patient evacuation and general nursing. It was also necessary to be able to diagnose many illnesses and injuries and to be able to gauge whether to treat the casualty and/or refer them to a doctor.

In my down time from this relentless learning, I located

a nearby running club called Rangers AAC. I was soon engaged in track races with a group which included the Barralet brothers, Richie Bourne, Eric Brown, Trevor Newton and Paul Circosta. My running ability seemed to be right in line with many of these runners, and enjoyable competition ensued. One weekend I made a trip with them to an inter-club meeting at the athletics headquarters of Lang Park. In the five kilometres, I ran against the Queensland State Champion, Ron Irwin, and was left well behind. I am not sure if he ran that day, but there was talk of a young kid named Gerrard Barrett who had the potential to be the best runner Queensland had seen.

Of course, there is a long journey from youthful potential to fulfilment of your dreams as an adult. Around this time, Queensland had teenagers who had set world best times for ten kilometres for their respective ages. Richie Bourne and an even younger David Wilkinson had put up outstanding performances, but that is the only time I heard of David. Perhaps he gave it away and took up cycling!

I am not sure what it says about me, that I can remember the names of all the Brisbane runners that I met briefly on a few occasions; however, I cannot recall the name of a single fellow course member that I studied and worked with for three months. To be fair, some of the runners mentioned or their reputations made an impact at later stages of my running career. During this period, I also kept an eye on the Public Schools (GPS) Championships. Richie

Bourne and, in particular, Steve Colbourne, were regular stars of schoolboy athletics in Brisbane.

So, by years' end, I had succeeded in passing my course and was a fully trained medical assistant. I had also absorbed the reality that, while I was a top runner in Townsville and in the Australian Defence Force, there were many with more ability out in the wider world. Once more, it was onto the *Sunlander* for the long haul up the coast to my unit and home at 4 Camp Hospital.

On arrival, I resumed my hospital duties, albeit with much more expertise now I had qualified. Our patients had in common that they were young and fit before acquiring an illness or sustaining an injury that required hospitalisation. They were a mixture of national servicemen (Nashos) and regular soldiers, as were the medics providing their care. We Private and Corporal Medical Assistants carried out tasks allocated by our superiors, who were civilian, qualified, state registered nurses, who entered the Army with an officer's commission in Nursing Corps (RAANC).

We did regular monitoring of a patient's condition, dispensing medications and injections and venipuncture (under supervision), physiotherapy, urine analysis, wound care and dressing changes. As there were no medical orderlies, we also provided all the meals, body and teeth cleaning, bed pans and urinals, as well as regular cleaning and polishing of the ward area.

Our roster had us regularly swapping between day and evening shifts and occasionally a complete week of night shift was performed. Night shift was pretty relaxed once the patients settled for the night; however, at dawn when you were ready for bed, there was a frantic rush to get the morning medication and Temperature, Pulse and Respiration (TPR) rounds completed in time for handover.

Our medical officers were unlike any Army officers I had encountered at this stage in my career. They were both young captains who had become doctors with the financial assistance of the Army. In return for this, upon graduation they signed up for a number of years as an Army Medical Officer. They were even less interested in military skills than I was, something I really enjoyed about them. I would encounter both Captain Peter Wilson and Captain John Wainwright again.

They made all the medical decisions and part of my job was to assist them or carry out tasks they set me. I well remember that Captain Wilson had a regular outpatient clinic where he specialised in wedge resections. Assisting in these minor operations to remove part of a patients' ingrown toenail was my introduction to the blood and gore of surgery.

Most of my workmates seemed to be Nashos who had varying levels of enthusiasm for participating in life as an Army Medic. A couple could have signed up for a further period as a commissioned officer but preferred to stay in the ranks and just get it over with. An example was qualified pharmacist Private Colin Stone, who got my attention by driving around in a white MGA sports car. Another was Private John Granata who was an optometrist.

While I had been absent down south, I had missed competing in the only non-track distance running event I was aware of in the local area. The annual Army cross-country was held on a five-and-a-half-mile course from the beach at the entry to 4 Camp Hospital to Kissing Point, Rowes Bay, the home of another Army Base called Jezzine Barracks. I was pleased to see that an Army Nasho medic called Alan Browne, from 2 Field Ambulance at Lavarack Barracks, had defeated all the gung-ho soldiers from the Arms units.

I had in mind that I would be well suited to this event, and I was motivated to attempt it this year. It was the wet season when the weather was always hot and humid, with a regular evening downpour coming as some relief. I commenced doing some running training, often a very early run along the beach before it became too hot. My first encounter with the extremes of Townville's weather came in the form of Cyclone Ada, which brought strong winds and heavy rain. I recall one day when we just sat indoors, the downpour dumped twenty-four inches of rain in twenty-four hours.

My regular Friday evening visits to Corcoran Park

resumed, and I usually won whatever distance event they were holding as the final event on the program. There was a very good runner from out of town named Bill Dodd and a hugely talented schoolboy named Steve Gannon. Occasionally they would turn up, and in events from 800 metres to 5 kilometres, I would have to settle for a minor placing.

In January 1971, a group of TAAC athletes journeyed down to the Sunshine Coast to compete in the Country Queensland Championships. It was the wet season and the Maroochydore track was submerged. Still, as runners had travelled from all over the state, the program of events proceeded.

I was placed second in both of my events. After an Under-19 1500 metres placing in 4 mins 33 secs, I backed up for the open 5000 metres where I crossed the line just behind my Townsville nemesis, Bill Dodd, in 16 mins 52 secs. On a sodden track, this was a big personal best (PB) for me.

In March I returned to the rough grass track at Lavarack Barracks for the Queensland Army Inter-Area Championships. In the 1500 metres, I ran a big PB of 4 mins 21 secs but had to settle for second behind a 1st Battalion (I RAR) national serviceman named Bernie Smith. I backed up in the 5000 metres and won clearly, in the same time that I had set for an Inter-Service record last year over the shorter three-mile distance. This year

Chapter 4 Townsville

Major Jim Goodwin was an interested onlooker, as he held the event stopwatch.

I commenced a training diary and recorded lots of long solid runs and many more rest days between them. During May, I averaged over forty miles a week and was running much more regularly.

I was still playing football and basketball. A big reason for the success of Hermit Park Australian Rules Club was their fitness advisor, Bill Caulfield. He had apparently been a professional runner and had competed at the Victorian athletics mecca, the Stawell Gift. Bill must have been keeping an eye on me, as one day he had a quiet word in my ear: 'Give this football away, son. You are a runner.' I think I already knew, but with Bill's advice ringing in my ears, I concentrated solely on running.

There was a purpose behind my build-up of training miles and that was the Queensland 10 Mile Championship, to be held in the sugar city of Bundaberg in June. For some reason, I always believed that I would perform better at long distances, so this, my first Queensland Championship, would be a test of that theory. The course took us from beachside Bargara through the tall fields of sugar cane to the Bundaberg athletics track. All I remember was that it was a long way, and it was very hot. Joe Patterson, an accomplished milkman from the Gold Coast, won clearly (56 mins) from Toowoomba's

Ross Clarke (59 mins 20 secs). I held on for third placing, recording 60 mins 15 secs.

Meanwhile back at my day job, my CSM, WO2 Robert Allen, with whom I played football at Hermit Park, called me into his office. I must have been performing well enough at my job, as I had been promoted to Lance Corporal. To my surprise, he strongly suggested that I attend a course that was necessary if a soldier wished to be considered for a posting to the Australian Army Training Team Vietnam (AATTV). He added that I would not receive a posting to the unit as it was all winding down; however, I would learn a lot and it would be good for my career.

I knew nothing about any AATTV and the CSM didn't elaborate; he just waited for my decision. I was completely unaware that a Meritorious Unit Commendation on his uniform was a clue that he had served with the AATTV. He must have been a high flyer as he seemed very young to be a warrant officer.

In the end, it was nothing to do with the Army that influenced my decision. The TAAC had a fine group of young female runners, and the best of the lot was sixteen-year-old Barbara Willis. Barbara ran the 400 and 800 metres and was the first junior Queenslander to win a medal at an Australian Championship. The same young lady was also attractive, came from a well-to-do Catholic family and was a straight-A student. We had done some great training together, been out on a few dates and I had visited her at the family home. Basically, I was head over heels in love with her, but coming from my background, I was perhaps an unsuitable match, and it was her senior year of study.

It ended before it had begun, but it took me a long time to accept the reality. My solution was a bit like the old story of a man joining the French Foreign Legion to recover from a broken heart. My 'Foreign Legion' was to accept my CSM's kind offer and dedicate my next two months to improving all aspects of my hated military skills.

So, one day after returning from Bundaberg, I packed my gear and journeyed down to Ingleburn on the outskirts of Sydney for a month's course at Infantry Centre. Here I was back doing what I hated – and I had volunteered for it! All that remains is a blur of lessons and constant activity, though not as harrowing as recruit training.

What was instilled was a basic knowledge of the military skills necessary to function adequately in a war zone. We were taught many infantry skills, being exposed to a variety of weapons and their care and use. There were also tactics, field craft, operation of radio sets and coding, how to set a Claymore mine and the calling-in of artillery support. All of this would be easier for an 'Arms' soldier who had regular exposure to all this information. In contrast, I had been serving in a very relaxed and non-military setting. My usual uniform at 4 Camp was a set of white overalls, we never saw weapons and we had one brief parade a week.

Anyway, the time passed and before I knew it, we were off to Queensland for the remainder of our training. The venue for this was even further from my comfort zone. The small town of Canungra is in the hinterland jungle, inland from the Gold Coast and well south-west of Brisbane. It is the home of the much-feared Jungle Training Centre, which has in more recent times been re-named Land Warfare Centre.

In I went with my course companions for another month of the same. We were accommodated on a cleared ridgeline in a row of four-man tents. There was much emphasis on keeping our fitness up and refining our new-found skills in a jungle environment. There were many forced marches and navigation through the hilly terrain. A few incidents that remain clear in my mind are a small example of our activities.

At the grenade range, we were seated in a concrete bunker that was exposed to the sky above, while we waited for our turn to throw a grenade. There was plenty of noise as the explosive devices were hurled as far as possible before they exploded. There would be a few activities that led to such anxiety for both the novice grenadier and his instructor. One miss-throw, or if a student was to 'freeze', then death or injury were the likely result.

My companion in the bunker was Corporal Kevin

Mulligan, the only other RAAMC member on the course. We heard an explosion even closer than usual and some loud noise above us. Chaos ensued as a tree branch fell between us, smashing the wooden stock of my SLR rifle before it landed on Kevin's lower leg. Talk about realistic training! He received a fractured tibia and fibula (lower leg), but was allowed to complete the course, though in a limited fashion.

There was also the 'Sneaker Range' where we practised patrolling through the jungle while being constantly surprised by pop-up targets that we had to rapidly aim at and hit. This was followed by crawling across a field under barbed wire obstacles while a 50-calibre machine gun was being fired just above us. A 50-calibre is a very loud and powerful weapon.

One of our final activities was to complete an obstacle course, which included going through a deep, smelly, water obstacle we had long dreaded, called the Bear Pit. Once we survived this, there was a long climb up a ladder to a platform sited high above a lake. Fully clothed and with webbing and rifle, the only choice offered was jump, or be pushed. If you were unable to surface and get to the shore, there were generally staff willing to perform a rescue.

Eventually, this course also came to completion, and I could return to the familiarity of my home at 4 Camp Hospital. I had passed and was totally happy if that were the last such course I ever attended, a testimony to my ability to just get through each day, knowing that all things must end.

On my arrival back up north, having not run a step for two months, it was straight back into athletics training. I managed ten sessions before my first competition, the North Queensland Championships, held at the North Star track in Townsville. My results were all I deserved, having been down south, away from the tropical heat and not training.

I managed third in a 400 metres and 800 metres before trying distances more to my liking. In the 5000 metres, I finished second to Maurice Creagh from Mount Isa in a disappointing 17 mins 33 secs. My 1500 was another second, although my time of 4 mins 27 secs was an improvement. I was disappointed, as these were events I should have been capable of winning.

A further month of training brought improved fitness, and my only defeat in local races was by star schoolboy Steve Gannon in an 800 metres. No problem, as he was very fast and I was nobody's idea of an 800-metre runner. Near the end of September, I ran a PB of 4 mins 20 secs for 1500 metres.

A week later, it was time for the Army cross-country. Most of the Townsville Army units entered teams, and civilians were also welcome in this, the only non-track run held each year in Townsville. The large units from Lavarack Barracks were always hard to beat, especially

1 RAR. The course was again set along the sand of Cleveland Bay foreshore, from Cape Pallarenda to Jezzine Barracks at Kissing Point. In the second half, we deviated through the mud and mangroves of the Town Common.

For the first three miles along the sand, I was close behind the pacesetter, a runner from 1 RAR whom I didn't know. The large field of 198 was spread out for miles behind us. After we left the beach, I assumed the lead and as I went by, the leader told me he was Andrew Grady; he asked me to let him win, as it was very important to his status back at 1 RAR. That was all the incentive I needed: I gave it everything to distance him over the final miles. I was all alone as I crossed the line in front of a large crowd at Jezzine Barracks. I had set a record of 29 mins 28 secs for the five-and-a-half-mile course. Grady was next in, followed by 1 RAR's other fine runner, Bernie Smith. Many of our 4 Camp Hospital staff were there and there were wild celebrations when it was announced that our small unit had also won the team event. I got the impression that our doctors had placed a few bets with officers from other units when visiting the Lavarack Officers' Mess and had made a killing.

On the downside, I had badly strained my calf muscle. Luckily, I had very attentive doctors to get my leg straight into an ice bucket. Being presented with a large trophy from the Brigadier had this kid from the poor side of Woodend North wondering at the momentous change of lifestyle. In another case of 'what a small world it is', Andrew Grady had just a year earlier placed second in the Kyneton High School mile race behind Robert Falloon. I had even ridden off the same mark with him in a road race with the Kyneton Cycling Club. I managed to beat him home on that occasion also and he was absent from any congratulations.

There was a big write-up in the local paper and I did an interview on the Townsville television station. Meanwhile, I had three weeks off to try to recover from my first running injury, then I had a few weeks of alternating painful runs with rest days.

During this period, I was approached to participate in a fundraiser for some new clubrooms at the Police Youth Club. The PYC had varied sportspeople in their membership but realised they needed an infusion of runners to conduct their event. The ideal recruiting ground was the recent Army cross-country. The event planned was a relay run from Cairns in Far North Queensland to Townsville.

I am not sure if I gave my leg injury any consideration, as I enthusiastically agreed to take part. The relay was scheduled for mid-November which, as the lead-in to the wet season, is way too hot and humid for distance running. By this time, I had met some local distance runners, including Peter Lahiff, Rowan Carr, Dave Wharton and Malcolm Allan. We sometimes trained together and raced at TAAC in track events.

Chapter 4 Townsville

Leading up to the Cairns–Townsville Relay, team members had some training runs at Anderson Park and a large photo of the group appeared in the Townsville *Daily Bulletin*. Although only half of the team were runners, all were fit sportsmen and this photo became a base document in the history of the yet-to-be-formed Townsville Marathon Club (now the Townsville Road Runners). It is here I met relay organiser Peter Hone and boxer Bob Down, and renewed acquaintances with Rowan Carr and fine Army runner Bernie Smith. Dave Wharton, also a boxer, was unavailable due to his final year of school exams.

On the drive to Cairns, I became aware of the sporting background of some of our PYC members. They included Ray Dennis (a boxer), Dennis McMinn and Bill Cook (gymnasts) and Dave Smith. Late inclusions were a young Mark Adams and Terry Lee who was an Army cook from my unit. Our team also included a couple of physiotherapists and drivers.

At 10am on Saturday, 13 November 1971, I shook the hand of the Mayor of Cairns and set off on the first leg of our epic journey. We had ten runners rotating and each leg was approximately thirty minutes. In the intense heat, day and night, we ran every five hours as quickly as we individually could. Levels of fitness and running ability were quite varied and after halfway, some team members were having difficulty. There seemed no hard and fast rules, so gradually those of us still going well took on more of the load by running further or doing extra legs. The following day, we formed up as a group and ran a final lap of the oval at the PYC, having set a record for the 216 miles between Cairns and Townsville, of 25 hrs 32 mins.

My calf was still giving me trouble, but as it had survived the relay, I went back to training about 40 miles a week. There were just a couple of TAAC 1500-metre events to complete the year. In one, the placings were myself and future local legends Peter Lahiff and Bob Down.

CHAPTER 5
Townsville to Vietnam, 1972

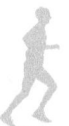

As I recall while writing fifty years later, 1972 was a huge year in my life and it warrants its own chapter. It began with my annual Christmas leave being spent down south in Kyneton. Early in the trip, I stayed with my older brother Garth, his wife Pam and newborn Laurae. As January wore on, we had a falling out and went our separate ways. I caught up with other family members and my old cycling mates.

When I had first landed in Townsville in 1970, it was in the aftermath of Cyclone Ada. While I was enjoying Victoria's summer weather, up north, Townsville was being smashed again by Severe Tropical Cyclone Althea.

Late in January, I flew back into the tropical heat of Townsville. There were many trees down around town and plenty of property damage. The most obvious was the foreshore along The Strand, where there was bad erosion and many fallen trees. I settled back in work at

4 Camp, which was saved from bad damage, nestled as it was in its semicircle of hills.

A few days after arriving, I went to Friday evening athletics at TAAC. I had a new runner to compete against, Army Engineer Captain Graham Moon. After he had given me a sound thrashing, I learned that he had a 10-mile race in fifty-six minutes to his name and was one of the top orienteers in Australia – whatever an orienteer was!

A few of us, including Dave Wharton and Bob Down, started to meet up with Graham for training runs. The weather was oppressive, and we all looked forward to the daily evening downpour for some relief. Early in February, Graham Moon went to Victoria and came second in the Australian Orienteering Team selection trials. At the same time, I was off to 3 Cavalry Regiment at Lavarack Barracks for another dreaded stint of rehashing my military skills.

Each Army promotion requires a pass in Subject A (Military Skills), Subject B (Corps specific skills, medical in my case) and Subject C (Military Law). I was sent on my Subject A and C course for promotion to Corporal; I found the constant marching while giving and receiving drill lessons very tiring and stressful. Somehow, I dragged myself to TAAC athletics on Friday evening and paced Barb Willis to a PB of 400 metres in 58.2 secs, a great run by her in those weather conditions.

Chapter 5   Townsville to Vietnam, 1972

The next week on course was even worse as I attempted to give coherent lessons on handling weapons with which I was totally unfamiliar. I was convinced I would fail this course but did not really care. I just wanted it to end so I could return to my comfortable environment at 4 Camp. Somehow, in the midst of all this effort and stress, I found time to run, and recorded a fast 4 mins 20 secs. Before returning to Lavarack Barracks, one afternoon I had a six-mile run with Graham Moon and we had a discussion regarding the formation of an orienteering and cross-country running club. I was averaging about thirty miles a week in training, and whenever Graham was in a track event, I was consigned to second place.

As my time at 3 Cavalry Regiment wore on, I gave my final lessons and managed to do enough to pass. After a fortnight, I was thoroughly over it, and though I didn't have my results, I headed back to Cape Pallarenda. I am not sure of my frame of mind at that time but the first thing I did was volunteer to go to Vietnam to serve in a Regimental Aid Post (RAP) with the AATTV.

Meanwhile, down in Brisbane, some of our young TAAC runners were putting in outstanding performances at the Queensland Championships. Barbara Willis won the Junior 400 metres and was nominated as Vice-Captain of the Queensland team for the Australian Championships. Jill Sager was also in the team, having won the Junior 200 metres and a second in the 100 metres. Barbara also won the Junior 800 metres but was disqualified before a second in the Open 400 metres. A couple of very fine runners indeed.

It was very busy at work and the wards were overflowing. Early in March, I had a week of night duty. Night duty completely throws the body clock out and it is also difficult to sleep during daylight due to the stifling heat. I had been promoted to temporary Corporal and was to be on permanent day shift in future. I had been told that I would be in charge of running the canteen which served the other ranks. This was in addition to my usual medical assistant duties.

I also had a few social outings with Jennie Christensen, the daughter of Joe, our RQMS at 4 Camp, all the while still carrying a torch for Barbara Willis.

One day, I picked up the Brisbane paper and there was a runner splashed all over the front page. Trevor Newton was one of the Rangers AAC runners with whom I ran when down in Brisbane on my Medical Assistant course. It seems he had hacked out a running track around his property boundary. Once constructed, he started running and did not stop for twenty-four hours. In doing so, he became the first Queenslander to run a hundred miles in twenty-four hours. I thought, what an amazing feat of endurance, but who would want to do such a thing?

Chapter 5 Townsville to Vietnam, 1972

During March, we had a couple more meetings regarding the formation of a distance running/orienteering club. These were usually held at Graham Moon's married quarters in suburban Vincent. I was aged nineteen but thought I was a fully formed athlete; Graham, on the other hand, was thirty and I thought him a bit 'long in the tooth'. An example of our track running exploits at TAAC follows:

800 metres:
- 1: Graham Moon, 2 mins 7 secs
- 2: Greg Wilson, 2 mins 8 secs.
- 1500 metres
- 1: Graham Moon, 4 mins 22.1 secs
- 2: Greg Wilson, 4 mins 30.4 secs.

I never defeated Graham in a track race, and I never competed against him in my more favoured road or cross-country races. I did hold on to the hope that I would keep improving as he was surely on the downhill slope from his peak. Having said that, Graham was a champion orienteer and would surely have given me a test in cross-country.

Late in March, I ran my final race against my former schoolmate, Andrew Grady. In a 1500 metres, I won easily in a solid time. Our local champions went off to Perth with the Queensland team for the Australian Athletic Championships. Meanwhile, training with Graham had me pretty fit and I prepared to join other TAAC runners on a trip to Bundaberg for the Country Queensland Championships.

While Barbara was winning bronze in the Junior Australian Championship, I finalised my training with a narrow 1500-metre victory in 4 mins 20 secs. That was up with the best I had done and augured well for my chances at Bundaberg.

On April Fool's Day, I was back for my second visit to the Bundaberg sports ground. Unfortunately, Cyclone Emily was also visiting. There was torrential rain and the track was under water; however, athletes had travelled from all over the state and the show must go on.

It was a top day of running for me, which commenced in the 800 metres. I came a distant second (2.06.8) behind Max Warmington; he was state champion and ran 1 mins 59 secs on the soggy track. I won both the 5000 metres (16 mins 41 secs) and 1500 metres (4 mins 26 secs). On both occasions, I had revenge on Mount Isa's Maurice Creagh, who had cleaned me up last year when I was unfit following my AATTV course.

I caught up with some Brisbane runners I had met previously, notably the Barralets, Steve Colbourne and Ross Clarke. Their Invitation events were washed out on the Sunday. The road north was cut by flood waters south of the 'horror stretch' and so we all spent a few days down in Brisbane, until it was passable.

Back at 4 Camp Hospital, there were a bunch of new

officers, and the relaxed early days became a distant memory. The Commanding Officer (CO), Lieutenant Colonel John Taske, was a former Medical Officer with the Special Air Service (SAS). He went through the place like a dose of salts and it became an unpleasant environment to serve in. A couple of the other officers upset me as well until I was all set to apply for a transfer. Then news came through that in July, I was to be posted to South Vietnam.

On Saturday night I went to see the movie *Doctor Zhivago* accompanied by Barbara and Jill Sager and her sprinter boyfriend, Peter Kelly. The next day was a 'runathon' at TAAC where I completed my longest run yet, covering a hundred laps or twenty-two miles. I spent a week sore and tired as my body recovered. It had become obvious that Barbara and I were not 'an item'. Later on, there was a party to which I invited Barb and she seemed reluctant. When it was over, we were over. We had been going out together for a year.

Similarly, Jill had broken up with Peter. Jill and I really got on well and kidded around about going steady. However, I was soon heading away, and we never followed it up. I often wonder what may have been.

The day after the runathon, 15 April, was scheduled to be the first event of the Townsville Marathon Club, even though it had not been officially formed. As it was, only Graham Moon, Bob Down and I turned up and the event became an eight-kilometre training run around Task Force Hill at Lavarack Barracks. At training during the week, I met Malcolm Allan for the first time. He was a handy runner with Western Districts in Adelaide before being called up. He was serving with 2 RAR.

It was then time for the TAAC Championships, and even though I was Country Queensland Champion, 'normal service' resumed. I managed to win the 400 metres in a 55.8 secs PB and the 1500 metres in 4 mins 25 secs. What about the 800 and 5000 metres? Well, Graham was in both of them! I ran a PB of 2 mins 4 secs in the 800, but still behind his 2 mins 2.5 secs. In the 5000 metres, I ran a respectable 16 mins 23 secs, equalling my PB from Bundaberg; however, this time I was thirty seconds in arrears. I left the meeting with mixed feelings. I was pleased with my performances, but as the track season was over, I was aware that they would be my final events with TAAC.

A few things happened in the final week of April. Graham organised the first orienteering event held in Townsville. It was very hot, and the event was in rugged jungle at the base of Mt Stuart. The maps used were photocopies of Army topographical maps and were difficult to read while trying to run flat out through the scrub. I think Peter Lahiff may have attended, but I felt I was there solo. I finished, confused, heat-exhausted and suffering many cuts and scratches. My only words to Graham were, 'Thanks, but never again!'

Chapter 5 Townsville to Vietnam, 1972

Around this time, the 3 Task Force Inter-Unit Championships were held at Lavarack. In the 1500 metres, Bernie Smith (1 RAR) defeated me by one second in a very respectable 4 mins 21 secs. I gained my revenge in the 5000 metres, running 17 mins 21 secs to beat him by 40 seconds.

On the last day of April, I flew out to Victoria to attend an Instructor's Course at SOAH Healesville. I seemed to be attending too many courses, but this was Medical Corps and there were few drills and weapons compared to previous courses. Nevertheless, here I was and the weather leading into winter was beautiful.

On my weekend off, I travelled to Kyneton and caught up with family. On Saturday, Rob Falloon picked me up and we travelled to Albert Park Lake to compete for Rob's South Melbourne Club. It was my longest race so far and I was pleased to finish twenty-seventh of one hundred and two starters. I ran the first lap in a solid 17 mins 30 secs with Olympic track runner Jenny Orr; after that, I let her go and continued at six minutes per mile, covering the twenty-five kilometres in 1 hr 37 mins 39 secs. I also met Jenny's brother, Robert Orr, who ran at my speed. I learned that their father was one of Australia's top Veteran runners. This year was the year when Victorian Veterans Athletic Club was formed, giving older athletes the chance to compete with similar age groups, starting at thirty-five years.

The second week of training passed quickly, and I

was pleased to be one of only six to qualify in a course numbering fifteen. There was another run, but the good weather was just a memory as winter had set in. The race was a King of the Mountains over twenty miles from sea level at Point Leo to Arthur's Seat and return. I went too hard and did an uphill ten miles in 1 hr 2 mins 30 secs, lasted only a few more miles and pulled out.

I had a couple of weeks of leave and spent some time with an ex-4 Camp Hospital friend, Paul Jensen. I also visited Kyneton again and caught up with my cycling club friends. Late in May, I went to Festival Hall in Melbourne where I attended the only concert performed in Australia by the American brother-and-sister music duet, The Carpenters. I will never forget the crystal clear and powerful singing of vocalist Karen.

On the downside, the cold and wet weather got the better of me and I came down with what I thought at the time was a heavy cold. It was influenza, but even with the flu, I joined the other South Melbourne runners for a relay from Craigieburn to Gisborne, where I ran 2.1 miles in 10 mins 51 secs. The next day I was back on a plane for a four-hour flight to Townsville. My long day finished with an evening shift.

I was informed that a run had been organised by Jim Goodwin and Graham Moon as a feature of the Townsville Pacific Festival. It was titled The King of the Castle and the course was from The Strand to the top of

Castle Hill via a steep goat track before completing the loop down the access road.

In hindsight, this is the 'one that got away'! I was still quite ill with the flu. However, they were not going to postpone the race on my behalf. Suffering nausea and dizziness, I took myself up the course, three days in a row. On one, I was accompanied by Graham Moon, Bob Down and Mike Phillips. My time was better each time, with the final attempt being 36 mins 30 secs.

On race day, I had to work a morning shift, before lining up with seventy-three starters at the waterfall on The Strand. A large crowd of spectators saw us off on a solid climb through the streets and then on to a rough and ever steepening goat track. Towards the top, there was no running, as progress was a rock scramble using hands and feet.

I must have been in second place throughout. I didn't see anyone else throughout the race, understandable as a sneak peek while on the goat track would mean falling instantly. Back on The Strand, I sprinted for the line through a blur of spectators. The first time I saw Mike Phillips was when we shook hands after the finish. His winning time for the 5.5 mile course was 34 mins 11 secs and I was a scant four seconds behind. The ever-consistent Bernie Smith filled third placing. To this day I wonder what Graham Moon would have done if he had not been busy as an organiser.

A bare week later, it was time for the Army cross-country. I guess the organisers were not going to give me a home ground advantage, as this edition was moved to Lavarack Barracks. It was ground very familiar to all Townsville soldiers, except the residents of Cape Pallarenda. The ten-kilometre course provided a fitting farewell victory for Bernie Smith, who was about to complete his national service. In a desperate sprint finish, he ran 38 mins 42 secs to pip me by two seconds, with Mike Phillips well back in third.

My posting to Vietnam was rescheduled to August. Working conditions at 4 Camp were deteriorating, as Lieutenant Colonel Taske and the nursing officers made life difficult. Still, I had some pleasant distraction during outings with Jennie Christensen.

Late in June, Graham Moon and Dave Wharton organised a team of runners to conduct a relay from Townsville to Charters Towers. It was held to celebrate the centenary of Charters Towers, which had been the second-largest city in Queensland back in the gold rush period. The strong team of eight runners – Graham Moon, Dave Wharton, me, Peter Lahiff, Bob Down, Ross Christophis, Kevin Hawke and Merv Uren – completed the eighty-five miles in 8 hrs 30 mins. This team of top runners consisted of many future foundation members of the Townsville Marathon Club. We all ran about ten miles, split into five segments. I was very satisfied to total 56 mins 50 secs and I held my form to the end. In my final leg, I ran faster than Graham, which would be the only time. I had met Peter Lahiff earlier, but he had only met Graham and Dave ten days before the relay. They were in running gear when he had dropped in to sell some insurance to Graham. Conversation turned to running and soon Peter was running a lap of Lavarack cross-country course with Dave. Yes, he could run and, bingo, he was in the team.

A few days later, I received letters containing the incorporation papers for Townsville Marathon Club (TMC) and on 3 July, I mailed them. The following Sunday, the newly formed TMC conducted its first event. It was a ten-kilometre road course in the grounds of James Cook University. There were only seven starters, and I had the honour of being first over the line.

- 1: Greg Wilson, 35 mins 48 secs
- 2: Mal Allen, 37 mins 45 secs
- 3: Dave Wharton, 40 mins 7 secs
- 4: Otto Geryge, 40 mins, 20 secs
- 5: Bob Down, 41 mins 9 secs
- 6: Mike Pugh, 41 mins 20 secs
- 7: Mike Henderson, 51 mins 28 secs.

We were lacking officials, so a stopwatch was left at the finish line; first home had the responsibility of recording all the results. After the event, I must have put the result sheet in my pocket, and when I left Townsville, it went with me.

It is only in writing this fifty years later that I notice that in four weeks, I had improved my best time for ten kilometres by almost three minutes. I was most fortunate to even be in this inaugural race as my departure from Townsville was imminent. Perhaps I should have been rated a 'frequent flyer' over the next month.

Just over a week later, I received word that I was detached to 3 Cadet Battalion for a month. I did the rounds and said goodbye to my Townsville friends in case I never saw them again. On 23 July, I boarded an RAAF Caribou aircraft and was flown south to Rockhampton on the central Queensland coast. A very slow and rough flight gave me my worst ever case of travel sickness.

I jumped in a Land Rover and was driven sixty miles north-east to Shoalwater Bay Training Area. On arrival, I found a vast tent city and discovered I was to be in charge of four medics and run a Regimental Aid Post (RAP) for 3 Cadet Battalion's annual camp. It was ten days until the cadets arrived and this time was spent on preparations, such as setting up an RAP and constructing showers and latrines.

In August, it became much busier when 400 cadets arrived and all had to have medical examinations. Then many of them became sick with a virus. I received notification that I was to attend a Physical Training Instructor's course – whatever! I remember chatting to the Physical Training Instructor (PTI) on my last trip to

Chapter 5 Townsville to Vietnam, 1972

Healesville, where Sergeant Ken Baker and I had become friends and had done a few runs together, which led to me applying for the course.

On the evening of 13 August, I was on a plane back to Townsville. Two days later, I flew down to Sydney and marched into the School of Artillery at North Head to commence a Battle PT Leaders Course. It was a disaster!

I soon realised that I did not want to be a Battle PT Leader in a battalion, but a 'normal' PTI like Ken Baker. After a day of two involving such things as rifle exercises and gymnastics, every muscle in my body was aching. It could have been the physical activities, but it was also apparent that I had picked up a dose of the flu from my cadet patients. On day three, I spent hours at the RAP before being sent to bed to recover. I was dragged out of my sick bed and abused by the course staff for wasting their time. 'You must have known you were posted to Vietnam and should not have attended the course.' What?! I was a soldier and just did what I was told when I was told. Cadet Camp – yes, sir! PT Instructors Course – yes, sir! Nowhere was there any word of a posting to a war zone. Oh, I suppose some time back I was informed that it was postponed until August. It was now August!

On the evening of 19 August, I was back in a plane and returning to Townsville to march out. The next day happened to be the second day of the North Queensland Championships. With little training and a bad dose of the flu, I ran in the 800 metres. Graham Moon was first with 2 mins 2.6 secs, with me in third (behind Maurice Creagh) in 2 mins 8 secs.

The next day was spent at Lavarack Barracks collecting some pay, having a dental check and being issued some clothing and equipment. On Tuesday, I flew again to Sydney and spent the night at the Eastern Command Personnel Depot at South Head. My head was spinning as I lay on a bed a couple of miles across the Sydney Harbour from North Head, where I had been in my sick bed four days earlier.

Three days later on 25 August 1972, I joined three companions on a Qantas flight to Singapore, arriving at 11 pm. What was left of the night we spent at a luxurious Equatorial Hotel. It was hot and humid as we returned to the airport in the morning for a two-hour flight to Saigon, the capital of South Vietnam.

At that time, Tan Son Nhut Air Base was reputed to be the busiest in the world as the civilian flights shared it with military missions. It was a strange feeling to have landed on a civil flight at an airfield teeming with military activity and then walk into a large terminal which resembled a railway station.

We had received no instructions and there was no one to meet us. The four of us sat down and thought it through. I spotted a Pan Am counter and figured they would speak English. They contacted an American provost (military police) who arranged for us to be collected by the Australian Forces. Welcome to a war zone!

Saigon seemed a ramshackle and very busy city. The city centre had some grand buildings which dated from the French Colonial era. We were accommodated at the Miramar Hotel in Tu Do Street, which was a hub of activity and the city's red-light district. My first impressions were of chaotic traffic with no discernable rules, pedestrians dicing with death to cross the road, motorbikes and little blue-and-white taxis.

Next morning, we walked around to get a feel for the place. We found some breakfast at the United Service Organization (USO), an American club for servicemen. We also ventured to the Vinh Loi Hotel, protected by a sandbag wall as it was where the Australians who worked in Saigon were accommodated. I took a lift up a few floors and walked into a room. My welcome with the first Australian I encountered was, 'Get out of here now!' I had accidently entered the Sergeants' Mess and was most certainly not welcome. On finding the correct floor, we stayed for a film and lunch.

The next day, we had a Jeep ride to the Free World Building, which was large, white and had a row of flags of the Allied nations participating in the conflict. As most Australian Forces were no longer in South Vietnam, we were supplied with everything by the US.

They provided us with documentation to show we were part of the Military Advisory Command, Vietnam (MAC-V). I was also issued with a 45-calibre pistol and an M16 automatic rifle. Then it was back to the Miramar, lunch at the USO and an evening movie at Vinh Loi. I attempted to walk back alone to the Miramar but I lost my way in the dark and did a large circle back to the Vinh Loi. On attempt two, I found my way to the USO and from there to the bustle of Tu Do Street. It was a daunting experience to be lost, wandering around a city where no one spoke English, and where the war zone dangers were a complete unknown. No mobile phones in those days!

We had been told we would be transported to our units by a Bell UH-1 Iroquois ('Huey') helicopter (chopper) as it was too dangerous to travel by road. We were collected and taken to the Free World Building before boarding the chopper at 11 am. There was a short flight to the town and base of Long Dien to pick up some rations, but once they were on board, the chopper had too much weight and we were offloaded! We were then transported by road back to Saigon and stayed the night at the Vinh Loi.

Take two! Once again off to the Free World Building and then by Land Rover to Ton Son Huit Air Base. From there, we had a flight to coastal Vung Tau on a C-130 Hercules transport plane and then a road trip in an AATTV Jeep, north to the provincial capital of Phuoc

Chapter 5 Townsville to Vietnam, 1972

Tuy Province, Ba Ria, where Headquarters (HQ) AATTV was located at Van Kiep. We had lunch and were greeted by the Commanding Officer.

That afternoon the four of us reinforcements went our separate ways. Corporal Kevin Mulligan was my companion on the grenade range when his leg was broken during training. Now he was in a Jeep with me as we headed east to the coastal fishing village of Long Hai. The nearby Long Hai hills were a notorious Viet Cong stronghold, and we kept a vigilant lookout with our M16s cocked.

Approaching Long Hai, I was dropped off at Long Hai Training Battalion (LHTB) where I was to assist Warrant Officer 2 John Nolan in teaching first aid to Cambodian troops. Kevin continued through the village to an old French fort at Long Phuoc Hai, where he was to perform similar duties.

My unit was in a large compound with high wire perimeter fences, watchtowers and lots of concrete and sandbag protection. An outer compound contained living quarters and training facilities for the visiting Cambodian (Kymer Serei) trainees. An inner compound with a further layer of protection was home for the fourteen AATTV members and the US Green Berets that we were attached to.

I was shown to a plywood-and-tin room in a row behind a concrete bunker wall. Welcome to my new home! I was introduced to some of my fellow team members, in particular my mentor John Nolan, the only other Australian Medical Assistant. There was a bit of March-In administration where I was issued with ID Cards, US Special Forces badges and a treasured Green Beret with a distinctive AATTV hat badge.

I had just turned twenty and was on my first full day in a training unit in South Vietnam. Meanwhile on the other side of the world, a fifteen-year-old Shane Gould was creating history with five gold medals at the Munich Olympic Games. I went back and forth to Van Kiep, manning a mounted machine gun on the back of our team Jeep, driven by Warrant Officer 2 Jock Clarkson. No road trips were allowed without this protection for the vehicle driver.

As I was the only Australian Corporal at Long Hai, I was at least ten years younger than my Warrant Officer teammates. The exceptions were young officers Lieutenant Ross Harvey and Lieutenant Rod Margetts. A few days before my arrival, our Company Sergeant Major (CSM), and Warrant Officers 2 Ken Dunn and Bruno Carbone had been on patrol with a Cambodian battalion near Nui Dat 2 (now known as Nui Thom) when they were ambushed by the Viet Cong. Four of the enemy were killed; this was the final contact our element of the unit had with the enemy before it ceased to function.

I commenced giving lessons, alternating half-days

with John. This involved going to classrooms or outside areas within the Cambodian compound. I would impart the lesson in English and then the Cambodian interpreter would hopefully pass on the information accurately.

On Saturday, I assisted John in setting an exam for the current battalion medics. In the afternoon, I took off out of the compound and ran right through Long Hai village to where Kevin Mulligan worked – a fruitless enterprise as he was absent on a field exercise. When I returned, a rather large Afro-American US member came up and asked me if the run was such a good idea. He pointed out the risk of getting shot and that the roads were mined. Strange the decisions you make when you are twenty and bulletproof! I took his advice and limited my exercise to inside the protection of the compound after that. I guess doing something so silly was the result of going from Australia by plane, and with little direction flying straight into a war zone. Many of the AATTV members were veterans of multiple tours to Vietnam, and as they knew the ropes, they assumed I did also.

The US Special Forces were elite troops and knew their stuff. They were also way more relaxed and enjoyed better facilities than Australian units. An example was a Saturday night at the Long Hai base club. The members of the band were brought in from the Philippines and a bunch of local young ladies were allowed onto the base to join in the fun. I could not imagine this happening in an Australian unit.

Sunday was a day off. I played basketball in the morning and during the afternoon, seven Aussies and four US members formed a soccer team and played against a team from the Taiwanese troops, who guarded the camp perimeter. Apart from losing seven to five, wrecking my shoes, then damaging my feet playing without them, a good time was had by all.

Monday, I assisted John with lectures before heading out to the rifle range with Alan Frisby to 'zero' my weapon. Perhaps we did get it firing accurately, and while it was easier to handle than a SLR, my scores were nothing to write home about.

Most days now we seemed to get a tropical downpour of rain. Being hot and wet was a nice change from just being hot. The weeks rolled by with preparation and giving lessons and some Jeep shotgun trips; reading and movies filled in spare time. On the weekend, the guards gave us a thrashing at soccer, but my toe was so painful I only watched.

In mid-September, Kevin Mulligan came up from Phuoc Tuy Training Centre and took me back for a look around. I attended Sick Parade with him and had lunch before returning for guard duty. This involved climbing up into a watchtower high above the perimeter and using a Starlight Scope (night vision apparatus), watching to see if any Viet Cong were sneaking up to attack the camp. I will admit to feeling vulnerable up there in plain sight, but it was probably quite safe as they would have needed a large force to overrun our compound. All around the jungle had been defoliated (with Agent Orange!) and it was a flat 'killing ground' right out to the Long Hai hills.

The following day, I had a trip to Van Kiep and in the afternoon, we had a rare visit from the Commanding Officer of AATTV, Brigadier Ian Geddes. There was an alert which turned out to be a false alarm but entailed sitting behind a concrete wall wearing a flak jacket and helmet for half an hour.

On Saturday, we held an exam and Voeurn, who spoke good English and became a friend, received top marks. The same trainee managed to teach me how to count in Cambodian. In the afternoon, it was good to listen to Radio Australia and catch up on the football and horse racing from back home.

The next day, I was once again manning the machine gun as an escort to Van Kiep for Ken Dunn and Graham Haupt, who were off for a spell of rest and recreation leave (R&R). I managed to get a few runs in by doing laps inside the compound and the lessons continued, among them stretcher drill and burns.

On 22 September, we were informed that we were forbidden to train of any Cambodians aged under sixteen years. There must have been adverse publicity back in

Australia and political pressure was applied. The only advisors still working were myself and John Nolan, Bruno Carbone and Alan Cleasby. A US Colonel from Forces Armeé Nationale Kymer (FANK) Headquarters arrived, and John heard that all training would cease when the final Cambodian battalion graduated on 22 November. Both Long Hai and Phuoc Tuy would close on 30 November.

On 24 November, I was awarded my South Vietnam Medal for twenty-eight days of active service in the Vietnam War. It was Sunday, and that saw another trip to Van Kiep as well as some running and weightlifting.

The following day, we had an alert at lunchtime when automatic gunfire was heard close by. We hurriedly got into flak jackets, with steel helmets on, and took shelter. The shots came from inside the Cambodian compound, only fifty metres away. It seems there were problems with pay and morale among these Cambodians. One of their platoon commanders tried to kill his Commanding Officer. There were five casualties and I rushed off to the dispensary in case the US medics needed further assistance in treating multiple casualties.

Another week of lessons and some final exams for the medics of 43 and 44 Battalions. They did very well, averaging 75 per cent, with a couple of perfect scores. Some dignitaries visited us from faraway Canberra. They had the Cambodians parade and in Long Hai alone they detected 190 soldiers aged under sixteen years. They were sent back to Cambodia without completing training so that the Australian Government could say, 'Look we are not training under-age Cambodians!' No problem that they were being returned home to fight the vicious Kymer Rouge and that our relations with our US allies were now strained. Two Cambodians from Recon Platoon were 'fragged' by a land mine; one had jaw injuries and the other lost a foot. It was still dangerous out beyond the wire.

During a couple of trips to Van Kiep, I met George Hooper and Terry Jennings who had both been on the Mobile Advisory Training Team (MATT) course with me in 1971. On Saturday evening, we attended a formal dinner at Van Kiep. There were more high-ranking officers there than I had seen in a long time. As the youngest soldier, I had the honour of being Mister Vice for the dinner. This entailed being in charge of the evening's dining activities once the 'top table' had left.

Early in October, Brigadier Geddes visited with an American Naval Rear Admiral. They totally ignored any US training but paid close attention to all AATTV advisors. John Nolan figured they might be trying to sell us to the US Navy!

I held the fort for a few days while John, accompanied by Roy Chamberlain and John Grelk, had some R&R in Bangkok, Thailand. On Sunday, Roy took me for a drive around Long Hai village. The best part of it was the hotel with a swimming pool and beach front views over the South China Sea. In mid-October, 44 Battalion left for their return to Cambodia. Lovely young people, with a French-influenced love of life. I now reflect on the hell on earth they returned to.

Towards the end of October, a peace settlement was imminent. We were informed that we would be leaving South Vietnam as soon as possible after the peace deal was signed. I worked afternoons and had a day off, lolling around the pool in Long Hai. The next day, it was back to the beach as troops were put through a water crossing exercise.

The rest of the Cambodian medics did well in their final exam. We took them into Long Hai to celebrate and in the afternoon, I helped clean the dispensary. Ken Dunn left for Van Kiep. In November with no trainees left to teach, I commenced work in the dispensary.

In the afternoon, it was a trip out to the 30-calibre machine gun range with Roy. The Aussies put on free beer, a bit wasted on non-drinker me! The celebrations continued the next day, so there were some pretty sore heads. I imagine the out-of-character celebrations were to do with the end of our involvement with the FANK training program.

For myself, it ended on 4 November as I marched out of Long Hai Training Battalion to fill the duties of running the RAP at Headquarters AATTV in Van Kiep. After I had gone, John made the following comments on LHTB: 'All uncertain, miserable. Everything being packed up. Club closed and unable to get a beer! Expect worse conditions and food has really deteriorated.'

My first days at Van Kiep started with a weekend of swimming, reading and lazing around. My accommodation was now a stretcher in a communal dormitory building. Then I rode shotgun on a Jeep trip, at first north to the site of the departed Australian Task Force at Nui Dat. The place had been thoroughly ransacked by the Vietnamese. There was no infrastructure and the location was reverting to jungle. The only proof that we were in the correct location was a long strip of tarmac that had been Luscombe Field, the airstrip.

We then travelled south back through Ba Ria and down to the large coastal city of Vung Tau. This bustling place is on a peninsula and was formerly Cap St Jacques. It had been an R&C centre for the Allied Forces and the Viet Cong! We drove to the top of 'Radar Hill' to take in the view and get some photos and then drove to the coast where we located the former Badcoe Club which had long been our R&C centre, named after Peter Badcoe, AATTV's first Victoria Cross recipient.

My month at Van Kiep was not as enjoyable as Long Hai had been. John Nolan had been great to share the workload with so I could just do my job with no interference. Now I had a bunch of higher ranks who grabbed me for whatever dirty fill-in job they could find. Early on, I had the pleasure of being on duty all day and night. We heard the Melbourne Cup, won by a despised Tasmanian outsider called Piping Lane. I really should have had a bet on it, as it was ridden by Adelaide jockey John Letts. His brother Daryl had been a cook at my previous posting in Townsville. In late November, the final Australians left Long Hai, which meant John Nolan, Bruno Carbone and Rod Margetts were now at Van Kiep also.

Part of my duties were to run the Regimental Aid Post (RAP). The previous incumbent was Peter Hulsing, the same man with a broad Dutch accent, who had been my instructor back in 1969, when I attended my first Medical Orderly course. There were very few casualties, but I did get to put a few sutures in a scalp wound. I also did lessons for MATT 1.

The contrasts were huge. On duty all night patrolling the perimeter while armed with an automatic shotgun, followed by a formal dinner where, as the youngest member I had to again assume the duties of running the activities once the head table had departed.

I remember meeting Don Targett; we had cycling, rank and youth in common. I took a photo of a huge cake they baked for him for his twenty-first birthday. There was also a road trip down to a very quiet Long Hai Training Battalion. We collected stores and attended a FANK Training Command dining-in night, which was a farewell as the unit closed for good.

My future in South Vietnam was uncertain. There was talk of a posting to MATT 1, but I was also due for R&R, which could be taken back in Australia. Perhaps I am fortunate that the MATT 1 posting didn't happen. On 20 November, they were engaged in the last enemy contact by Australian forces for the ten years of war. On the last day of November, I packed up and travelled to Saigon where I stayed at the Vinh Loi. After a day off in Saigon, I flew out on Singapore Airlines. From Singapore the next day, it was up the Malayan Peninsula to Penang before a ferry ride across to Butterworth.

After a night at RAAF Butterworth, I boarded a RAAF Hercules for a slow, noisy and boring flight to Darwin. By the time I landed on 3 December, a new Labor government had won the election. The next day, it was another eight and a half hours by Hercules to RAAF Richmond on the outskirts of Sydney. After a bus trip to Mascot Airport, I just made it in time for a flight to Melbourne.

During my few days of leave spent at Kyneton, I still had hopes of returning to Vietnam as the news stated that advisors would be returning to Australia by the new year. By 12 December, this had changed to 'all troops out as soon as possible (ASAP)'. At the same time, national servicemen were released to the freedom of their civilian life.

Meanwhile back at Nui Dat, John Nolan had been

conducting a training course for Vietnamese officers. As soon as the election result was announced, a Jeep collected him. They just had to leave the students on patrol in the Long Hai hills. He was on the last Hercules flight out and arrived at Richmond on 20 December.

I was only on leave from Vietnam. On 18 December, I flew to Sydney to be officially returned to Australia at the Eastern Command Personnel Depot. By the time the Hercules from Vietnam had landed, I had taken a train ride back to Melbourne and then all the way out to the School of Army Health, Healesville, where I had been posted as an instructor.

CHAPTER 6
Marathoner and marriage

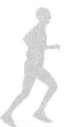

I headed off on leave until mid-January when I commenced work at the School of Army Health (SOAH). I had got back into running and training and renewed my acquaintance with the South Melbourne runners. On New Year's Day, I attended the Maryborough Gift meeting where I met some of my old cycling mates. It was also the professional running debut of Olympian Tony Benson, who won the 1600 metres in brilliant fashion.

In the first of many dubious career decisions I made regarding my Army career, I arranged a swap with the corporal in charge of the Regimental Aid Post (RAP). He wanted to be an instructor, and I much preferred to work as a medical assistant rather than tell others how to do it. Following active service a posting to a training unit is the path to rapid progression up the rank structure. I just didn't enjoy it and when permitted chose a different path. So, after a week of marching students around and doing lessons, I was in my own facility, way up the hill at the other end of the camp and was living in a room in Summerleigh Lodge.

At my nearby RAP, I conducted a sick parade each morning. I would then transport to Healesville Hospital any patients I considered needed to be seen by a doctor. I ordered medical stores, took blood samples, conducted immunisation parades and medical examinations, with a visiting doctor. My only exposure to military nonsense was a weekly Commanding Officer's Parade.

I got back into running, training and competition with the South Melbourne runners I had met in Victoria a year earlier. I let my Army unit know that I wished to attend the 3MD (Victorian) Inter-Service Championships. In mid-March, I competed for the Army against Navy and Air Force runners. My results were pleasing with a second in the 1500 metres, with a personal best (PB) of 4 mins 14 secs. I followed this up with victory in the 5000 metres in a PB and record time of 16 mins 2 secs.

The next month, a group of South Melbourne runners journeyed to Bendigo for a big amateur handicap at the Easter Fair. I had competed at this meeting as a juvenile cyclist and loved the atmosphere of the huge crowd. The race was 3200 metres; I am unaware of who was responsible for the handicapping. Young local champion Bruce Petts was off the back mark and I had forty seconds start on him. I had never been given a start in a running event, and nobody knew if I could even run.

Just go as fast as you can for as far as you can. The result was that I won in a time of 9 mins 23 secs. One of the top Melbourne runners was walking around post-race, shaking his head and saying, 'There's always one!' I think this event may have influenced the decision I later made on my future running career.

One of tasks at the RAP School of Army Health was to collect prescriptions for my patients from the local pharmacy. A bonus was that there were three attractive young assistants working there. One day I built up my courage and, as well as some pills, I came away with a date. Sandy Richards responded positively when I suggested we attend a dinner in Lygon Street, Carlton with my South Melbourne running mates. The only downside for her was the requirement to watch me run a ten-mile race around Princes Park. It was memorable in that I was so ill after the run I threw up my dinner – not sure that was the best date to invite a girl to!

In July, after two weeks of training at forty-five miles per week, I ran my first marathon in the Victorian Marathon Championship. These were the days when, if a runner couldn't go quicker than three hours for the marathon, they were unlikely to attempt the distance. Hence, the fields were much smaller than in later years, but they did not lack quality. The race was held over 26 miles and 365 yards, by far the longest running event I had contested. I was thirtieth out of a hundred and twelve starters, with a time of 2 hrs 49 mins 18 secs. As most of my running had been in Townsville or in military competition, this was a bit further from the front than I was used to, so I decided to do another one! A month later, and with no extra training, I entered the Victorian Country Marathon Championship in the hope of an improved result. I did improve – by a meagre 28 secs.

I finished an exhausted eleventh out of sixty starters. When I was passing the twelve-mile mark, the winner was on the return trip at fourteen miles. I guess the marathon just wasn't my event, being so far behind at the halfway mark. Little did I know the winner was the current holder of the world record, Derek Clayton. My respectable 2 hrs 48 mins 50 secs was about half an hour behind his winning time of 2 hrs 17 mins.

With the advent of spring, athletics interest turned to the track season. I spent a couple of weekends sitting around for hours before running nowhere in a D Grade 5000 metres. The thought niggled away that the professional running and cycling carnivals I had grown up on were much more exciting and enjoyable. I was also aware that with my marathon efforts, I was not up to the standard of the top runners in Victoria.

Over the Christmas holidays, I spent a couple of weeks visiting Graham Moon who was now living in Canberra. I

Chapter 6 Marathoner and marriage

got in some really good training with him in preparation for professional track running. Graham was also coaching a pair of attractive young runners and I asked one out for dinner. Safe to say, there was mutual attraction, because Pauline Bensley and I spent a week together at a house she was minding in Belconnen. We enjoyed the moment as we both knew I was just visiting, and it was a long way from Canberra to Healesville. All too soon, I had to return to work and step into the world of professional running.

The track meetings were held all over the state and involved a lot of travel for races that lasted only a few minutes. In January alone, I attended eight meetings and soon won a restricted 1600-metre handicap. A week later at Trentham, I came a close second in my first open race. My handicap mark was mid-field; this was adjusted depending on your performances.

At the end of the month, I ran at the big Wangaratta meeting that was held over three days. I wasn't able to get close to the winners, but I may have been a little distracted. Pauline had come down and we spent the days renewing acquaintances at the Council Club Hotel in Wangaratta.

With all this regular racing, I was improving my PBs almost every run. A warm-up for the Army Inter-Area 5000 metres was held in February where I won in record time, dipping under sixteen minutes for the first time (15 mins 59 secs). A few weeks later, on a bad track at Puckapunyal, I won a treble of Victorian Army Championships: 800 metres, 1500 metres (by half a lap in 4 mins 20 secs) and 5000 metres (by a lap in 16 mins 23 secs).

Three days later, I competed in a professional 3200 metres at Bendigo. I again ran a PB of 8 mins 52 secs but finished only seventh as I had to give the winner, Phil Hassel, a fifty-metre handicap start. A week later, I discovered he was a member of the Royal Australian Air Force (RAAF).

In the Victorian Inter-Service Championships, held on the Melbourne University track, I came second in all three distance events behind three different RAAF athletes. After running the 800 and 1500 metres, I had to run against a fresh RAAF runner in the 5000 metres. That runner was Phil Hassel who had cleaned me up in Bendigo. He went like the wind. I just clung on lap after lap, right at my limit until eventually I was cut adrift in the final laps, unable to sustain the pace.

I had seldom been defeated in military running events, so I wasn't sure if I were happy or sad with the result. I had run a PB by a huge twenty-five seconds and smashed my previous Inter-Service record, with 15 mins 35 secs. However, a fresh Phil was too good on the day and finished ten seconds in front, setting a record that stood for many years.

My first track season culminated with a visit to the

Stawell Gift meeting. Pro runners cultivate a handicap and set themselves for this meeting. Not me; I go flat out every race and at Stawell, I couldn't get near them.

In autumn, the pro athletics scene switched to cross-country, which I felt I would be better suited to. As a new runner, I was put on a fairly tight handicap which, if I was uncompetitive, they would gradually increase. In my second event, I ran a PB of 26 mins 25 secs for eight kilometres. The next time out, I followed up with a ten-kilometre PB of 33 mins 4 secs. Neither of those runs got me in sight of the handicap placegetters, as I was conceding nine minutes to some runners.

It was enough, though, to earn me a place in the select field for my first Australian Professional Championship, held over ten kilometres at Flemington Racecourse. The best I could do was thirteenth in a field of fifteen. The winner in dominant fashion was former Olympian and world pro record holder, Tony Benson, whom I had watched thrashing a 1600-metre field at Maryborough a year earlier.

A week later, I attempted another marathon, this time at Traralgon. It was a disaster, with me recording terms such as 'exhausted', 'stitch', 'cramps', 'vomiting' and 'dizzy' instead of a finishing time. Common sense would have seen me pull out, but that seemed to be lacking on the day.

Just a week later, I recorded fastest time in a novice ten kilometres at Princes Park. Then it was the Victorian

Country Championship over ten kilometres at Creswick. This was very hilly and I improved to come sixth of a hundred runners. It goes without saying that the winner was the star, Tony Benson.

In July, I further improved my eight-kilometre time and in doing, so won my first pro race at Warrandyte, also recording the second-fastest time. The event was sponsored by 'Jock' Logan, a former champion pro distance runner. Jock offered to train me, and while I did my own thing, we remained firm friends and he followed my career with interest. A week later in the Australian pro 10 Mile Championship, I improved my PB by more than five minutes from my debut at Bundaberg back in 1971. It was only fast enough for eleventh in this quality field.

The big event for the season was in early August, the Kilmore Feature Race of fifteen kilometres. It was very cold and the course was sodden. It involved two laps of a very heavy racecourse, with two ascents of a rough and muddy Monument Hill in between. What nobody knew beforehand, including myself, was that this was my ideal course. I conceded two minutes start to the race favourites, caught them up halfway and just cleared out to win by forty-eight seconds. It was a huge upset by a first season runner who had already been re-handicapped after the earlier win.

The fastest time of course went to Tony Benson with 50 mins 8 secs and I recorded second-fastest, just two minutes behind, with a PB of 52 mins 11 secs. Earlier, I had been five minutes behind him over just ten kilometres! On the plus side, I won $500 and the respect of my opponents. However, there was a price to be paid. The following week, I was running off the back mark with the multiple Australian pro marathon champion, Ted Paulin. Back to a flat, fast course, and I never saw which way they went.

There were a couple of championships to finish off my first cross-country season. In the Victorian 15-mile championship, I ran a PB of 1 hr 23 mins 33 secs to finish sixth behind Tony Benson's 1 hr 19 mins 23 secs.

In my first Australian pro marathon championship, I came third in a PB of 2 hrs 42 mins 1 sec. Ten minutes in front, Ted Paulin continued his winning streak, narrowly defeating Phil Bateman, with both recording 2 hrs 31 mins.

In between all this running, my personal life took a dramatic turn. With much regret, I terminated my long-distance romance with Pauline and resumed going out with Sandy Richards. As it was nearing the time when the Army could repost me, I got in first with a request to go back to Townsville. With a move from Healesville pending, I proposed to Sandy and we were married on 30 November 1974 in the Uniting Church at Healesville.

The first night of our honeymoon was at the Marylands Guest House in scenic Marysville, followed by a road trip of eastern Victoria. We camped at Fraser National Park, drove through the high country on a back road through Matlock and Walhalla. Then it was Wilsons Promontory and a week on the beach at Carrum.

A month later, I was posted to District Support Unit (DSU) at Lavarack Barracks in Townsville. In February 1975, it took three solid days of driving for us to reach Townsville. For me, I envisaged a return to a location I had enjoyed and was very comfortable in. For Sandy, it was being uprooted from all she had known in her hometown, leaving family and friends, her employment and the tennis club where she was champion, to travel 2000 miles to North Queensland for an uncertain future as an Army wife. I imagine it was a huge leap of faith for her to decide to marry me and move away.

CHAPTER 7
Townsville champ

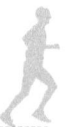

I was back training with my Townsville Marathon Club friends, old and new, right from the start. Peter and Ann Lahiff were amazing with an offer of accommodation in their North Ward home until we were able to find a place to live. I am sure this helped Sandy settle into an alien environment, up in the tropics where she knew nobody.

Running-wise, I took up where I left off with a Townsville Amateur Athletic Club (TAAC) 3000-metres victory over Jim Hartnett and Peter Lahiff. As it was the summer wet season, the Townsville Marathon Club was having a break, but we met each Thursday evening at Peter's for a lap of North Ward, which invariably became an unofficial race.

Sandy and I rented a unit in Mitchell Street, North Ward, an area I enjoyed with its proximity to the beach and Castle Hill. It meant a bit of a commute out to work at Lavarack Barracks, but that was a small price to pay. Sandy picked up a job as an assistant at Dawn McFadden's pharmacy, in nearby Garbutt.

Three weeks after arriving, I flew down to Brisbane to compete in the Queensland Army (1MD) Orienteering Championships. (I recall swearing back in 1972 that I would never orienteer again, but a couple of events in the gentler environment of Victoria had been more enjoyable.) The map of suburban Daisy Hill was rather sub-standard, but I must have done something right. After navigating the six-kilometre course in fifty-eight minutes, I was crowned 1MD Orienteering Champion. I guess it just shows that running ability will take you a fair way in orienteering. Barry Hitchens, my Townsville teammate, was runner-up.

While down there, the next day I competed in a 3000 metres at Lang Park. I came sixth with a PB of 8 mins 59 secs. Way out in front, setting a Queensland record, was Gerrard Barrett (8 mins 20 secs). The barefoot fifteen-year-old I first met in 1971 had come a long way. He was to continue to excel as one of Australia's champion international athletes.

Back in Townsville, the TMC events commenced and there were also a few TAAC track events remaining. The highlight of the TAAC events was that they hosted the Country Queensland Championships in a two-day meeting at the end of March. On day one, on a sodden grass track, I came second in the 1500 metres

Chapter 7 Townsville champ

to Toowoomba runner Rob Stone. This was followed by a 5000 metres where I led throughout, defeating Mike Phillips and Jim Hartnett by half a lap.

By day two, persistent soaking rain had turned the track into a quagmire for the 10,000 metres. I ran barefoot for the first time in my life, as my shoes just stuck fast in the mud during my warm-up. During the race, I ran on an outside lane white line, trying to find somewhere where I only sank ankle-deep. It must have worked or, again, mud which slowed others down more suited me. I defeated two Gold Coast runners by a hundred metres and managed to lap Mike Phillips, who had beaten me in the first King of the Castle.

During April, 3 Task Force had a ten-day training exercise at Tineroo Falls on the Atherton Tableland. As the Task Force medic, I was required to be there. I sat there in the rain forest, unable to train and with a lonely, unhappy wife back in Townsville. It was an integral part of my job, but one I had not been exposed to in previous postings. It interfered a lot with my first love and my running career.

Following a discussion with Sandy on my return to Lavarack Barracks, I informed my superiors that I would resign from the Army on the completion of my six-year enlistment period in August. I said I didn't want to spend long periods out bush, as I was newly married. They reluctantly agreed, but followed up with, 'To be consistent, you will of course not be attending military sporting competitions'.

Ouch! I could do nothing but agree to their terms. A week later, the Australian Defence Force sent their first ever team to the US for the World Military Orienteering Championships. The Australian team was Major Graham Moon, Captain Dick Mountstephens and Corporal Barry Hitchens. The latter had been behind me in the 1MD Championship but won an overseas trip when I was not allowed to attend. For better or worse, I had made my decision.

Over the next two months, I built my training up to average 250 miles a month and my performances reflected it. Most TMC events were handicaps, which gave everyone a turn at winning a race. For me, the important aim was fastest time honours, which I managed to achieve in every event.

In May, the fourteen-mile Woodstock run was held in hot conditions. I led with Dave Scully until he tired at nine miles. I went on to break the record by three minutes in 82 mins 12 secs. Then in June on the Town Common, I ran a PB for ten kilometres (32 mins 50 secs) ahead of Dave Scully and Jim Hartnett.

A week later, a few of us travelled down to Sarina for the Utah Marathon, held over 16.8 miles. It was a class field and I made the mistake of going too fast early. English runner Ian Brotherton won from Keith Canard and Rob Stone. I held third place until pulling out with four miles to go. I had raced and been beaten by the minor placegetters on a previous occasion.

My six months back in Townsville were wrapped up in fine style. Firstly, a win in the Charters Towers Goldfields Fun Run of six miles; another PB of 31 mins 13 secs saw me three minutes clear of Dan Clyne and Jim Hartnett. A week later and it was time for the annual King of the Castle. I was confident that I was a much better runner than when I was narrowly defeated in 1972. My confidence was well founded when I broke the record by over two minutes with a time of 31 mins 14 secs. That was also the margin back to runner-up Mike Phillips, who had won on the first three occasions. My final run in Townsville (for now) was a one-hour run. This I won covering 10.95 miles from Dave Scully (10.6) and Dan Clyne (10.5). Though my performances were mainly in my own small pool of Townsville, I will own up to being very satisfied with the results.

A few days later Sandy and I packed up and left Townsville for the long drive south and my discharge from the Army. A part of Sandy's unhappiness in Townsville was that she found her boss at the pharmacy a tyrant. She had resigned and was at a loose end, which was aggravated by my trips out bush.

We just happened to be passing through Caboolture, north of Brisbane, as they were hosting the Queensland

Marathon Championship. I was in second place throughout, behind my nemesis Keith Canard (2 hrs 38 mins). Unfortunately, the effort took its toll and I was unable to go on, although only four miles from the finish. After my 'demise', Keith was left almost half an hour in front of the placegetters. Both second and third had a link to Townsville: Graeme Barralet competed up there a bit during this period and Paul Circosta had won the first Townsville Marathon back in 1973. For me, it was a learning experience and a certain second place that got away.

A few days later we were back in Healesville. I had completed my Army career.

CHAPTER 8
Civilian life

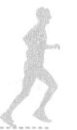

We rented a house in Lilydale and I took a job as a postman in suburban Croydon. Sandy was also employed and happily settled back into tennis and enjoying having her family nearby. With the big lifestyle changes, I had not been able to train enough and my running results deteriorated.

At the end of August, I ran in the Australian Pro Marathon Championship at Pakenham. Ted Paulin clocked up win number six from a Queensland pro named Kevin Fisher, whom I had heard about from our shared pro running mentor, Jock Logan. Kevin had won a couple of Mareeba Rodeo Road Races and the Great Pyramid Race at nearby Gordonvale. I was destined to follow in his footsteps, but today I was only capable of seventh place at 2 hrs 48 mins 17 secs. I was one place behind champion ultramarathoner George Purdon. I was back to where I started with marathons in 1973, but to be fair, I had trained even less than then.

The track season was no better and I couldn't get near the placings, even with a 3000-metre PB of 8 mins 46 secs. The only run I was satisfied with was a big Melbourne Fun Run, where I came fortieth of 900 entrants. I ran a PB of 38 mins 40 secs for twelve kilometres. I trekked off to Stawell at Easter and again ran a PB of 4 mins 4 secs for 1500 metres, which only got me ninth – a pretty hard game and a lot of talented runners. Enjoyment of my running had disappeared, and I pined for the enjoyable times I had back in Townsville.

We decided to purchase a caravan and set off on a lap of Australia, though I am not sure how we planned to fund it while being unemployed. Early in May, we headed off travelling through Yass and Coonabarabran. On the third day we entered Queensland at Goondiwindi and visited Dave and Cathy Scully at their navy bean farm at nearby Yelarbon. Dave had also left the Army and it was great to catch up with our good ex-Townsville friends. On we travelled and after a few days in Brisbane, we worked our way up the coast until we arrived at Townsville. Jim and Patsy Hartnett were kind enough to let us park the van in the driveway of their Wulguru home. I jumped straight back into running with the Townsville Marathon Club.

Three days after arriving from a long drive and on minimal training, I ran in a two-person relay from the base of Mt Stuart to the summit. I ran the fastest of the first legs on the steepest section of the climb. This had no right to be a memorable performance, but subsequent results show that it was. My 17 mins 38 secs was thirty-two seconds in front of John Temby and Steve Colbourne who almost dead-heated. I had not previously raced either runner, but I knew of Steve's record as a schoolboy. He was Queensland's public schools track champion, whereas I'd come second in the Woodend Primary School eighty-yard dash in Five Mile Creek Park!

On reflection, I was very surprised to beat him, and John Temby narrowly pipped him for second. Perhaps it was an indication that I was at my best running up steep hills. The most amazing fact is that the record time I set has not been surpassed in all the years since. After all that, we only came second in the relay, as I had been deliberately paired with one of the slower runners, Gary Zylmans. Gordonvale visitor Ian Leet and local Mansell Blakeley finished twenty-four seconds in front of us.

The following week after a heavy training load, I ran in the 15 kilometres from Nathan Plaza to Ross River Dam, a race I had won last year. For ten kilometres, I was locked in battle with John Temby before I finally shook him off. The effort in doing so pushed me to a PB of 51 mins 2 secs, an improvement of 1 min 37 secs over last year.

Early in June, it was time for this year's King of the Castle. The local paper had me favoured to win as defending King. I was not so sure, as I knew about Steve Colbourne.

In the end, it was a one-horse race. Steve led throughout and sliced another 1 min 15 secs from my record, becoming one of the few in the race history to break thirty minutes with 29 mins 58 secs. I didn't see him at all, which is normal for this race. If you were to look anywhere except at your feet and the next foot hold, the treacherous Goat Track would bring you down. On reflection, I am sure the reason I couldn't get near thirty minutes was that you have to run back down. I was second at 31 mins 32 secs, with John Temby fifty seconds back.

As you will be aware, I had been running as a professional down in Victoria. In those days, a pro was forbidden to run against amateurs. Apparently, news of my Kilmore Feature Race win had reached the hallowed halls of the Queensland Amateur Athletic Association. TAAC and TMC were informed that I was not to run in their events. TMC had their own issues with Brisbane and were happy for me to compete but suggested that perhaps I shouldn't run in high-profile events.

One such event was on a week later, a ten-kilometre Around the Hill Fun Run in Townsville. Instead, I was on my way down to Sarina to have another crack at the Utah Marathon after my DNF (did not finish) the previous year. The results speak for themselves, and I rate it as the best race ever held in Townsville. A now grown-up Gerrard Barrett won clearly in an outstanding 29 mins 22 secs, from another international in John Stanley (30 mins 30 secs). Our own champ, Steve Colbourne, was not disgraced, but a further two minutes back.

You will have an idea of the class of these runners when reading the result of the Utah Marathon (16.8 miles). First was John Stanley who backed up with a 1 hr 36 mins 42 secs from another NSW runner, Kev Skelton (1hr 40 mins 6 secs). I got to the finish intact, though perhaps I was a bit conservative after last year. My third place was in 1 hr 44 mins 6 secs and next, of course, the ever-reliable John Temby about three minutes back.

Sandy had started a job at the new high-rise Travelodge on The Strand and I did a bit of cleaning work at Townsville High School, but mainly I ran. In June, I covered 306 miles; by July, it was up to 338 miles, and in August 388 miles, culminating in a series of results that I have equalled only once in my running lifetime. It commenced with a couple of defeats behind Steve Colbourne and I assumed that would continue no matter what I did. However, at the end of June, Steve travelled to Brisbane for the Queensland Marathon Championship. I had run well against most of the top five finishers, but they usually had my measure.

- 1: Gerrard Barrett, 2 hrs 24 mins 15 secs
- 2: Richard Bourne, 2 hrs 36 mins 36 secs
- 3: Keith Canard, 2 hrs 37 mins 16 secs
- 4: Rob Stone, 2 hrs 38 mins 27 secs
- 5: Joe Patterson, 2 hrs 39 mins 38 secs.

Steve came over the line in seventh place with 2 hrs 43 mins. We never spoke about the result and whether he was satisfied with it. If his outstanding ability at short distances had been maintained over the marathon, I would have selected him for second placing. It is likely that the marathon flattened him, and combined with my increased fitness, he was no longer in front of me in races.

We had a five-mile race and my run of seconds continued. Although I ran a PB of twenty-six minutes, Dan Clyne finished ten seconds in front. John Temby narrowly beat Steve for third, but it was only a week after the marathon.

The next week, we trekked out to Dave Wharton's family farm for the annual Woodstock 13.6 miler. In 1975, I had taken five minutes off Mike Phillips' course record. This time, John Temby forced the pace and tried everything to drop me off. He was unsuccessful, but at the line, he was only twenty-seven seconds back after a stirring duel. The outcome was a winning time of 1 hr 17 mins 51 secs, which took another huge slab off my own record (4 mins 21 secs).

It was on again the next weekend as Ian Leet had invited a few of us up for the Mareeba Rodeo Road Race. This annual event was over ten miles from Walkamin to Mareeba, where it finished at the rodeo grounds. John Temby was straight into it again, running what I felt was an unsustainable pace. However, I had firmly in mind

Chapter 8 Civilian life

how close he had come last week and clung on for dear life. Ian Leet held on also, but halfway he eased back and ran his own race. In the later stages, John fell victim to his own tactics and I stormed to the finish almost two minutes clear. My time was a huge record and lifetime PB of 52 mins 40 secs. As John weakened, he was just able to hold off Ian for second place. An indication of what John's pace had done to the field was that fourth placegetter Ray Clitheroe was over five minutes away. I doubted the course measurement, so we checked with the car odometer – it measured 10.3 miles!

Striking while the iron was hot, my winning run continued with a Town Common ten-kilometre race in 33 mins 3 secs, with Steve more than 1 min 30 secs back. It was hot, with a loose, sandy surface and I lost thirty seconds retying my shoelace.

On the first day of August, I lined up with nine others at Weir State School on Ross River Road in Kirwan, a suburb of Townsville. It was the fourth running of the North Queensland (Townsville) Marathon, held on an out-and-back course along Hervey Range Road. It was hot, but I was determined not to repeat the error of going out too fast and being unable to finish. Even so, I was out in front by myself for the whole distance. My first half was run at 6 mins 30 secs per mile, but a strong second half had me recording miles of five to five-and-a-half minutes. Halfway was achieved in 1 hr 22 mins 58 secs, and I came home with a huge negative split of 1 hr 15 mins 38 secs. Behind me, the weather and distance took their toll on the field.

This fine run improved my marathon PB by 3 mins 26 secs and sliced a huge nineteen minutes off the course record, with 2 hrs 38 mins 35 secs. As they later changed the marathon venue, this is the other record that I still hold at time of writing. Peter Lahiff was already aged in his forties and ran a great race for second in 2 hrs 52 mins 23 secs. A few hours later, Alan Stanbrook hobbled over the line, having earlier removed his shoes due to blisters. He was the only other finisher!

It was an awesome feeling to finish a marathon so strongly, but we will never know what I could have done at a more even pace and in temperate conditions. It was a memorable finale to my Townsville Marathon Club career. I had decided to abandon the rest of the around-Australia trip.

I must have been fit and thus had recovery powers of a young man. Four days later, I was up in Gordonvale and staying at Ian Leet's cane farm. The Great Pyramid Race was invented years earlier by drunken cane cutters betting against each other about who could race to the top of Walshs Pyramid and return to Gordonvale the fastest. As this race had prizemoney, it was not an event the other Townsville runners would dare attend. It was a daunting prospect, as Walshs Pyramid was well named and would not have been out of place in Egypt. The course was eight miles, with the first and last two flat through the heat of the cane fields. The main problem was navigating across the Mulgrave River on a large, round water pipeline. A fall would mean the end of your race – and there was the small matter of crocodiles!

Two miles brings you to the base of the climb and then it is straight up the northern ridgeline on a rough and indistinct path. So, four days after the marathon, Ian took me for a run of over an hour from home to the base of the climb. The next day, we climbed halfway up, the return trip being 1 hr 30 mins. The view even from halfway was superb with Cairns to the east and the Atherton Tableland on the opposite horizon. I am glad I saw it then, as there was definitely no sightseeing on race day.

It should have been a simple race, as I had proven a very strong hill runner and I didn't know anything about my competitors. I used my superior speed to clear out on the flat, so I wouldn't have trouble passing on the rough and narrow climb. I reached the top a long way in front and now all I had to do was get back to town. Running flat out downhill is not one of my strengths, as I don't like injuries and try to stay safe. The trail was hard to follow, especially as you had to watch every foot placement to prevent falls. I lost the trail three times and told myself to just keep going down, even if I had to 'bush bash'. Finally, back on a flat gravel track, I was advised that I was in second place.

I managed to get my body moving in some semblance of normal running and picked the new leader off before we reached town. He must have been moving slowly as I won by five minutes. After all the misadventure, my time of 1 hr 19 mins 19 secs broke the course record. I have no idea how much time I lost out there, but nowadays the Great Pyramid is a big race on the Queensland trail running calendar and attracts hundreds of runners. The record is now about 1 hr 15 mins, and I think that would have been within my capabilities had I not got lost.

An unfortunate sequel was that Ian took me to Cairns Show the next day for a two-mile race. The organisers had heard of my Pyramid result and since I had won easily, they said no, it was only open to locals who played a ball sport. Talk about make it up as you go along! They flung a $25 shop voucher my way, which I handed to my kind host.

Two days later, back in Townsville, we hitched up the caravan and headed west. My plan now was to return to Victoria and see if my current form held up in the stronger competition down south. At the little town of Prairie, I turned south, following a faint brown line in my map book. Four days and 1400 kilometres after leaving Townsville, we finally arrived to spend the night at the outback town of Cunnamulla.

Chapter 8 Civilian life

With the wisdom of hindsight, it was a foolhardy adventure, but we got through almost unscathed. Towing an overloaded sixteen-foot caravan, behind a three-litre Torana was really hot, slow and bumpy. The worst of it was that bulldust had filled the huge potholes on the road so they were impossible to see. No consideration was given to fuel usage in these conditions and whether we could make the next open garage.

All I remember, when stopping at tiny Muttaburra after an empty desolate 200 kilometres, was seeing a dilapidated tennis court absolutely jam-packed with galahs. Then it was Aramac before we finally hit the bitumen at Barcaldine. As soon as we did, an oncoming car sent up a stone which broke the windscreen. Once that was replaced, it was on through Blackall and Charleville to the last town before the NSW border, Cunnamulla. We pulled up in the main street of Cunnamulla and one of the locals, on noticing my track suit said, 'You must be here for the big race tomorrow!' Well, no, but tell me more! We stayed overnight and the next day I competed in the Opal Festival Mile.

A week after running up a huge mountain and I am attempting a mile race on a track in the middle of nowhere – what could possibly go wrong? After three laps, I had a good lead and just had to plug through to the finish. In the last lap, an 'express train' picked me up and left me in the dust. I had no idea what I was doing running at Cunnamulla and even less on how I managed to bump into the world professional record holder for 400 yards, one John McDonald!

So we left Cunnamulla with a sash, some prizemoney and a stray kitten that had adopted our car while we were absent. She was a little tortoiseshell we named Paroo after a far-flung tributary of the Darling River that flows through Cunnamulla's nearby sister city of Eulo. There is a saying, 'Back of Bourke', and after another desolate 250 kilometres, we eventually reached civilisation at Bourke. Three days later, we parked our van beside a rippling brook in the vibrant, green surrounds of Healesville's Badger Creek Caravan Park.

On arrival, I got straight into heavy training with my mate from Chum Creek, Wally Butler. I averaged over a hundred miles for each of the next two weeks. Without easing up, in the middle of it, I fronted up for the Victorian Pro 15 Mile Championship at Whittlesea. It had traditionally been a flat, fast, out-and-back course, on which I had run 1 hr 24 mins 20 secs last year when finishing fourth behind Tony Benson. They had changed the course, but I went in ignorant of what that entailed.

At the halfway point, the road turned both into gravel and steeply uphill to circumnavigate Yan Yean Reservoir. Yippee! I stormed past the pre-race favourite, Gary Robertson, and marathon champ Ted Paulin, and even with a downhill run into the finish, they were unable to reel me in. I had run exactly the same time as last year, but the hills slowed the others much more than me. Gary Robertson was more than a minute back in second, with Ted Paulin close up.

I recall Ted's young son, Dean, calling out to me on crossing the line, 'You can't beat my dad; you aren't good enough!' In general terms, he was correct, but on the day, on the hills ... I advised him to look at the scoreboard. Fast forward a dozen years and Dean became a four-minute miler!

But the day belonged to me. I had brought my Townsville form to the 'big time' and won my first (and last) Victorian Pro Championship. I scooped the pool by winning the sealed handicap, by a huge three minutes. Oops! Another hill course, another big win and there went my handicap for a few more years. I should also thank Tony Benson for being absent in the US, chasing the pro riches over there.

A fortnight later, it was down to Pakenham for another attempt at the Australian Pro Marathon Championship. The handicapper had well and truly fixed me up, as only the previous winners, Ted Paulin and Phil Bateman, were still waiting to go as I set off with Ray Riordan from the two-minute mark. I am not sure if any teamwork was in play, but Ray shot off at a ridiculous pace and I clung on as best I could.

By the halfway mark, he suddenly pulled out and left

me very vulnerable to anybody who was running a more sensible, even pace. That someone was six-time champion Ted Paulin, who loomed up at twenty miles, and I had no answer. He finished off a great run for a forty-year-old, winning in 2 hrs 27 mins. I battled on to finish second in a new PB of 2 hrs 33 mins 18 secs, narrowly in front of NSW runner Richie Robinson. The handicap? Forget it! A bloke named Cormick had eighteen minutes start on me and ran 2 hrs 35 mins!

Around this time, I enquired at Army Recruiting about re-enlisting in the Army. I had been doing a lot of running and very little work, which wasn't sustainable. They said, 'Sure, come back and go through Kapooka recruit training again.' The conversation ended right there. I had been a corporal with two promotion subjects for sergeant, overseas active service and six years' experience. I was not going through the hell of Kapooka again!

I started work as a storeman at Rotary Tableting, a pharmaceutical company in Croydon. Not long after, a pro running mate, Kerrie Beattie, convinced me to have a go at selling life insurance. Sandy and I moved down to Warragul in the caravan, and I began my new career. That lasted a couple of months; money ran short as no policies were sold – definitely not my type of job. I had a few races with the locals, including my first and last steeplechase. My only losses were seconds in the steeplechase and in a five-kilometre race behind local champ John Duck.

Chapter 8 Civilian life

So, 1977 commenced with us back in Healesville, tail firmly between the legs. I tried a bit of sawmill work but found it way too heavy. Then I drove laundry trucks for French's Laundry in Healesville. We were still living in the caravan and Sandy's parents decided that was not an ongoing option. They kindly donated the deposit, and we purchased our first home in Blue Gum Drive, Badger Creek.

On the running front, I was all over Victoria competing in pro track events. I was only training lightly and doing interval work to increase my speed for these short races. I won a 1600 metres at Korumburra and then ran a 3000 metres PB of 8 mins 39 secs when second at Wangaratta. Another PB of 4 mins 1min 8 secs for 1500 metres followed, so my form was pretty good.

In March, the Moomba 1600 metres was a rare excursion on to a proper synthetic running track at Olympic Park. I didn't waste the opportunity and although unplaced, I broke four minutes for 1500 metres for the first time.

Danny Furlong, a running mate from Castlemaine, got in touch with a novel suggestion. He wanted me to join him in a relay event being held to celebrate the centenary of the gold rush in Castlemaine. All that was required was to take turns at pushing a wheelbarrow from Melbourne to Castlemaine. There was a field of a dozen teams, and we were accompanied by a stagecoach as we departed the city. From the early stages, it was obvious that our team had a distinct class edge and, barring accidents, had it in the bag.

We won each stage until on the final day, we held an unassailable lead. I think Danny must have been embarrassed, because without informing me, he didn't turn up for the final stage. This left me struggling on against fresh runners. If his plan was to share the spoils by having someone else win the final stage, all I can say is, it worked! Anyway, the prizemoney of $275 was more than I had collected for many 'professional' races, so it was well worth doing.

Danny had been the race favourite when I won my first cross-country back in 1974 and was a handy runner. In a sad sequel, a few years later, he had a massive stroke and spent his short life severely incapacitated.

My pro track season wound up with a trip to the big ones at Stawell and Bendigo. I was close up behind the placegetters after running well, but it is difficult to beat runners who cultivate their handicap and peak for one event. When the cross-country season began, it was more of the same. I was a bit tired, flat, ill and just not on top of my game. A twelfth in the Australian Pro 10 Mile (54 mins 25 secs) and third in the marathon (2 hrs 41 mins 52 secs) saw me going okay, but down from my best form.

With a mortgage now to pay, I needed a well-paying and secure job. I knew where to find one but would not do recruit training again. I had a brainwave: I would try the 'old boys' net. I contacted my first CSM, Bob Allen, with whom I had played football in Townsville and who sent me on the AATTV course. He had since done a 'knife and fork' course and become an officer and a gentleman. He was now in charge of Medical Corps postings.

The result was positive in that if I passed the recruiting tests, then I could be posted directly to 2 Military Hospital. I guess it's not what you know but who you know. I discussed the option with Sandy. Having lived through the insecurity of the past two years, she was happy for me to re-enlist.

By September, I had re-enlisted in the Australian Army and received a date to report to 2 Military Hospital at Ingleburn on the south-western outskirts of Sydney. I was driving my hugely overloaded laundry truck around the slippery, tight bends of the Black Spur on the Maroondah Highway when the brakes failed. I managed to keep from driving off the road and into a gully, but when I returned to the depot, I informed the owner of what I thought of his truck. It was just as well I had a future career lined up as we agreed I was finished.

My final pro run was a 5000 metres on the Melbourne Showgrounds trotting track. I was unplaced but my time of 15 mins 38 secs showed I could still run. The fastest time was the remarkable Tony Benson who clocked in at 14 mins 3 secs!

Going back into the Army meant both of us understanding it involved both good and bad aspects. We both considered that the good outweighed the bad and it was just a matter of enduring the latter.

CHAPTER 9
Back in the Army

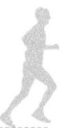

At the end of September, I drove to Ingleburn and commenced work at 2 Military Hospital, working in the ward as a trainee under supervision. I leased a modern townhouse a couple of kilometres away in the suburb of Ingleburn. Sandy joined me a month later after leasing out our house and was soon able to find a position at the hospital as well.

I checked out the Sydney running scene and soon decided the pro competition was unsatisfactory. So, I would run amateur instead, but I didn't want a recurrence of what had happened in Queensland. It was just running to me, and the top amateurs were paid far more than I had ever won as a professional. I solved it by checking my birth certificate, which was adorned with the name 'Greg Harvey'.

For two years, I had a dual identity: running as Greg Harvey and working under my accepted family name of

Wilson. It was the middle of the jogging craze and there were a couple of fun runs available each weekend, as well as organised amateur competitions. There was no option but to take the organisers' word that their course distance was accurate. I say that because my first event on little training was a ten-kilometre fun run in Liverpool. I came fifth of 200 and ran a PB of 32 mins 20 secs.

In our local area, the biggest fun run was the Fisher's Ghost Run at Campbelltown. It was thirteen kilometres and I came thirty-second of 2000. I had never before experienced a field of that size, and the depth was amazing too. I was the first Army finisher. A couple of days later, I had my first Army competition in a couple of years. At the 1 Task Force Championships, I won both the 1500 metres (4 mins 28 secs) and the 5000 metres (16 mins 17 secs).

I would often travel over to Cabramatta with some local runners I had met to run with Western District Joggers. At Christmas, we drove back to Victoria for a leave break at Healesville. This would become a regular visit from wherever the Army had us located. I got plenty of good training in with my Chum Creek mate, Wally Butler, and it was great for Sandy to catch up with her family.

Prior to leave, I had been required to take trade tests to ensure I was competent as a medical assistant. I guess I hadn't forgotten much, as I attained almost perfect scores. When I returned to work, it was as an Instructor Private on Training Wing. After escaping from duties as an instructor at Healesville, I was now leading a syndicate of trainees, and I was of the same rank as them.

Early in 1978, I ran fifth in a Sydney ten-kilometre fun run and recorded a PB of 32 mins 15 secs. The winner was a fun run whiz kid called Andy Lloyd who was about sixteen. A few years later, he would win three Melbourne Marathons and a Commonwealth Games 5000 metres gold medal. A couple of weeks later, I won a six-mile fun run at Plumpton from a field of 150 in 30 mins 41 secs – they are very difficult to win.

I had registered with Western Suburbs Athletic Club and next competed in the NSW Track Championships. A PB of 15 mins 30 secs in the five kilometres was only good enough for thirteenth behind John Andrews (14 mins 1 sec). Similarly in the ten kilometres, a solid 32 mins 52 secs only got me eleventh behind Lawrie Whitty (30 mins 40 secs). I was running well, but the standard was a bit above my best.

The Army now sent teams from most states (Military Districts) to an orienteering event called MIL-O. It meant a week away each year at a variety of locations, being paid to run around in the bush. That sounded right up my alley! The main problem I had was getting selected for my state team. I was considered fast but erratic as I had a tendency to get lost. I narrowly scraped into the team of ten, although in the competition, only three were required for a team.

We were based at Puckapunyal for a series of events in Central Victoria. ACT were running short of orienteers for their team, so NSW gave away their most expendable member, and that was me. I was very happy, as my new team captain was Graham Moon, the founder of the Townsville Marathon Club. I had not seen him for five years and it was great to be on a team with him. We had only one other member – Sergeant Ian Nolan who had served with Graham in Vietnam – so nobody could afford to get lost.

It was no surprise that Graham won each of the four days' competition from Captain Dick Mountstephen. The shock for NSW was that the third placegetter was one Greg Wilson. This result meant that the ACT won the teams event, and on the final day, we also won the relay. A pleasing result, in what is very much a second sport for me. I suspected that NSW might not be so keen to loan me out in future.

A big May followed with a bunch of non-podium PBs: a half-marathon (73 mins 4 secs), a 25 kilometres (1 hr 27 mins 56 secs), a 22 kilometres (1 hr 13 mins 13 secs) and a 33 kilometres (1 hr 57 mins 22 secs). The latter event was Mt Pritchard to Warragamba and was solidly uphill towards the end. There was a pretty handy trio in front of me. Dennis Nee defeated young Andy Lloyd, and third was my old nemesis from Queensland, Keith Canard. My only placing that month was my only non-PB, a second in the Newcastle Marathon in 2 hrs 40 mins 51 secs.

Two more marathons followed in June, and both were just over 2 hrs 40 mins. In the Parramatta 25-kilometre race, I was able to take four minutes off my PB with 1 hr 23 mins 45 secs.

A month later, it was back to the track as the NSW Army (2MD) Championships were held at Singleton. Midway through the meeting, an aeroplane flew over and we had a parachutist land in the middle of the track. I discovered that he was the Commanding Officer of the Parachute School at Nowra and I was to run against him in the distance events.

That was my first meeting with Lieutenant Colonel Alan Batchelor, a man who had quite an influence on some of my later military athletics. In the one afternoon, I chalked up wins in all three of my events: 1500 metres (4 mins 39 secs), 3000 metres (9 mins 32 secs) and 5000 metres (16 mins 47 secs). When you are running multiple events in one day, it is wise to spread the effort and not attempt to go flat out.

A couple of weeks later, I represented the Army in the Inter-Service Championships. Again, I won the 1500 metres (4 mins 15 secs) and the 5000 metres (15 mins 46 secs). After not quite being up with the top liners, it was nice to be able to have the occasional race in a restricted field and manage a win.

During my work on Training Wing at 2 Military Hospital, there was an incident that might have brought my Army career to a premature end. Even though I was now at the lowest rank of Private, I was in charge of trainees. One day, I was marching them around when the Quartermaster, a Captain who was a former Regimental Sergeant Major, abruptly commandeered them and directed them off to do a job for him. He was so arrogant that he didn't even ask! However, in the Army, if an officer says, 'Jump', all you do is ask, 'How high, sir?' Nevertheless, I was offended by his actions and told him, a crime for which I could have received a whole range of punishments. Over the next week or so every high rank in the unit told me to apologise to him. I just kept on refusing and stated he should apologise as he had been in the wrong. I had no idea what action they would take, but obstinately I would not back down, no matter what the repercussions. In the end, it just went away. I think they decided I was way too difficult as a Private so, once the dust settled, I received a promotion to Corporal.

I also had periods of working eleven-hour days and a detachment to run the Regimental Aid Post (RAP) at the School of Engineering. This time around, I happily accepted what the Army required and got back into training later.

I think my running performances picked up some more in the first half of 1979. The newly named

Chapter 9 Back in the Army

Australian Services Orienteering Championships (ASOC) were based in Adelaide. Graham Moon was absent, but never fear, another engineering officer appeared on the scene to win the event – Major Peter Rose. In an event that seemed mainly the domain of officers, I was one of the few enlisted men competing. Peter Rose won the first two days, but on the final day, I managed to beat him to the line. I did it under duress, as I ran into a stump halfway through and badly lacerated my thigh. This result won me second place overall, in front of Captain Dick Mountstephens. When I stopped, they saw my damaged leg and called for a medic. I sat under a tree and said, 'That would be me!'

A week later, I journeyed out to Parkes in the central west of NSW and won their twenty-kilometre road race with a PB of 1 hr 10 mins 38 secs. A highlight was an unplaced run in Sydney's biggest half-marathon at Sutherland. It is held on an undulating gravel road through the Royal National Park. I ran the first half in 35 mins 25 secs and came back a minute faster. It was hugely competitive and although I placed sixth, I was only twenty-one seconds behind third place! My time of 1 hr 9 mins 38 secs was by far the fastest half-marathon I ever ran. In the field behind me were a Warragamba winner, a state marathon champion and a 2 hrs 25 mins marathoner.

In May, I clocked up 338 miles in training and competition, including returning to Newcastle for another marathon. A local star named Brian Morgan won by ten minutes but it was a riveting contest for the minor placings. I was locked in battle with Sydney doctor Hugh Dearnley. Periodically, he would stop running and lie down on the road to perform stretching exercises – I had never seen anything like it! The first time it happened, I dashed away and thought I had broken him. A few minutes later, a patter of feet and he was back with me. The fact that he could keep getting back on was telling, and when Hugh crossed the line in 2 hrs 37 mins 18 secs, he was ten seconds in front.

I went back to Warragamba, and in another solid effort, I repeated my fourth placing in a time of 1 hr 57 mins 3 secs and shaved a tiny nineteen secs off my PB. Winner Robert Squirrell was two mins 30 secs in front of me after finishing the same distance behind me at Sutherland. Only two seconds behind him was Alex Watson who would later become known Australia-wide. Alex was a head taller than all the other runners and solidly built, so it was a top performance.

What set Alex apart was that he was equally adept at four other sports. They were swimming, fencing, horse riding and shooting. In later years, he represented Australia at the Olympic Games in the Modern Pentathlon. In contention for a medal, he came unstuck after the fencing competition. It seems he drank too much Coca-Cola to keep himself fuelled and alert. He tested positive to caffeine, was immediately disqualified and sent home in disgrace. He fought for years to clear himself of what he (and I) felt was an unfair decision.

The competition was so tough that results depended on how an individual was feeling on the day. The NSW Marathon Championship was a case in point. The best I could do was tenth (2 hrs 36 mins 23 secs), some ten minutes behind the winner. Behind me, though, was Alex Watson and a top-class runner in Gary Hand. More than happy with those scalps.

In July, I had a couple of 'Andy Lloyd' moments. The first of these was in the Great NOSH Footrace, held over fifteen kilometres through the bushland of Lane Cove National Park. As befitted an event organised by an orienteering club, it was rugged cross-country on technical trails. This was right up my alley! I led the field of 240 throughout and won by 2 mins 48 secs, recording 58 mins 36 secs. In doing so, I broke the event record by seven seconds. The record had been set the previous year by Andy Lloyd! I should add that Andy had been just seventeen; when he came back as a nineteen-year-old, he took it straight back.

A week later, I was down in Nowra attending to some unfinished business. The previous year, I had been leading their King of the Mountains but had to pull out three miles from the finish. This time, I had a bit more respect for the climb and was fitter. I led the twenty miles throughout and finished with a negative split, winning by four minutes in 2 hrs 4 mins 48 secs.

Fun Runs often had teams competitions. In the local Liverpool Fun Run (ten kilometres), I combined with two local friends, Paul Curley and my training partner, Glyn Cox. We also recruited Andy Lloyd! He won in 32 mins 10 secs, with me coming fourth again (33 mins 32 secs). We won the teams event to the chagrin of a vocal second-placegetter, Horst Wegner. His opinion that Andy should not have been allowed to team up with us gained no traction whatsoever!

In August, it all started to fall apart running-wise. I was tired and flat and unable to train much. During this period, I ran my first Sydney City to Surf. I finished sixty-second of many thousands of starters, with a PB for fourteen kilometres of 47 mins 16 secs. An amazing experience, but so slow early, locked in the huge crowd of jam-packed runners.

I had enough residual fitness and perhaps a class edge to win our 2 Military Hospital cross-country in record time, almost four minutes in front of our physical training instructor, Mike Connor. The next day, I followed up with the 5/7 RAR cross-country but took it a bit easy by running with Kel Wakefield before edging away in the later stages.

A couple of days later, Sandy had some pregnancy-related abdominal issues and was hospitalised at

Liverpool. Soon after, she was transferred to a specialist maternity hospital in Sydney. On 18 August 1979, our son Daniel was born ten weeks premature. My wife and child were confined there for many weeks before it was deemed safe to let them come home.

I had long drives into the city to fit in around work. I also attended promotion and education courses to make me eligible for promotion when the time came around. I got another marathon in, but as you would expect, my performances over that distance were slipping. I had enough in the tank to easily win the NSW Army cross-country covering nine kilometres in 33 mins 6 secs.

The Fisher's Ghost twelve-kilometre race saw me twelfth in a PB of 40 mins 20 secs while achieving first Army and second local. Then at the end of November came the first of my duels with a top RAAF athlete whom I had not encountered before. It must have been five years since I had been defeated in Inter-Service competition, but at Narrabeen in the 5000 metres, that streak came to end. I led at a fast pace but tired in the final stages and Ian Hamilton came past to finish nine seconds in front. As happened five years ago with Phil Hassel, he had to set an NSW Inter-Service record of 15 mins 32 secs to bring me undone. A couple of hours later, I gained revenge in the 1500 metres where I sprinted from the 300-metre mark and just managed to pip Ian on the line after a stirring duel (4 mins 11 secs).

Annual leave had us back in Healesville where a new maternal grandmother had a great time spoiling Danny. Then in March 1980, I was back to Healesville for a Medical Corps promotion course. As this was medicine and not military skills, I was able to breeze through.

With that out of the way, I found time for some training and another marathon, where I was seventeenth of six hundred in 2 hrs 43 mins 39 secs. It was incremental but continued my slide away from peak performances. In orienteering, I slipped back to seventh and Graham Moon suffered a rare defeat at the hands of the other engineering officer, Major Peter Rose. I managed a fun run win at Camden, but at Sutherland Half Marathon I was ten minutes slower than in earlier years. In June, it was more of the same at Warragamba when my hill running strength deserted me and I had to do some walking.

The writing was on the wall – I was in trouble. For months, I had been feeling flat with dizziness, nausea and weakness. Somehow, I managed to put in a couple of weeks of heavy training, unwilling to face facts and succumb to the inevitable. On the strength of that, I disappeared from the Sydney running scene with a bang. My final race was a thirty-kilometre race from Palm Beach to Manly. Although the winner was well clear, setting a record, I was content with another fourth in a PB of 1 hr 46 mins 1sec, only 16 seconds behind Alex Watson.

Chapter 9 Back in the Army

Where I pulled that one from, I am not sure, as I was diagnosed with glandular fever a few days later and ordered not to do any exercise. A day later, we were on the road again as I had been posted to 1st Armoured Regiment, based at Puckapunyal in central Victoria. In less than three years, I had been promoted from private to corporal and was now marching into a new unit as a sergeant. A meteoric rise but not so surprising, when you consider my original six years of experience.

CHAPTER 10
Retiring from running

I marched into my new unit with some trepidation, as it was the first Field Force unit I had served in, except for my active service in Vietnam. This was an establishment full of armoured vehicles and gung-ho fighting soldiers. I was also newly promoted to run the Regimental Aid Post (RAP) under a Regimental Medical Officer (RMO). I also had three corporals, with one allocated to each armoured squadron. On top of all this, I was entering my new challenge on medically restricted duties.

I had a month off from running as I figured that should do it as far as glandular fever went. After a week of training, I went in an orienteering event that took me 2 hrs 26 mins, leaving me very tired and ill afterwards.

A week later, I drove to nearby Bendigo where the Victorian (3MD) Inter-Service cross-country was being held. On a rugged six-mile course at One Tree Hill, I led and after a tough battle, I prevailed over Chris Huppatz by thirty seconds. In doing so, I took two minutes off the course record, recording 33 mins 35 secs. So I was back in business, right? Wrong!

Three more weeks of training and feeling lousy; the RMO confirmed that I still had glandular fever. I had some other activities to entertain me, though. It was midwinter and that meant 1 Armoured Regiment's annual trip to Mt Buller for skiing. We stayed in forestry huts at Mirimbah at the base of Mt Buller and Mt Stirling. I was up there as medic but I did heaps of Nordic skiing and knocked myself flat again. What part of resting do I not understand!?

I had ten days on a mountain training exercise, where we played around with armoured personnel carriers (APCs) around Mt Matlock in the rugged high country between Woods Point and Walhalla north-east of Melbourne. I got a couple of tough runs in and lots of days just working. There was plenty of snow, rain and hail just to keep things interesting.

The Australian Inter-Service Marathon was on in Sydney, so off I went. I don't know what I expected with limited training and continuing glandular fever, but I got the result I deserved. I ran to the halfway mark in 1 hr 20 mins with a group that included a few old friends: Ian Hamilton, Alan Batchelor and Mike Connor. From here, I would expect to single out for a duel with Ian, but instead I stopped with every intention of pulling out.

After a few minutes, I decided to keep going and just alternated walking and running at a sustainable pace. I was the fifth Army runner over the line, twenty minutes behind the winning RAAF competitor. My time of 2 hrs 57 mins 8 secs was about the worst I had done in my career. That, and the way I felt, finally convinced me to retire – at least until cured. At the age of twenty-eight, my athletics career seemed over.

This time, I had two months off before I tried some training in January 1981. There is nothing like jumping in at the deep end. The Australian Six-Day Orienteering competition was held on a variety of courses throughout central Victoria. I competed in this event only once and came fourth in the Men's 21B field.

Glynn Cox, my running mate from Ingleburn, had moved to Griffith in southern NSW, so we had a road trip which started a tradition of an annual visit between the families. When I returned, I had another go at the professional track circuit. I performed reasonably but nothing to get excited about. My best run was when I went to the rich Lavington Gift meeting in southern NSW. In the 1600-metre handicap off the middle mark of 140 metres, I finished ninth, some seven seconds behind the winner. The next night in the 3200 metres (with a 260-metre handicap), I was third, only one second behind the winner. I finished in front of my co-marker, Geoff Molloy, who re-enters my story later.

Chapter 10 Retiring from running

During the week, I had a few trips to Melbourne where Sandy had been admitted to hospital. In the later stages of pregnancy number two, she was suffering pre-eclampsia. My first show of good form must have upset a professional trainer of some authority. When I turned up to run at Sebastopol the next week, I had been re-handicapped back twenty metres in the 1600-metre event, because 'somebody' complained that I had resumed competing on an incorrect handicap mark. Usually, a re-handicap only occurs after you win, but mine happened after a well-beaten ninth. Something a bit corrupt going on here, methinks! I had an argument with the handicapper about how unfair it was. Then I walked to my original 140-metre mark and ran from there, but I was so upset, I came nowhere. During the discussion, I said, 'Well, what about my 3200-metre handicap for tomorrow?' as it was still down as 260 metres. He assured me that would be adjusted also.

At Northcote, I had a lot of incentive to win after what I had been told. That's exactly what happened, and I paid for it with an unheard-of re-handicap of fifty-five metres! All this running had me going well enough to win all six Army events during the week, at the Inter-Squadron and Inter-Unit athletics competitions.

The next weekend at the rich Bendigo Gift meeting, I ran off my new mark. I had no choice but to run too hard early from way back there. As a result, I walked off the track at the halfway mark. The stewards suspended me for three weeks for an 'unsatisfactory performance'. I explained that the problem was an unsatisfactory handicap.

It was a busy time, as a few days later I ran in three events at the Victorian (3MD) Army Championships. I won the 800 metres but couldn't keep up with Captain Terry Fisher in the 1500 or 5000 metres. Times were slow and it was another indication that all was not well.

Two days later, Sandy was back in the Mercy Maternity Hospital and had an emergency caesarean. Our daughter Kimberley was delivered eight weeks' early. It was a difficult time for all, as I had work and a toddler to care for while Sandy and Kimberley were indisposed.

During all this, I had an appeal against my treatment by the handicapper heard. I presented all my results and with that evidence, the independent panel upheld my appeal. A hollow victory as on the way out, the handicapper told me that I could get stuffed. I was not getting my handicap back, and that was that!

There was always my military races to fall back on. The 3MD Inter Service was held late in March. Again I 'failed', with a second and two thirds in mediocre times. I went to the Stawell Gift at Easter and was way uncompetitive off my hard mark. That was it for pro track running as I was thoroughly disillusioned.

During May, I attended an Education Course for

Chapter 10 Retiring from running

three weeks and had to miss the annual orienteering competition. Having left Kyneton High School at fifteen, it was necessary to upgrade my education with a course run by the Army if I was to seek further promotion. I had struggled during my secondary schooling, particularly in mathematics and arithmetic. Now with maturity and teachers who could explain the lessons properly, I excelled. I received four distinctions and two credits in six subjects.

In May while being educated, I stepped my training miles right up with a view to competing in a new professional event called the Great Otway Classic. It was a three-day team race held in mid-winter over the rugged Otway Ranges. All the top pro runners were in it, and I was chosen as a number four seed in a team called Otway Traders. There were six teams, each with seven runners. All were required to run flat out two or three times a day.

Over-training had injured my right knee, but I ran anyway; it was very tough to back up on repeated occasions over three days. It was the hardest event I had ever done and my team finished fourth. I knew if I was to ever come back, I would need to be healthy, much fitter and not injured. Well, if I wouldn't rest due to illness, perhaps 'runner's knee' would force me to take a break.

Nothing to report for the next fifteen months. The little running I did was on minimal training and the results were substandard.

Three of the troopers who were in my unit warrant a

mention. Paul Winterton was one, whom I hadn't seen since I'd visited his house to play as a child in Woodend. Wayne Atkinson told me he was from Ballarat and had trained in a group of runners that included a promising young runner named Steve Moneghetti. I had stopped competing, so I didn't get to race him as he won the unit cross-country. Unfortunately, Wayne was killed in a traffic accident shortly after. The third trooper I did not meet personally until four years later and his name was John McCrystal. Upon meeting, I was surprised to hear him say that my running at 1st Armoured Regiment had inspired him to commence his own athletics career. My surprise was that I could inspire anybody with my unwell and relatively slow efforts at that time.

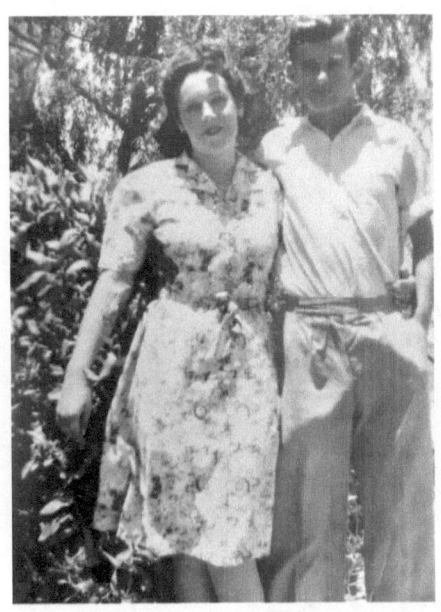

1946 Stanhope, Vic. Winifred Williams and Lloyd Tonks. Wini became pregnant and the young couple were required to marry, one day before the bride was put on a train back to Ayr, Nth Qld.

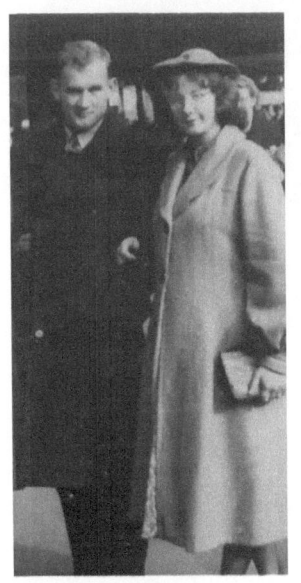

1948 Auckland New Zealand. Lloyd Tonks and a young Gwen Harvey prepare to leave for life as a couple in Australia. It is possible Gwen's coat is concealing my yet to arrive older brother Bryan? A future marriage is approved but, ... What about Winnie, the current wife back in Ayr Nth Qld?

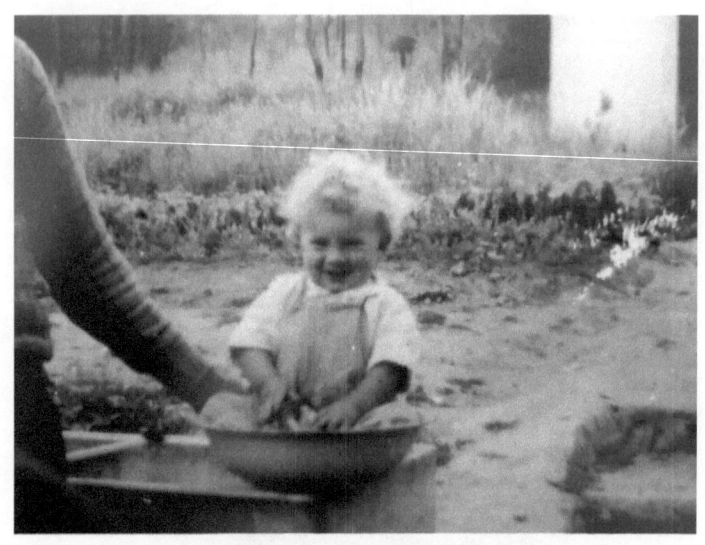

*1953 Edinburgh Rd Mt.Evelyn, Vic.
First photo of Greg and perhaps first bath also.*

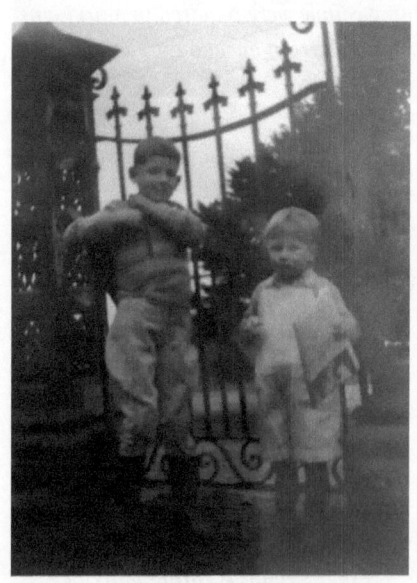

1957 Cemetery house, Woodend, Vic. A move from Woodend North and a name change for brothers Bryan and Greg Harvey. Now in a melded family they were Garth and Greg Wilson.

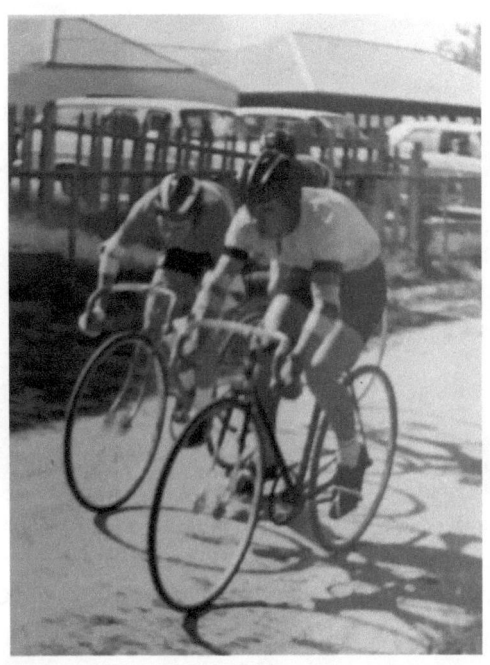

Mar 1969 Kyneton Cycling Track, Showgrounds, Vic. Greg aged 16 defeating fellow junior John Robinson and Geoff Cordy in a handicap race on the slippery gravel of the old showgrounds track.

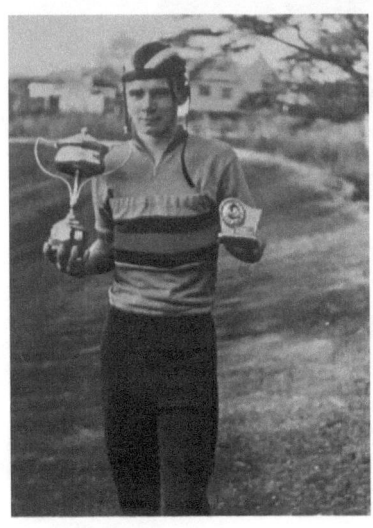

Jan 1970 Kyneton Velodrome, Vic. My first annual leave from the Army. On a visit back to Kyneton I was presented with the Kyneton (now Macedon Ranges) Cycling Club Track Aggregate trophy, for accruing the most points during the 1968-69 track season.

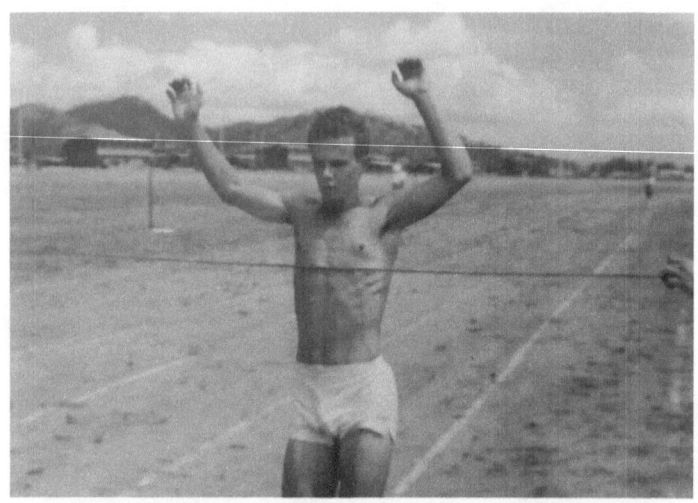

April 1970 1st Military District (Qld) Inter-Area 5 Kilometre Championship, Lavarack Barracks, Townsville. At age 17 Greg's second ever race was a was a big win from 42 year old Jim Goodwin.

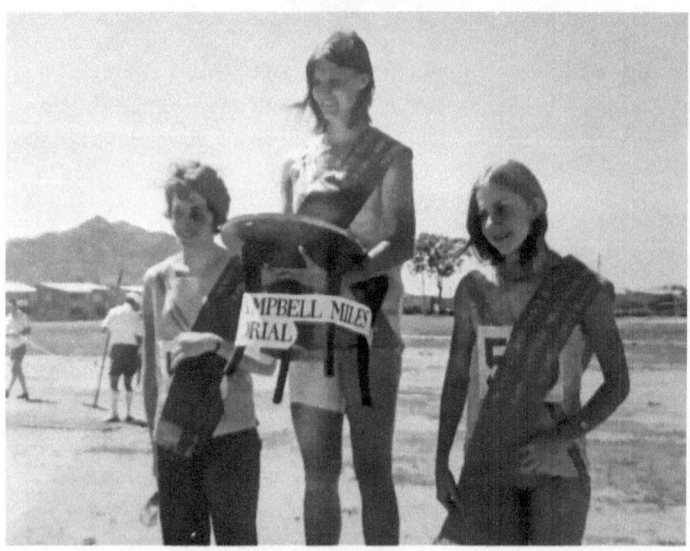

Aug 1971 North Queensland Athletic Championships, Northern Star Athletic Club, Townsville, Nth Qld. The Campbell Miles Memorial 100 metre podium with three stars from Townsville Amateur Athletic Club successful. L to R Barbara Willis, Jill Sager, Margaret Gilboy.

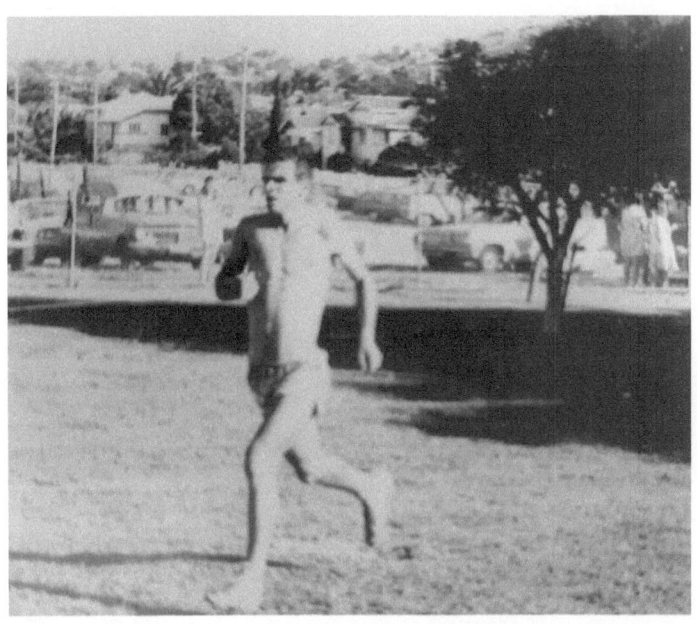

Sep 1971 3 Task Force (Army) Cross-Country Championship 5.5 miles, Pallarenda to Kissing Point, Townsville Nth Qld. Greg's first cross-country since high school and a clear victory in record time.

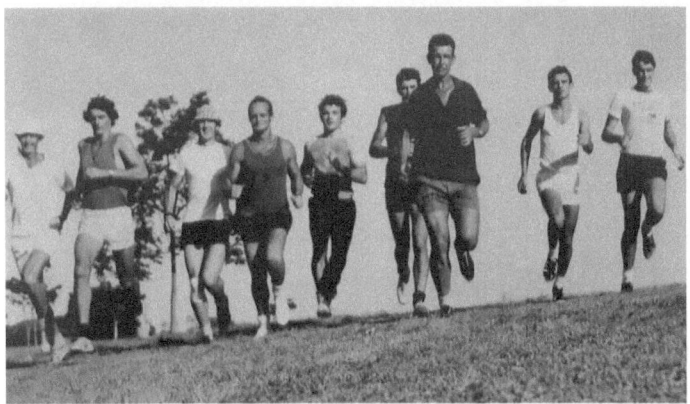

November 1971 Cairns to Townsville Relay, Anderson Park, Townsville Nth Qld. A pre relay training run. L to R Bob Down, Dave Smith, Peter Hone, Bill Cook (crew), Bernie McMinn, Bernie Smith, Ray Dennis, Greg Wilson, Rowan Carr absent Terry Lee, Mark Adams.

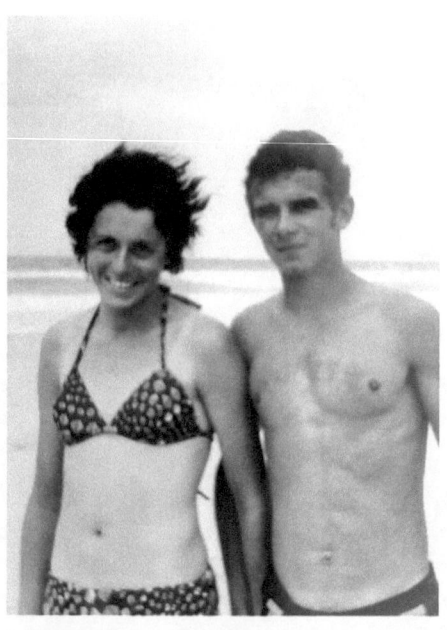

December 1971 Kirra Beach, Gold Coast, Qld. Barb and Greg caught up briefly on holiday visit to the Gold Coast.

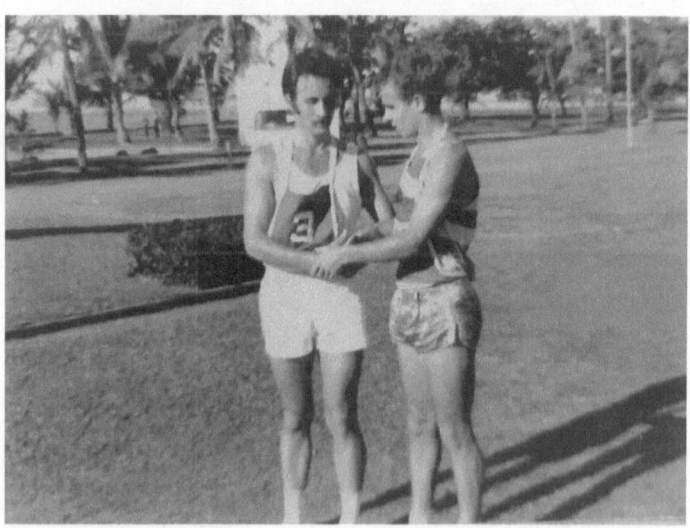

June 1972 Inaugural King of the Castle, Townsville Nth Qld. Winner Mike Phillips (L) being congratulated by runner-up Greg Wilson.

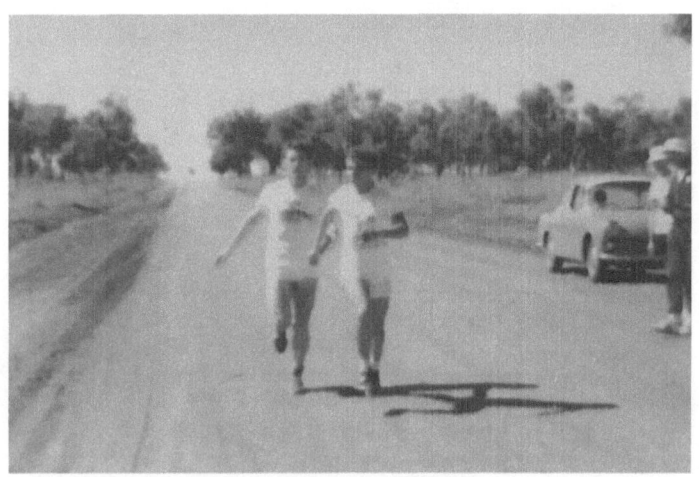

June 1972 Townsville to Charters Towers Relay, Flinders Hwy Nth Qld. Founder of the Townsville Marathon Club (now Townsville Road Runners TRR) Graham Moon hands over to Greg Wilson. Timing them are future Life Members of TRR David Wharton and Bob Down.

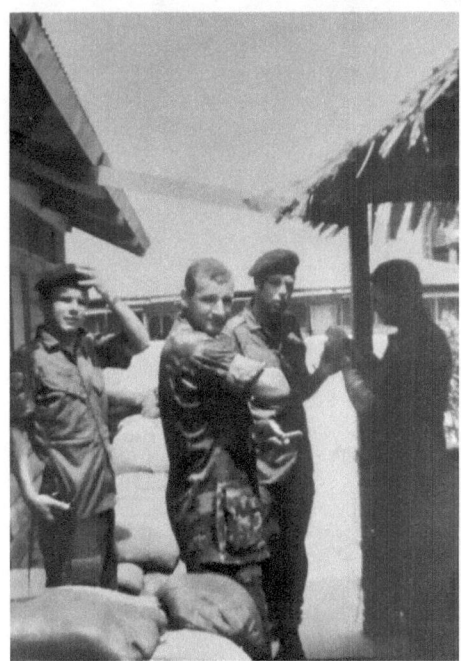

September 1972 Long Hai Training Battalion, South Vietnam. Cpl Greg Wilson (L) and WO2 John Nolan (R) chat with a US Special Forces member near our accommodation.

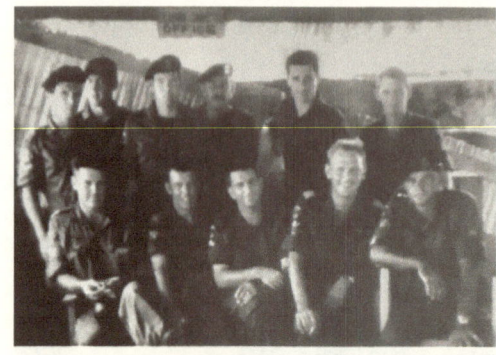 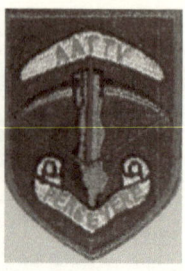

Oct 1972 Long Hai Training Battalion, South Vietnam. Members of the Australian Army Training Team- Vietnam (AATTV).

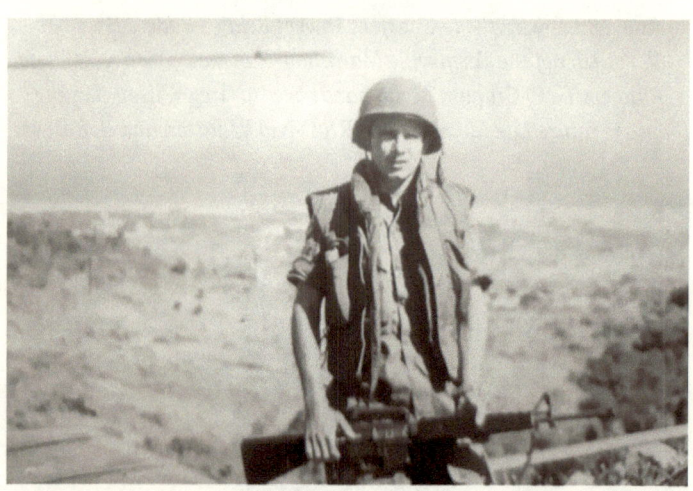

November 1972. Cpl Greg Wilson AATTV on "Radar Hill" above Vung Tau, South Vietnam, two weeks prior to returning to Australia.

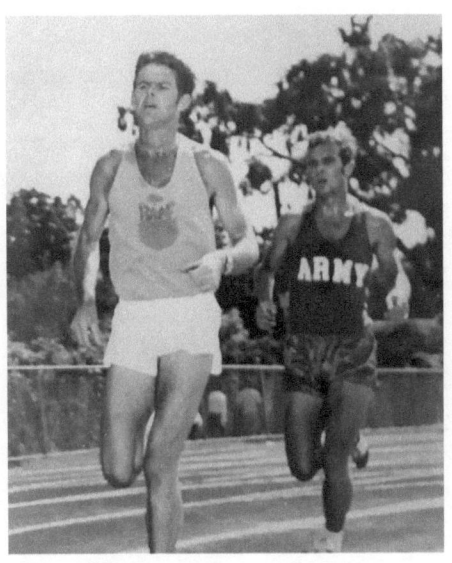

May 1974 Victorian Inter-Service 5 Kilometre Championship, Melbourne Uni Track, Vic. A 25 sec personal best of 15 mins 35 secs for Greg as he clung on to RAAF athlete Phil Hassel, but to no avail. Phil won by 10 secs and his record stood for a decade before Greg surpassed it.

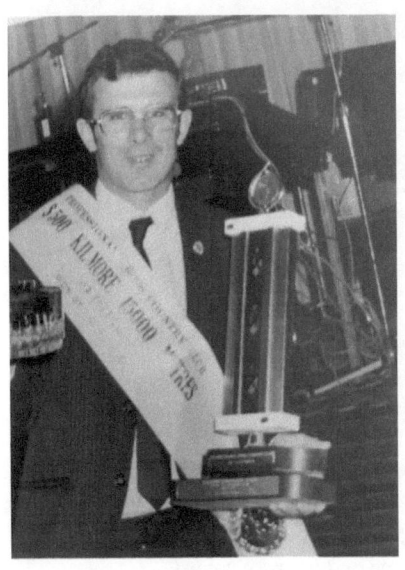

Oct 1974 Professional Cross-Country Club (PCCC) presentation night, Melbourne, Vic. A huge leap in Greg's first season, from novice to victory in the richest event on the calendar, the Kilmore Feature Race 15 Kilometres.

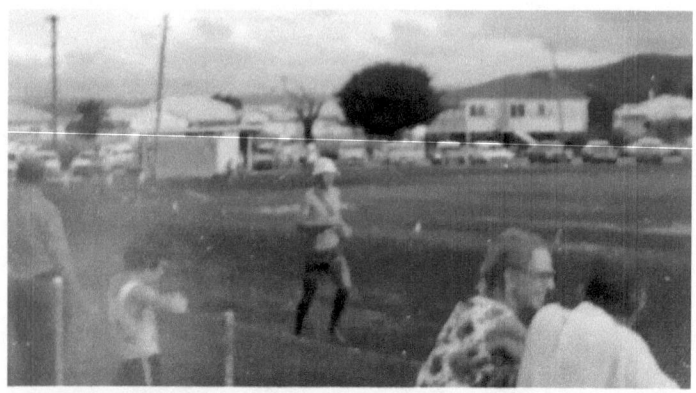

Mar 1975 Country Queensland 10 Kilometre Championships, Corcoran Park Townsville. On a "bog track" I ran barefoot on one of the widest white lines and still won by a lap. My final Qld amateur event prior to being banned as a "professional"

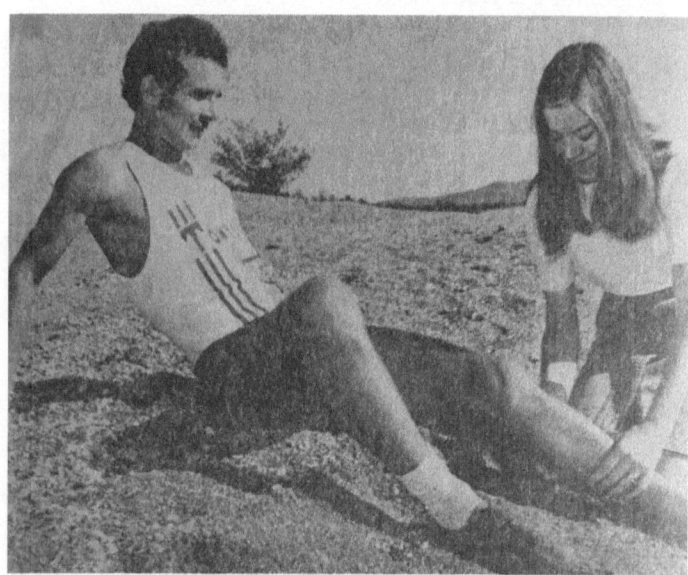

June 1976 King of the Castle, Rowes Bay beach, Townsville. Pre-race newspaper publicity has my wife Sandy pretending to massage my leg. Fame is ever so fleeting as Steve Colbourne broke 30 minutes and smashed me and my race record..

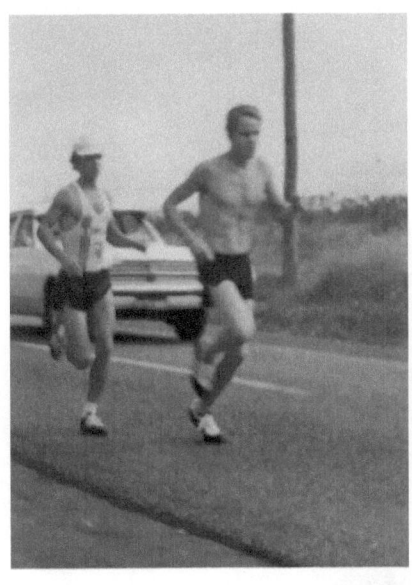

July 1976 Mareeba Rodeo Roadrace 10 Miles, Walkamin to Mareeba, Atherton Tableland, Nth Qld. John Temby forcing the pace as Greg clung on, then pulled away to win in record (career PB) time.

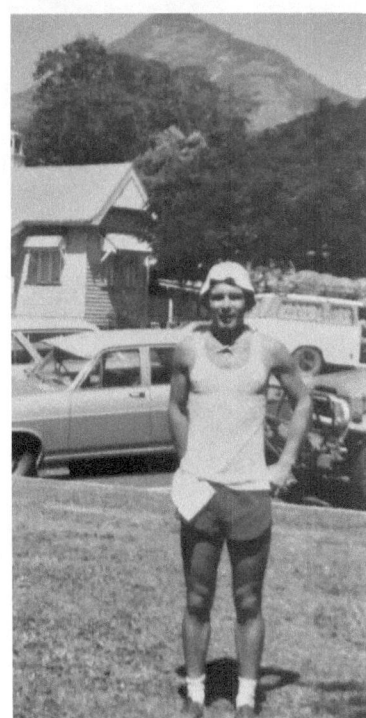

August 1976 The Great Pyramid Race, Gordonvale, Nth Qld. Pre-race Greg pictured with Walsh's Pyramid in the background. Won in record time.

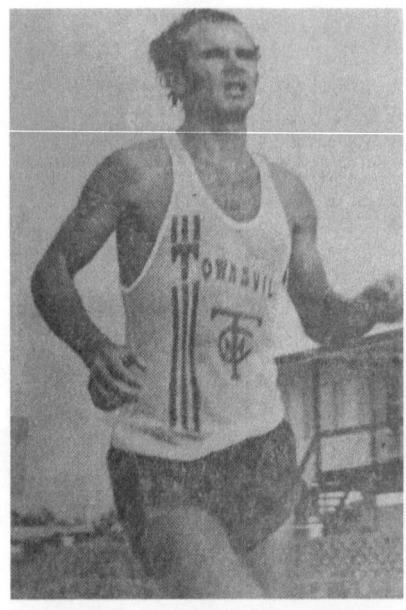

August 1976 North Queensland (Townsville) Marathon. Greg crossing the line in a personal best time, 2 hrs 38 mins 35 secs breaking the event record by 19 mins 33 secs. Second was 40 year old Peter Lahiff also surpassing the previous record.

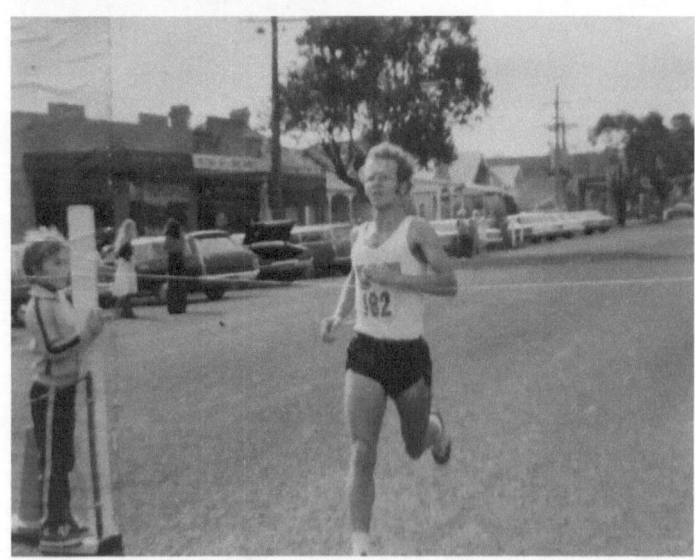

September. 1976 Victorian Professional 15 Mile Championship, Whittlesea. On return from Townsville, Greg's only professional championship victory.

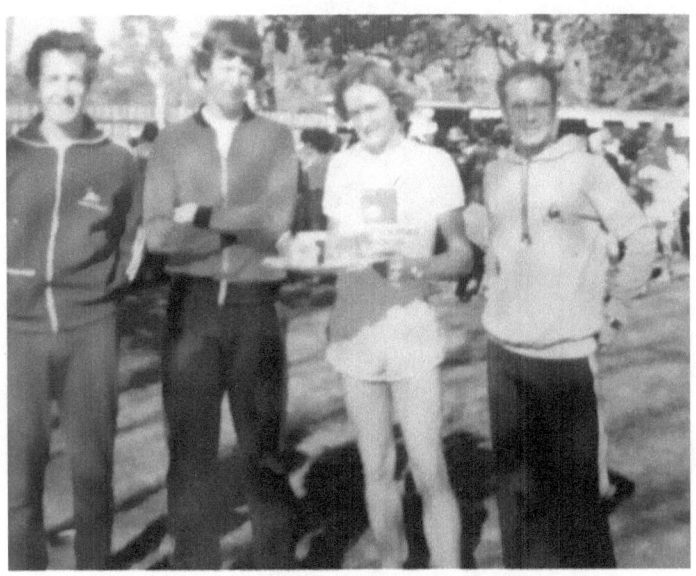

Jul 1979 Liverpool Fun Run 10 Kilometres, NSW. If you plan to win a team category in a fun run it helps to have a special team mate. L to R Glyn Cox, Paul Curley, Andrew Lloyd, Greg "Harvey". Andy was aged 18 and won the next three Melbourne Marathons and a Commonwealth Games 5 Km gold medal.

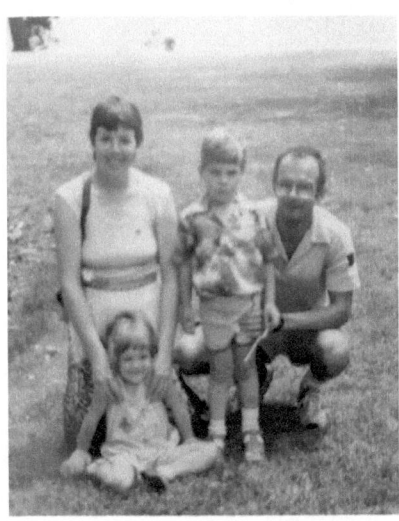

1983 Lake Burley Griffin, ACT. Sandy and Greg with Kimberley and Daniel

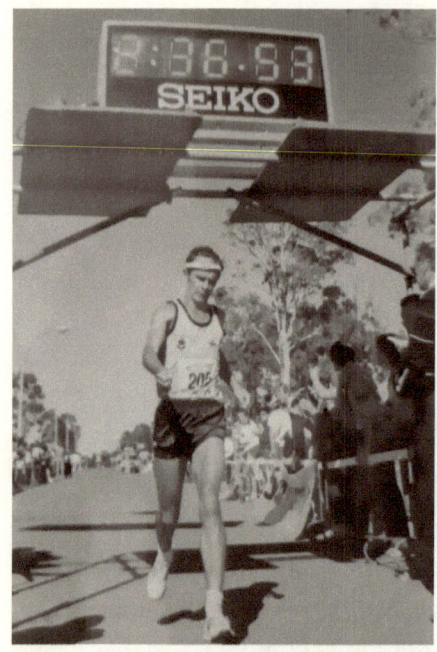

May 1983 NSW Marathon Championship, Holsworthy NSW. A successful comeback from years of illness with fourteenth placing and second in the Australian Defence Force behind Ian Hamilton.

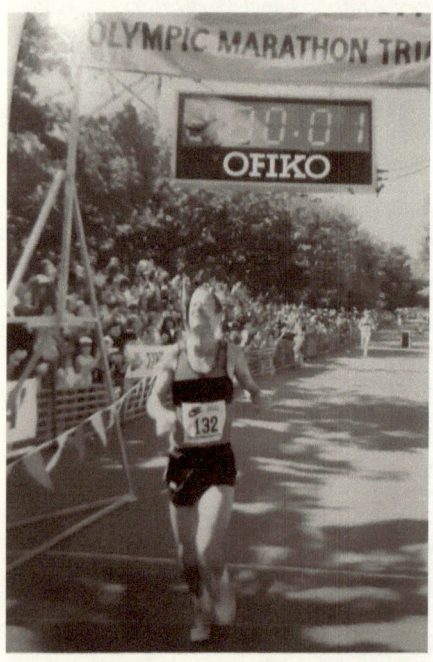

April 1984 Olympic Marathon Trial, Canberra ACT. Such was the quality of the field that a career personal best by Greg of 2 hrs 30 mins 01 secs in tough conditions only achieved 28th position.

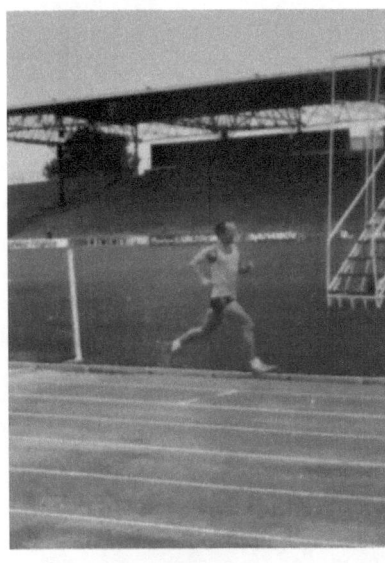

February 1985 3MD (Victorian Army) 5 Kilometre Track Championship, Olympic Park Melbourne. With one lap to go Greg is clear of John McCrystal. The time of 15 mins 17 secs was a career track PB, broke the record and was the only victory over John.

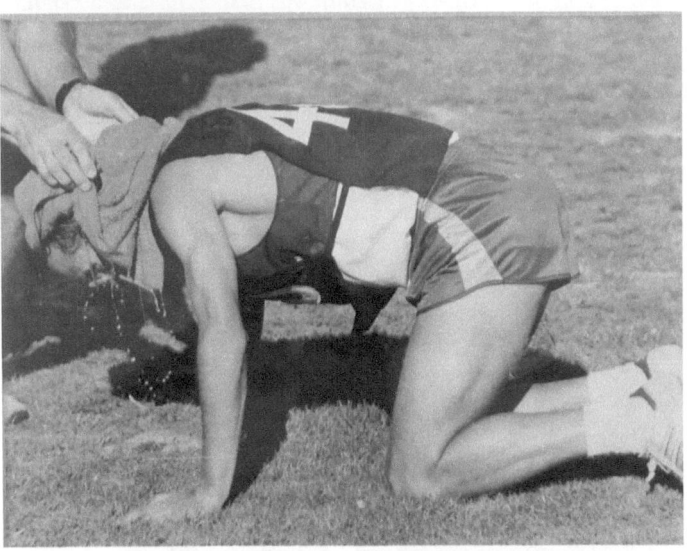

February 1985 Melton Vic. An Army posting back to Victoria, so time to resume professional track running. Greg pictured being assisted by training partner Brian Simmons after running in thirty eight degree heat and winning the Melton 3200 metre handicap.

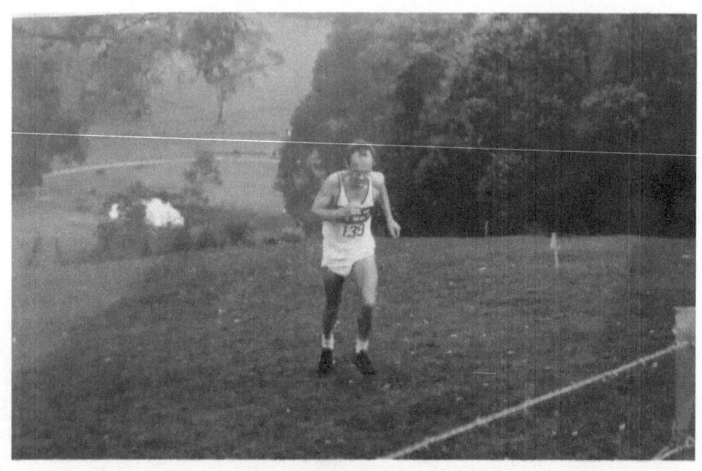

September 1985 3MD (Victorian Army) Cross-Country Championship 9.6 Kilometres, Healesville Vic. An event designed and organised by Greg, so it was fitting that he achieved victory and the host unit School Of Army Health was first team. Greg ascending "Heartbreak Hill" for the second time.

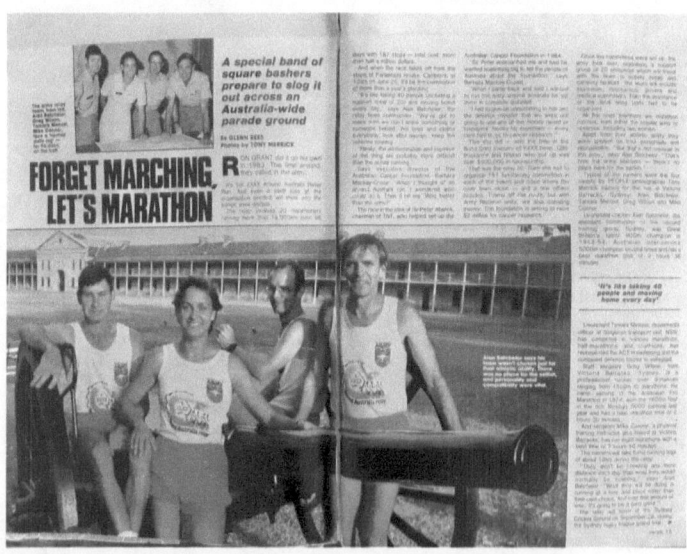

May 1986 XXXX Army Around Australia Relay promotion, Victoria Barracks, Paddington, NSW. PEOPLE magazine promoted the relay. L to R Sgt Mike Connor, Lt Tammy Menzel, SSgt. Greg Wilson, LtCol Alan Batchelor

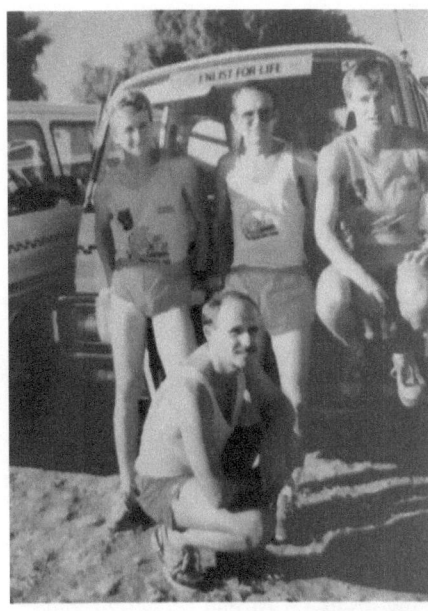

June-September 1986 XXXX Army Around Australia Relay Marathon.

Team Five L to R Pte Vic Perry, Sgt Ernie Stewart, SSgt Greg Wilson, Cfn Rob Combe

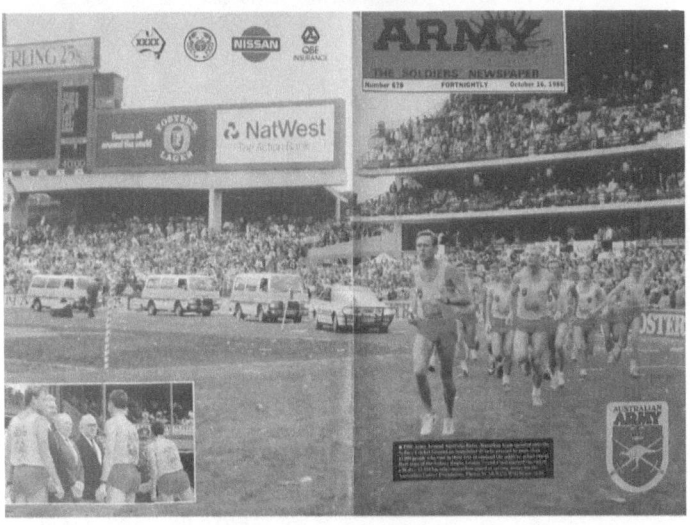

September 1986 XXXX Army Around Australia Relay, Sydney Cricket Ground. After 96 days twenty Army runners led by Lt Col Alan Batchelor finish off with a lap of the SCG at half time of the Rugby League grand final.

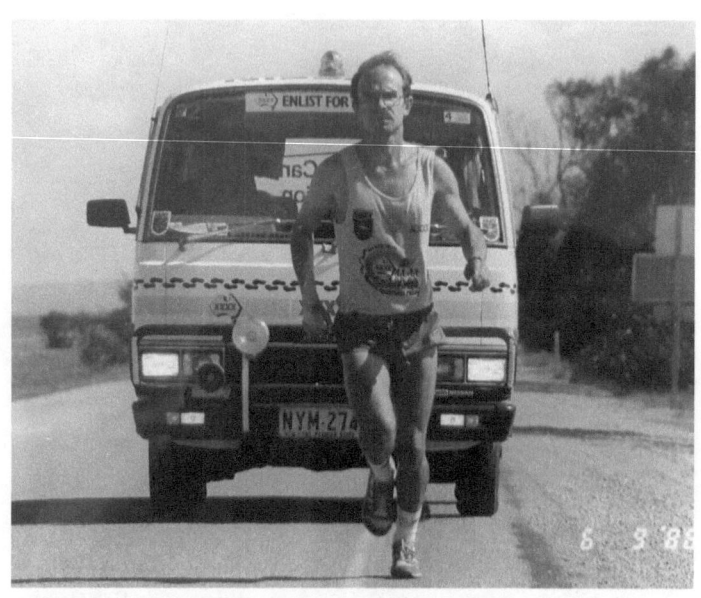

September 1986 XXXX Army Around Australia Relay Marathon. Greg running into a strong head-wind near Port Wakefield SA.

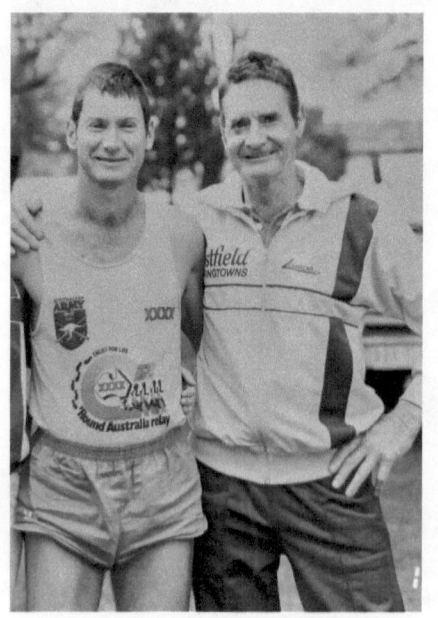

September 1986 XXXX Army Around Australia Relay. L to R Mike Connor, Cliff Young. The park in Colac, Vic was the venue for many of folk legend Cliff Young's ultra marathons. The relay "Cliffy lookalike" was Mike and a photo op was too good to pass up.

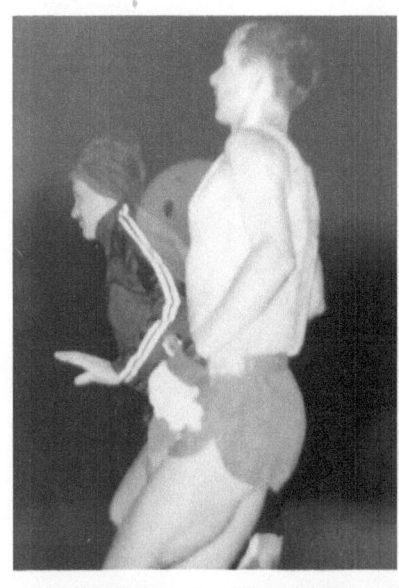

September 1986 XXXX Army Around Australia Relay, Queenstown, Tas. Almost midnight, no sleep, pouring rain and Gormonston Hill's 100 bends …some challenge there to remain on schedule! Job done Greg Wilson hands over to a "rugged up" Ernie Stewart.

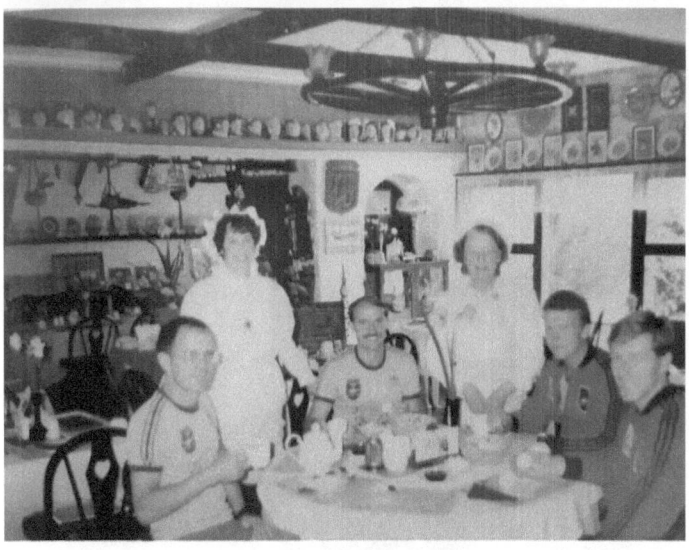

September 1986 XXXX Army Around Australia Relay, New Norfolk, Tas. Team 5 are feted with a Devonshire tea at The Colonial Inn, New Norfolk. A long night through the SW Wilderness now a memory as L to R Greg Wilson, Ernie Stewart, Vic Perry, Rob Combe enjoy the break.

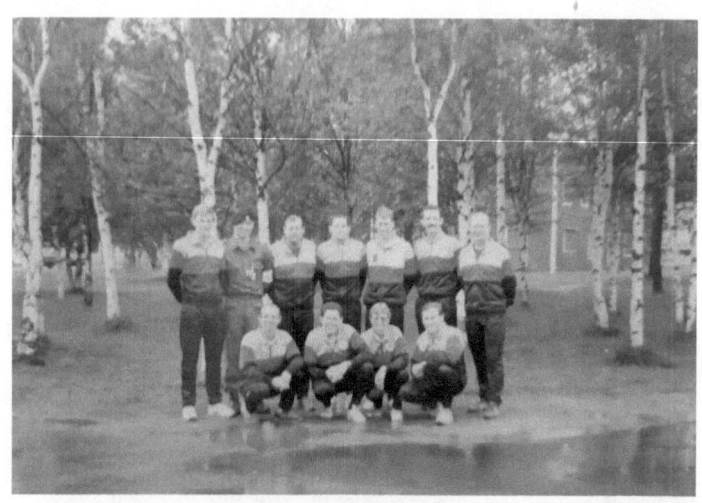

June 1990 Setermoen, northern Norway. The Australian Defence Force team at the World Military Orienteering Championships (XX111CISM) L to R Rear row: Lt Bill Gradden, Trond Hermannsen (Interpreter), Capt Dave Gratwick, Flt Lt Adrian Rowland, Capt Arnold Simpson, Maj Alan Clark, Maj John Suominen (Chef De Mission). Front row: SSgt Greg Wilson, LCdr Adrian Wotton, Leut Zoe Read, WO2 Mick Hodge.

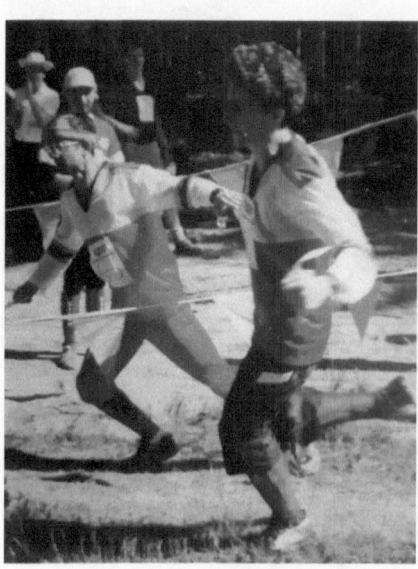

April 1991 Australian Defence Force Orienteering Championship, Camp Cable, Qld. Margaret Hatfield runs in to send Greg Wilson on his way for the final sporting event of a 20 year Army career. At age 39 he went out in style running second fastest relay leg and anchoring an Army team gold medal.

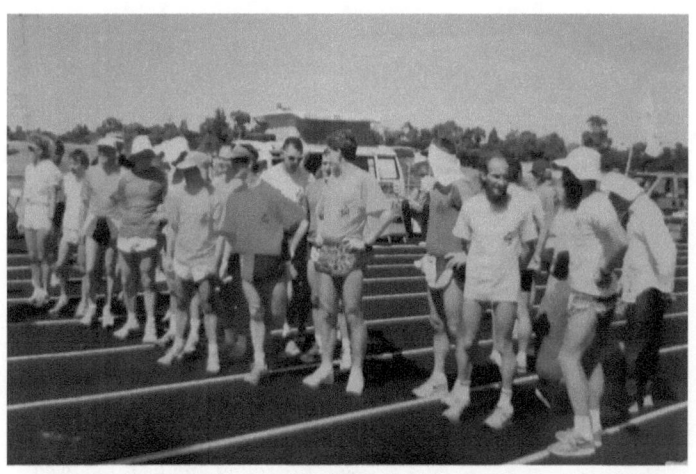

February 1992 Victorian 24 Hour Championship, Coburg, Vic. Front row from left are Helen Stanger NSW and David Standeven SA, male and female winners. Greg is centre between the green hats. Andrew Law TAS in red then Neville Mercer NZ in yellow, Michael Grayling and on the inside in white looking down is Cliff Young. A strong field and a very hot day.

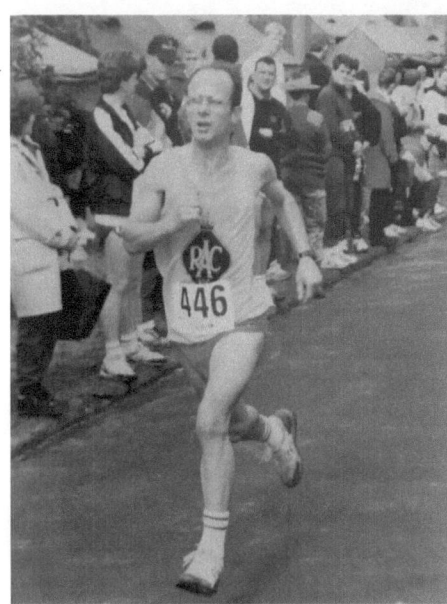

SEP 1992 Lake Relay, Albert Park Lake, Melbourne Vic. Greg striding out during one of three 5 kilometre legs. Joined mate Brian Simmons team for second placing

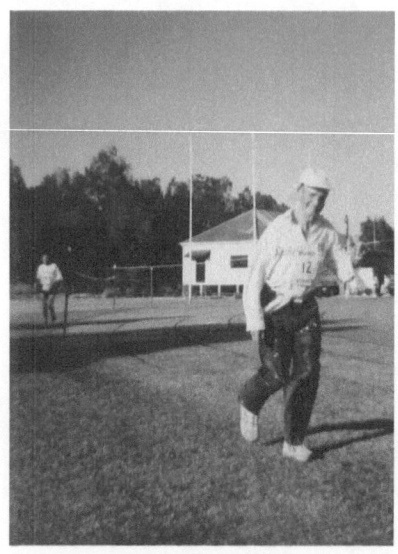

January 1994 Tacoma 12 Hour, Wyong NSW. Two giants of Australian ultra running. In the foreground is "Folk Legend" Cliff Young and he is followed by race winner the world class Bryan Smith.

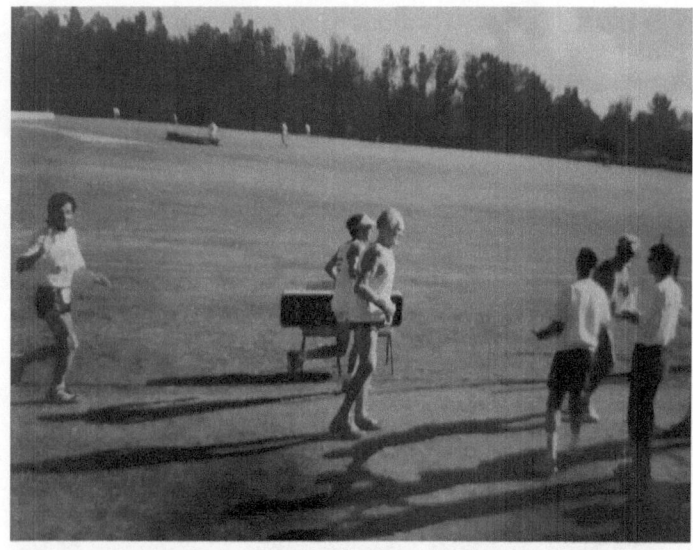

January 1994 12 Hour Ultra, Tacoma, NSW. Three male place getters passing a lapped runner and lap counters. L to R Bryan Smith 1st, Greg Wilson 2nd, Bob Channells 3rd.

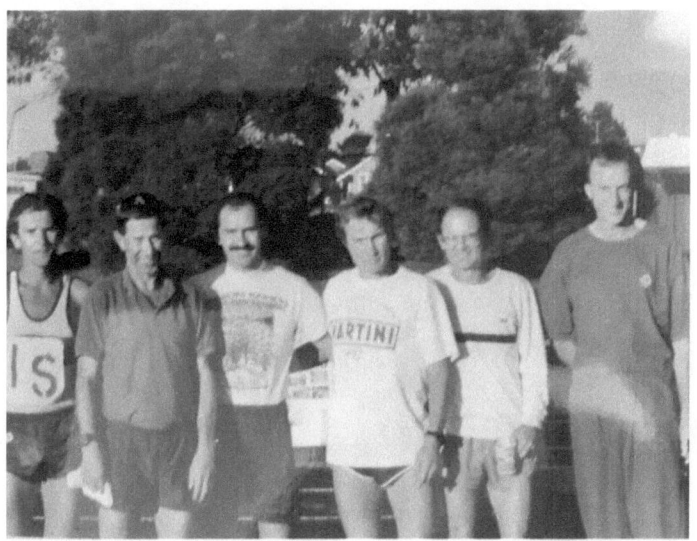

April 1995 Victorian 24 Hour Championship, Coburg, Vic. The Russians visited but suffered a rare defeat when they encountered the "Collosus of Roads" Yiannis. L to R Igor Streltzov, Leigh Privett, Yiannis Kouros, Gennardy Groshev, Greg Wilson, Geoff Hook.

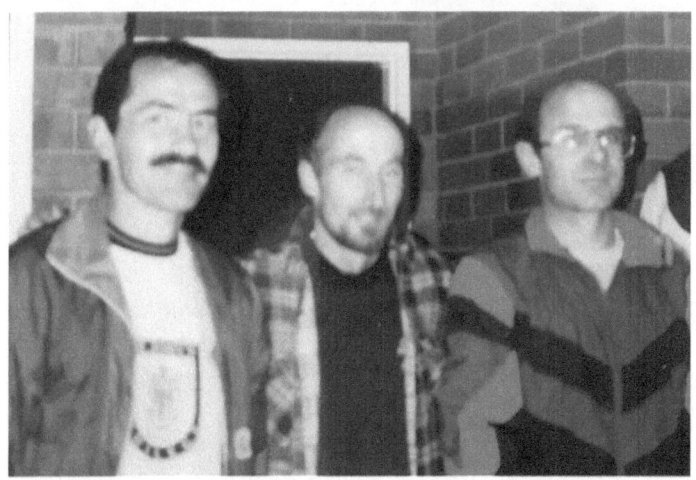

August 1996 Inaugural AA Australian 100 Kilometre Championship, Shepparton Vic. The winning Victorian team. L to R: Yiannis Kouros, Michael Grayling, Greg Wilson.

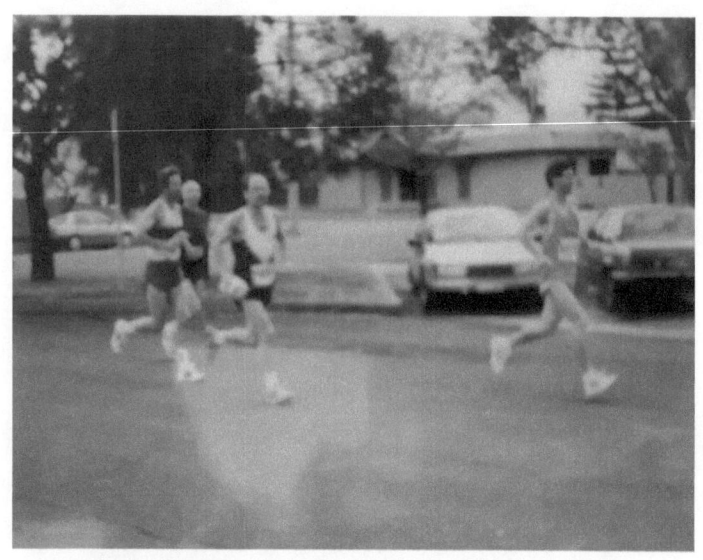

September 1996 Inaugural AA Australian 100 Kilometre Championship, Shepparton Vic. A full 5 kilometre lap behind Yiannis but the battle for third placing was close, L to R Asim Mesalic Qld 3rd, Greg Wilson Vic, 4th, Mick Francis WA who was third across the line but not AA registered.

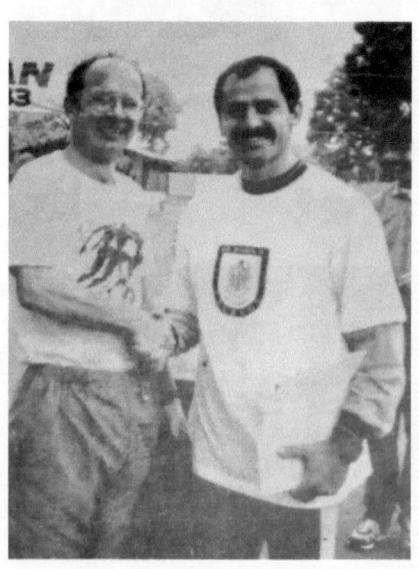

September 1996. Inaugural AA Australian 100 Kilometre Championship. A team gold medal to Victoria and a hand shake for Greg with the world's greatest ultra marathoner, team mate Yiannis Kouros.

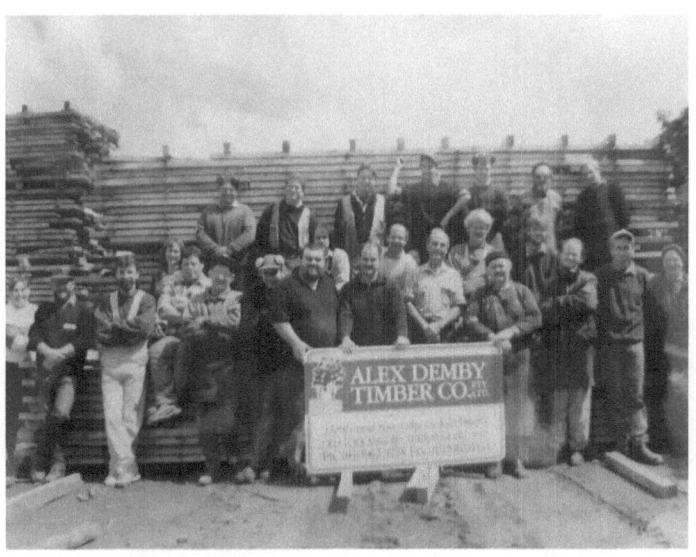

1997 Alex Demby Timber Coy P/L, Toolangi, Vic. A staff picture with Alex and son Gary Demby behind the sign. Just behind are timber workers and marathoners Brian Simmons and Greg Wilson (yellow).

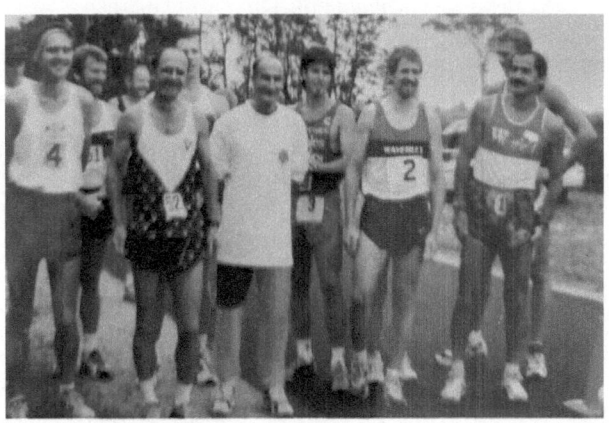

1998 Australian 100 Kilometre Championship. Top quality field at the start line and they almost finished in race number order. No 1 Yiannis Kouros, No2 Nigel Aylott, No 3 Ian Cornthwaite DNF, No4 Kelvin Marshall. Greg was unfit and ran second in the 50 Kilometre.

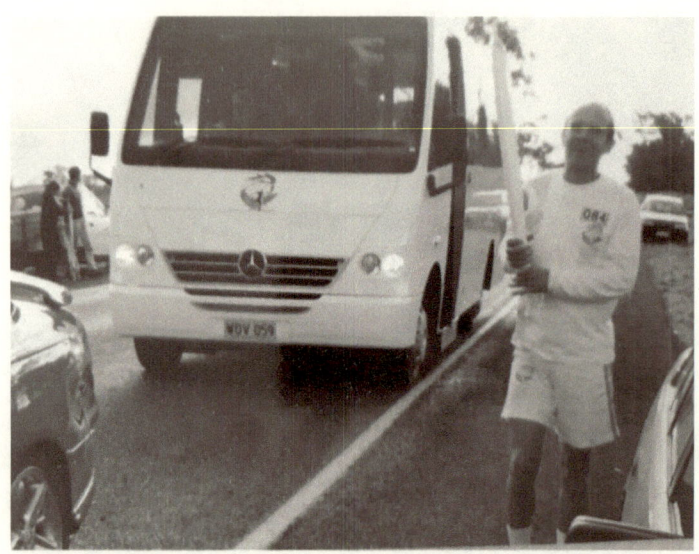

2000 I was not running and this in no athletic feat and dubious quality photo. However it is me carrying the torch during the Sydney Olympic Torch Relay. Near Mooroopna Vic. Ironically the town where my father and Winnie were made to marry post-war, ensuring he couldn't then marry my mother.

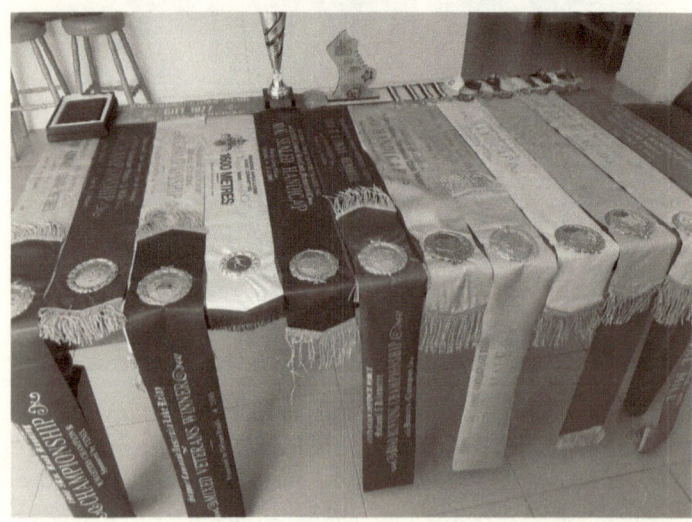

1974 to 2000 Greg's haul of winning sashes from professional track and cross-country races. These were only competed for during intermittent seasons of running in Victoria.

CHAPTER 11
My comeback

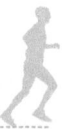

A highlight was that I had survived 1st Armoured Regiment and then received a perfect posting. In mid-1982, I was posted to the Directorate of Army Health Services (DAHS) in a medical/clerical position, for which I was perhaps not qualified but suited me ideally. The location of this department, which was in charge of all of the health services in the Australian Army, was in Canberra.

As is usual, the Army had removalists pack up the Seymour married quarter and store everything. Once we had driven to Canberra, we were accommodated in a motel until a new married quarter in Gowrie was allotted and we and our belongings could move in.

My unit was in Campbell Park Offices which were a series of modern, five-storey, very long buildings of concrete and glass, located in a bushland setting to the east side of Mt Ainslie. Its location was close to the centre of Canberra and had Russell Offices, Duntroon Military College and the Australian War Memorial as close neighbours. DAHS was located on the top floor and had a series of offices, all coming off a carpeted passageway.

It was a top-heavy unit in that I, as a sergeant, was probably the lowest rank working there. The man in charge was a Medical Corps legend. Major General 'Digger' James had come up through the ranks after being an infantryman and losing a leg. He then acquired a medical degree and went on to be in charge of all health services in the Army.

Directly under him was the man I was to work for, Brigadier Bill Rodgers, the Director of Medical Services (DMS). There were two Medical Officers, both majors, and I was basically their clerical assistant. Further up the passage was a Lieutenant Colonel in charge of all Army postings and promotions. He was Bob Allen, my first CSM at 4 Camp Hospital; the same man who sent me on a course in 1971 that led to my Vietnam service and had allowed me to directly re-enlist without doing Kapooka. He had also chosen me for this position eleven years later.

I think perhaps my reputation as a runner may have preceded me to my new unit. On day two, the Brigadier called me in and told me to get my running gear on and at lunch time he would take me for a run around Mt Ainslie. Sometime later, a sweating and short-of-breath

Chapter 11 My comeback

Bill Rodgers had learned what he needed to know and didn't invite me to accompany him again.

During September, I was doing a ten-kilometre run on Mt Ainslie every lunchtime. I saw the Medical Officer at Duntroon, but on hearing me complain that I was reduced to doing eighteen minutes for five kilometres, he couldn't decide between envy or laughter.

In the end, my saviour was the man I worked most closely with every day. Major John Wainwright had previously worked with me in my first posting at 4 Camp Hospital and he knew what I could run like. His job was to create replies to government ministers and ombudsmen, with raw data supplied by me, for the DMS to sign off on. It was most certainly not to cure his assistant's medical issues. However, when I told him I couldn't even climb the stairs without huffing and puffing, he listened. He had a word in the ear of Major Daniel at Duntroon and they got me over there for a series of tests. They suspected exercise-induced asthma, but that was ruled out when I was sent for a run and came back pale instead of hot and breathless. A blood test came back with a very low haemoglobin level of 9.5.

They had me admitted straight to the oncology ward at Woden Valley Hospital for investigations conducted by haematologist Professor Richard Pembury. He discovered that the iron stores in my body were almost totally depleted, indicating that I had been chronically iron-deficient for a long time.

The problem was that all tests for a cause came back negative. Professor Pembury came back to me with two alternatives. The first was exploratory surgery where they would open my abdomen from sternum to navel and have a good look around for the cause. It was likely this major operation would lead to many ongoing abdominal issues. Gulp! I wasted no time in asking about option two.

He suspected that it might be 'runner's anaemia', with the constant pounding causing iron loss through the blood vessels of the lower limbs. This sounded logical to me. Option two was to give me intravenous iron followed up with oral iron to see if that improved my condition and to eat red meat, not drink tea with main meals and take vitamin C with the iron. Yes, option two, thanks very much!

By the end of the year, my haemaglobin level was back to an acceptable level of 13.1. In mid-February 1983, I eased back into training and at month's end, my haemaglobin level was a healthy 15.6. After about four years, was it possible that I could get back to normal?

In March, I averaged around 70 miles a week with an interesting break in the middle. DAHS sent a group out on Adventure Training. We travelled down to the Snowy Mountains ski resort of Thredbo. From there, we put on our bush gear and set off on a multi-day hike. At first, it

Chapter 11 My comeback

was all uphill to Dead Horse Gap and Rams Head to Mt Kosciusko. From the highest point in Australia, it was across to Abbott Peak until a night spent at Byatt's Camp.

Day two was down Hannel's Spur which had been a pioneering stock route in the early days. Whatever it had been, it was a real challenge to find it and then stay on it. The track was overgrown and perilously steep. Pity help the cattle and drovers back then! Eventually, we descended to the river and back to Geehi. Day three was a rest and a search for some slow hikers. I then had three days off with Achilles tendinitis. Well, it was an adventure!

At the end of the month, I contested my first race in full health for a few years. It was the five-kilometres OPS Branch Fun Run, flat and fast on the shores of Lake Burley Griffin. In the early stages, I followed top local Army runner Mick Whybrow, before taking over for an easy victory in 15 mins 42 secs. It seemed that I was back in business. Around this time, I located the nearest amateur athletic club and became a member of Weston Creek AAC.

In mid-May, I travelled up to Sydney for the Inter-Service 5000 metres. I knew full well what I had been doing for the previous four years but had no idea of Ian Hamilton's activities. It turned out nothing had changed. In a tactical race, he was able to sprint better than me and won by two seconds (15 mins 57 secs).

I cranked my weekly mileage up to 100 miles for a

couple of weeks and took a trip to Victoria to remind the Great Otway Classic selectors that I was still around. I ran a 6.5-kilometre pro cross-country at Greensborough and won the handicap. My 22 mins 1 sec was also second-fastest behind new local star Leigh Patterson.

We took a bit of leave and spent two weeks in Healesville. I trekked off to Mt Beauty and won their six-kilometre fun run in a record 19 mins 20 secs. This was just a side trip as the next day at Wangaratta, I competed in the Victorian Pro 8-kilometre Championships. The leading pair dropped me in the middle stages, but I came back strongly at the finish. Result:

- 1: Leigh Patterson (24 mins 59 secs)
- 2: Daryl Butt (25 mins 35 secs)
- 3: Greg Wilson (25 mins 45 secs).

It was rewarding to run a PB and be up there with the top pro runners.

After an easy week, I drove to Holsworthy Barracks, south-west of Sydney, to make my marathon comeback. It was the NSW Championship and incorporated the Australian Defence Force Championship. I finished fourteenth in the State Championships with 2 hrs 36 mins 53 secs. In front of me was one runner from the Defence Force. Yep, you guessed it! Ian Hamilton ran 2 hrs 32 mins and won a Commodore computer, whatever that was! Second prize was a feeling of contentment and a set of sore legs.

Chapter 11 My comeback

A reader paying careful attention will note that I had just run in an amateur State Championship a week after placing in a Professional State Championship, and with no false name. I didn't even think about it, as it was all just running. Much later, I discovered that the ridiculous wall between the two codes was being broken down at last.

After recovery and a couple of solid weeks, I ran in the ACT 25-kilometre Championships. It was windy and I returned two minutes faster than my outward journey. I came ninth, which is about the spot I land in no matter what amateur state championship I compete in. My 1 hr 26 mins 32 secs was a PB for a course that I knew was accurate.

The first half of June was rather hectic, coming on top of right knee pain from doing too much. One further tough week and I bowed to the inevitable and took a day off running.

Instead, I flew to Adelaide for the Military Orienteering Championships (MIL-O). After averaging 1 hr 45 mins a day for four days of running flat out through the bush, I jumped on a plane to Victoria. One bare day later, I was competing in the toughest multi-day event of all, the Great Otway Classic.

Again, I was a number four runner and as history repeats, my team finished fourth of the six teams. Just a brief idea of the challenge follows. Sat am: 9.6 kilometres, pm 10.9 kilometres; Sun am: 5.9 kilometres straight up out of Apollo Bay, pm 10.9 kilometres (holding off Geoff Molloy – more about him later!); Mon am: 442-metre sprint on Colac Velodrome, then 7.9 kilometres; pm, 8 kilometres. All done as fast as you possibly can, and too bad if you don't recover for the next leg.

I now had a strained right thigh to accompany the knee, so I gave myself a week off. All of July, I was back to doing eighty miles a week. An idea of my fitness can be gauged from my mid-month Campbelltown Marathon. The race was won in 2 hrs 25 mins by Horst Wegner, the man who didn't like us recruiting Andy Lloyd for a fun run team. I finished second in 2 hrs 36 mins 15 secs and regarded it as a long, steady training run. I then did a thirty-minute run in the evening and took no recovery days.

In August, my first year back after illness culminated in the Australian Pro Marathon Championships, held at Lara, near Geelong in Victoria. I ran with the leaders at below 2 hrs 30 mins pace and was in second place at thirty-five kilometres. The rest was not pretty: I vomited, then fell to the ground with leg cramps. I struggled on for fourth with the body fine, but legs that would not function.

I then took a well-earned break – perhaps even a bit overdue! A couple of months later, I was having trouble with right-side sciatica, but on not much training, and had a couple of surprising runs. In the five-kilometre Defence Fun Run, I finished second to Mick Whybrow, but it was a PB of 15 mins 5 secs. Two days later, I was back in thirty-second place in the *Canberra Times* Fun Run 10 kilometres, but again it was a PB of 32 mins 8 secs. I assume my body was fit from the earlier hard training and fresh from the break.

CHAPTER 12
The Great Otway Classic

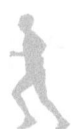

The year 1984 was special as it was the only time in my running career that I exceeded my achievements of Townsville in 1976. It only happened because I worked very hard to achieve it. However, that was not my intention when I started the year.

The previous winter when I had been down in Wangaratta for the Vic Pro 8-kilometre Championships, it happened to coincide with the first Sydney-to-Melbourne Ultramarathon. George Purdon was a top pro distance runner, although his advancing years had him running marathons in my ballpark. He was also the best Australian ultramarathoner I had heard of, with the exception of Bill Emmerton who raced predominately in the US.

George was the race favourite and was in a good position after a long day's running. So, job done for the day, he went to bed to recharge for day two. When he woke up, he soon found out that an unknown called Cliff

Chapter 12 The Great Otway Classic

Young, at age sixty-one, had reinvented the accepted ultra running customs. After a short nap, he just kept running and was not seen by the remainder of the field until they crossed the finish line ten hours or more behind him.

During my Wangaratta trip, I stopped on the roadside to cheer George on as he ran past in pursuit. Let's just say he wasn't up for a social chat as he was tired, irritable and out of winning contention. I had never considered running any further than a marathon. They were quite hard enough and, er, why would you?

Late in the year, I put in an application form to compete in the 1984 Sydney to Melbourne which was accepted. I knew I would need a support crew and I thought an Army unit could be ideal if they justified it as 'adventurous training'. I rang an officer at Sydney's RAAMC Field Force Unit and he was happy for 1st Field Hospital to undertake the support task.

Sorted, and so on New Year's Day, I commenced training. In January, I clocked up 316 miles with no days off. In February, I was sent to Healesville for a two-week promotion course. This would usually mean very limited running as I concentrated on passing the course. Not this time, as I managed a training run every day except one. That day, we were out bush and had an eleven-kilometre forced march while wearing heavy NBC (nuclear, biological, chemical) suits. All this activity had an unfortunate consequence when my course report came out. Although I had received excellent marks, I was marked down on 'attitude'. It seems that I didn't find enough spare time to attend the Sergeants' Mess regularly and get socially drunk with other course members – I was not a good team member! It seems that being the Army's top distance runner was not a scoring point when it came to career development.

The day after the course finished, I had my first race in the Healesville Fun Run of eleven kilometres. It was an exciting race with a good quality field of city runners. My 38 mins 28 secs got me second place, fifteen seconds behind Peter Nordhoff, with Maurice Hearn just eleven seconds further back. Well back in the field was a local nineteen-year-old runner whom I met for the first time called Brian Simmons – more about him later.

I returned to Canberra and after one day off when I was sick and vomiting, I totalled 291 miles for the short month. I was really pushing my physical limits and the first cracks began to show. Early in March, my left knee became sore and I had to take three days off. Did I get the message? Not likely! A week later, I clocked up my biggest week of running ever with 150 miles.

My right knee went out in sympathy, and as a consequence, I decided that my body would not tolerate the training needed for an ultramarathon. I also contacted my prospective support crew unit, and it seemed like they had never heard from me. I pulled out of the Sydney to

Melbourne. A few months later, the event was won by Geoff Molloy. We had been off the same handicap in pro running and I had beaten him during a leg of the Great Otway Classic. I will never know if I could have matched him over that extreme distance.

To tolerate such mileage, I had done no fast running at all. Who would need to on a race of nearly 1000 kilometres? So, what happened next was most unexpected. Two days after giving up on ultra running dreams, I ran in Canberra's West Basin 10 mile. It was a very classy field, and I went in with no expectations. The brilliant winner was Graeme Clews, brother-in-law of Robert de Castella ('Deek'), in 48 mins 27 secs. There were eleven finishers in under fifty-four minutes. I finished eighth in 53 mins 29 secs, less than a minute behind Queensland star Gerrard Barrett. I found it inexplicable that I could run at such a pace with absolutely no fast training.

I was still suffering leg issues and so had an easy month leading into and recovering from the Nike Marathon. The marathon was also the Olympic marathon trial and results would help determine the Australian team for the Los Angeles Olympic marathon. For the first time, the trial was open to the public, allowing anybody to enter. It attracted a huge field of approximately 2000.

The conditions were far from ideal, as it was humid and a strong wind was blowing. In the large field, it took me quite a while to just get past the start line, which would be significant later. The conditions were so tough that no male qualified for the Olympics in the event.

I started fast with a 5 mins 19 secs first mile, which I fully knew was not wise, but what do you do when there are about 1200 runners in front of you going even faster! I decided to throw caution to the wind. My Weston Creek Club mate Dan Dawes seemed to be on a pace that suited, so I stuck with him. Way out in front, another club mate Gary Hand was close to a 2 hrs 10 mins pace.

We continued on, covering each five kilometres in around 17 mins 30 secs. After the halfway point, Phil Aungles came past like he meant business and so I stuck with him. Turning for home the last time with ten kilometres to go, I was still feeling good but wary of really pushing in case the wheels fell off. From there, it was lonely and windswept. With no others around, it was difficult to gauge how I was travelling. I remember hearing a call of 2 hrs 14 mins with four kilometres to go, but short of oxygen, I couldn't work out whether I could go under 2 hrs 30 mins. At last, in the final stages, I saw Greg Sockhill and Bill Raimond in front. They were both 2 hrs 25 mins marathoners, and working to pass them kept me from plodding to the finish.

The effort to get past them told, and I had to ease off in the final kilometre as nausea was threatening to bring me undone in the final straight. Then through the

Chapter 12 The Great Otway Classic

cheering crowd, I could see the clock relentlessly ticking down, forcing me to sprint for the line.

The clock hit 2 hrs 30 mins as I stumbled to a halt under it. After I finished copiously vomiting on an innocent official's shoes, I found my official time was a lifetime PB of 2 hrs 30 mins 1 sec. Even that time was only good enough for twenty-eighth position. The placegetters – Grenville Wood, Rob Wallace and Graeme Clews – were excellent but the awful conditions prevented them from qualifying.

A couple of minutes behind me was the only qualifier, our world-class female Lisa Martin (later Ondieki). Two other great performances were put in by runners aged over forty, Roger Robinson (NZ) and Dot Browne (Vic). Roger was perhaps five minutes in front of me and for many years was the world's best Masters distance runner in his age group. Dot ran close to 2 hrs 40 mins and set an Australian age record that lasted for decades. The winning club team was Weston Creek and comprised Gary Hand, Alan Towill and me.

I spent the rest of April in recovery, as I came down with a bad dose of flu. I also reflected on how costly it was to lose thirty seconds across the start line with the clock already ticking. Morally, I was a sub-2 hrs 30 mins runner, and I was so confident that I would crack that mark in kinder conditions that I didn't order a finishing photo!

By May, I was acutely aware that the Great Otway Classic was looming. I took a month off using my annual leave and trained with some intensity two or three times a day. I had a few days off due to injury and being recalled back to work temporarily. In May, I tallied 325 miles, which included interval work and hills.

I was well aware of the peak form I was in. The only person I told down in Victoria was my Clifton Brick team captain from last year's Otway. Once again, I was selected as a number four seed. We were sure it would be important that I was running way better than my middle-of-the-pack seeding indicated, but would it be enough to improve on our fourth placing?

Last year's winning team, Sportsworld, was favoured, as well they might be, with the stand-out best pro runner in Australia, Viv Woodward, as their number one. Over the long weekend, I ran against their number two runner four times and against Viv twice. With me being so strong in the hills, the plan was for our number one, Frank Shevlin, to run fast downhill against lesser runners. We needed everything to go right, as Sportsworld were so strong that their number six seed was the seven-time Australian pro marathon champion, Ted Paulin! You may well ask how he was seeded two rungs below me!

We kept me fresh by ignoring the early morning time trial, which only required four from each team. My first run was 9.6 kilometres and in clocking 32 mins 20 secs, I

Chapter 12 The Great Otway Classic

retained the lead that our number one had set up. In the afternoon, I had one of the toughest legs on the course, 11.1 kilometres over very tough hills against the champion, Viv Woodward. I managed 5 mins 30 secs per mile up and over the mountain and came in with 38 mins 21 secs. My adversary had come past and had the lead in an outstanding 36 mins 30 secs. However, we still had Frank Shevlin to run the final leg, steeply downhill into Apollo Bay, against a low seed. Shevvy was sublime and at the end of day one, we had a well-earned sleep, sitting in first position.

On day two, we again saved me from the early dash up to Marriners Lookout and back. The second leg out of Apollo Bay was on Busty Road, which was winding gravel and steeply uphill all the way. Again, on this tough leg, I was competing against number two seeds and a number three, John Guerin, who had come third in last year's marathon championship. When I took over, we had been relegated to fourth on the road. Running strongly, I picked up and passed Rocky Quarrell and John Guerin and had us back to second behind Sallman's Bill Bedell. My time for over six kilometres was 21 mins 9 secs.

In the afternoon leg, I was feeling some accumulated tiredness, but I may not have been Robinson Crusoe! My undulating seven kilometres was covered in 24 mins 13 secs as I ran down Sportsworld's Rocky Quarrell again, beating him home by nine seconds, putting us in front once more.

On day three, my morning leg had just a few hills and I ran over them at 3 mins 15 secs per kilometre for 9.3 kilometres and I was timed at 30 mins 15 secs, leaving Sportsworld's number two Rocky Quarrell languishing forty-five seconds behind. During a sit-down lunch at Deans Marsh, we were joined at the table by Herb Elliott and were suitably impressed. For those unaware, Herb had a brief but excellent career as a 1500-metre runner in the '60s. He was undefeated in his pet event and won an Olympic gold by the length of the straight in a world record. What could he have done if he hadn't retired at twenty-two years old?

My final leg was a notorious 7.7 kilometres known as the Deans Marsh hill. It was steep, uphill, without a break, all the way to the top of the range above Lorne. Of course, on such a vital leg, my opponent was Viv Woodward. The good news was that we had hit the lead and so I had a start on him. I managed to hold him off for half the distance and then just put everything into not losing too much ground. By the end, I handed over to our final runner only 1 min 30 secs down.

It is difficult to compare various performances over the years and I don't even know the time I took, but that was the best I ever ran. However, it is a *team* relay and our number three seed had to gain 1 min 30 secs on Sportsworld's number seven for us to win the Great Otway Classic. It is beyond disappointing that at the end

Chapter 12 The Great Otway Classic

of 313 kilometres over three days, he was unable to close the gap at all.

After all that effort, we had broken the event record, but still been defeated by 1 min 30 secs. I thought I would be a shoo-in to be awarded best number four seed. I mean, what do you have to do? However, it was not my decision, and it went to a fine hill runner, Dennis Clarke. They did find something for me, though – Most Consistent! Hands down the best running of my career. Now it is unimaginable that we could keep backing up at that pace, when in the mornings we could hardly stand and walk. It was a mighty tough event and anything following would be an anti-climax.

In June, I had covered 225 miles, with pre- and post-Otway affecting my total. Three weeks later, the Army put a team in the Sydney Team Trot, one of the city's major fun runs. It was 11.4 kilometres and I finished seventh in 36 mins 21 secs. This equated to me running a career best of 31 mins 50 secs for ten kilometres and then continuing for 1.4 kilometres. Our strong Army team came third overall and was the first government services team. I was to rejoin these fine runners two years later for a relay run around Australia.

Shortly after I decided I would join Deek's group who were doing their final training hit-out, before he left for the Los Angeles Olympic marathon. It was a large group but I didn't know anybody and had no idea of the course through the Mt Stromlo pine forest. I didn't notice that the group was getting smaller, as runners decided they had done enough and returned to the start. Eventually, I realised that there was Robert de Castella, Dave Chettle, Gerrard Barrett and very few others. They were all international stars, capable of running around 2 hrs 10 mins for the marathon. They surged up every hill and then eased off. If I wanted to get home safely, I had to race flat out all the way and attempt to keep them in sight. I finally got back safely but exhausted. I never came back for a second run!

A week later, my good form continued in the ACT 15-kilometre race where I finished seventh in a PB of 49 mins 50 secs. Around this time, the award for first local in the Olympic marathon trial was offered to me. A few others had been in front of me but were unable to take the prize. It was a trip to New Zealand to run in their Hamilton Marathon in October. An international trip and not to a war! Yes, please!

My July tally was back up to 329 miles, but I had been to the well many times and body and mind were starting to fall apart. The problem was that I still had the Australian Defence Force Marathon Championship to contest. It was held in conjunction with the Gold Coast Marathon in early August. This was where I had intended to achieve my richly deserved sub-2:30 marathon, but it was not to be. The day was hot and humid and

Chapter 12   The Great Otway Classic

the best I could do on the day was 2 hrs 32 mins 15 secs. I was absolutely stuffed afterwards and could hardly walk. I was eighth overall and won bronze in the Defence Championship. In first place was John McCrystal (Army, 2 hrs 25 mins 30 secs) with Peter Bourgaize (RAAF, 2 hrs 27mins 28 secs) close behind. I was later informed by John that it was my running at 1st Armoured Regiment, where he was a non-running young trooper in 1980, that had inspired him to take up the sport. It sure worked, as he had won all three of his marathons and in times faster than 2 hrs 30 mins. At age thirty-two, it was surely time to hand over the mantle of top Army marathoner to this fine athlete.

I had done enough for the year. I was cooked and needed a break. However, there was the little matter of my first local prize from the Olympic trial. That trip to New Zealand for the Hamilton Marathon was due on 21 October. Then I found out the first ten finishers in the Defence Force Championship were chosen as a team to represent the Australian Defence Force in a marathon against the New Zealand Defence Force. It was to be held at Blenheim on the South Island of New Zealand on 25 October.

So I, who had never won a trip anywhere for anything, had now won two trips to overseas marathons. On the positive side, at least they were in the same country; a negative was that they were four days apart. What to do?

The other me, who wouldn't accept that this great season of running was over, came up with the obvious solution. Run them both!

It seemed reasonable as, back in 1978, I had run two marathons a fortnight apart, and the second one was faster. If I took Hamilton easy, then backing up should be achievable. My immediate preparation was to have five weeks doing absolutely nothing. Then I crammed in four weeks that averaged 85 miles.

Towards the middle of October, I ran in the five-kilometre Defence Fun Run flat and fast around Lake Burley Griffin. I led throughout and my 14 mins 57 secs was a new career PB. All seemed to be on track. Three days later on a dark evening, I ran along the bike paths to collect my plane tickets from Dave Cundy at Mawson. Some idiot had strung a trip wire across the bike path and I fell heavily, straining my left Achilles tendon. It was one week until I was due to run at Hamilton.

I had the week off, crossed my fingers and flew to Auckland, New Zealand. From there, it was a couple of hours on a bus through beautiful green countryside. Hamilton was the easiest marathon I have ever run. I coasted the first half at three-hour pace and felt I was jogging. On the return trip, I couldn't help but finish strongly. I passed about thirty runners in the last eight kilometres. As I crossed the line in 2 hrs 49 mins 50 secs, I heard a spectator say, 'He looks like he could go around again'. Just as well I suppose, as that's exactly what I had in mind. I had not felt any injury issues throughout the event.

When I woke up the next morning, I had trouble walking, let alone running. My body had been protecting my injured Achilles tendon and now my left thigh was badly strained. I got a lift in a car, enjoying New Zealand's beautiful scenery as I headed down to Wellington. From there, it was a very rough ferry ride across the Cook Strait to Picton on the South Island. A bus trip got me to Blenheim, which is located in a level valley in the Marlborough grape-growing region. At the RNZAF base, I met up with my marathon teammates.

The next morning, away we went and I hobbled to the halfway mark in a lot of pain. There was no point in continuing and so I withdrew. The race had the same result as back on the Gold Coast, with John McCrystal (2 hrs 28 mins) defeating Peter Bourgaize (2 hrs 32 mins). I was frustrated and didn't elaborate on any of my misadventures. The RAN Lieutenant Commander in charge of our team informed me that he would ensure I was never selected for another Inter-Service team. It was ironic that his threat, that I considered most unfair, was later totally irrelevant.

My well-earned rest was now injury-enforced. My memorable year of running in Canberra was over. During 1984, I had amassed 2693 miles while training and competing. In eleven years, I had competed in twenty-eight marathons. The majority were completed in under 2 hrs 45 mins. Only twice had I not been able to complete the course, even though I ran a couple while suffering illness. New Zealand was a disappointing way to finish my serious marathon running career.

At work, Lieutenant Colonel Bob Allen, had a change of scenery in mind for me. Towards the end of the year, I was posted to the School of Army Health with a promotion to Staff Sergeant. My new position was to be Training Development Warrant Officer (TDWO), for which I would be paid a higher duties allowance.

I had mixed feelings about leaving my wonderful current position and returning to the school. I was certain, though, that Sandy would be overjoyed to return to her hometown. I had an interesting phone call from Lieutenant Colonel Alan Batchelor during the later stages of my tenure at Campbell Park offices. He said there were plans afoot to have a team of Army runners run a relay lap of Australia. We tossed around the names of possible team members, and when I expressed scepticism about the venture happening, he replied that it was being considered at the highest levels.

CHAPTER 13
To Sydney

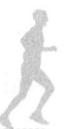

It was enjoyable to begin 1985 settling back in the familiar environs of Healesville. Located on the southern fringe of the Great Dividing Range, Healesville was all green grass, tree fern gullies and stands of majestic gum trees. A bonus was that we were able to move back into our home at Badger Creek, only a couple of kilometres from my work. Our block backed onto Badger Creek, which flowed through the famous Sir Colin Mackenzie Wildlife Sanctuary. At feeding time, we could hear the dingoes howling for their meal.

I was straight back into training with my good running mates Wally Butler and Brian Simmons. Just before Christmas, we were running up the range along the winding Chum Creek Road when we heard a voice calling from down in the gully far below. Once we established that it was a motorbike rider who had failed to take a tight bend and landed down in the thick bush, we tried to assist. While Brian ran to the nearest house to telephone for an ambulance, we did what we could with no first aid equipment. After some time, it came to light that he had had a pillion passenger on board. We located the injured rider's stepdaughter further down the hill. She was deceased – it was not going to be a merry Christmas in that household! That would have been the end of our training run except that we still had to make our very subdued way home. It can all end so suddenly!

When I had left Victoria almost four years ago, my pro track running career seemed over following a dispute with the handicapper. Upon entering some events, I was delighted to see that my handicap had been restored. I asked no questions but just enjoyed being competitive again. Right from the start, I was finishing in the top ten placings. Wangaratta was the first big meeting, and I was fourth in the 3200 metres. A week later at Melton, we endured a rough track and a temperature of thirty-eight degrees. I cleared out and won easily in 8 mins 46 secs. Re-handicapped for Northcote the next week, I still managed second.

My new job entailed working with a captain and two corporals to improve the training system. Tasks included syllabus, exam question writing and assessing the instructors giving lessons. Being the Army, there was also a week out bush on exercise up in the nearby Murrindindi Training Area. On my return from exercise,

Chapter 13 To Sydney

we locals tried to hold off a bunch of talented visitors in the Healesville Fun Run over nine and a half kilometres. In similar form to last year, I was close up behind Peter Nordhoff in 30 mins 39 secs, a six-mile PB.

The only problem was that there were a couple of other 'guns' just ahead of us. My training partner, Brian Simmons, was just fifty seconds behind me. I went all the way to Lavington NSW for another placing, and three days later, there were the Victorian (3MD) Army Championships.

In the 1500 metres, Jim Van Beek out-dipped me by the narrowest of margins, both of us breaking the record with 4 mins 13 secs. In the 5000 metres, I was up against the unbeaten marathon champion, John McCrystal. In one of my best runs, I led from the start and ran away to win clearly, which was probably a big shock to both of us. My 15 mins 17 secs broke the record that Phil Hassel had set a dozen years earlier when he beat me. It was also a career track PB for me and is the only time I was able to beat John.

When I cooled down, it became obvious that I had strained my left Achilles tendon again. Hoping that it wasn't too bad, I had an easy ten days and headed up to Bendigo for the second top pro running event of the season. On Saturday in the 3200 metres, I finished a close second in 8 mins 42 secs. The next day was a novel 1600 metres, as it involved a qualifying heat and then the final. In the heat, I ran a distant second behind Peter Cross and aggravated my injured leg in doing so. I would have pulled out of the final, except that I would have incurred a one-month injury suspension. As that would mean missing out on the Stawell Gift meeting, I decided to try to run. I sat in the stands for a couple of hours with an ice pack on my calf, before gingerly warming up. At the halfway mark, I managed to find another gear and, throwing discretion to the wind, I surged into the lead and cleared out. It was an unexpected move and caused me to take fairy-like footsteps in the home straight. I could hear my opponents rushing ever nearer, but I breasted the finishing tape a split inch in front.

How I managed the biggest track victory of my pro career, I will never know. My time of 3 mins 58.3 secs was another career PB and I had $600 and the winner's sash to remember it by. Just to bring me back to earth a bit, I will fully admit that these events are way too short and explosive for me to excel at. The stewards reinforced this when they questioned the minor placegetters. They were quizzed about why they failed to chase me when I took off in the middle stages, but no further action was taken. As you get re-handicapped for a win, it is possible they intended not to win in order that their handicap was not reduced before Stawell. The only comment I will make is that Peter Cross came out three weeks later at Stawell

Chapter 13 To Sydney

and ran 3 mins 52 secs in the fastest 1600-metre race seen at Stawell for many a long year!

Three weeks of nursing an injury and a dose of the flu were not ideal preparation for the 3MD Inter-Service Championship, but they were hardly likely to delay it on my behalf. In the 5000 metres, I set the pace, but when John McCrystal came past with three laps to go, I had no answer. I backed off to save myself for the 1500 metres but overdid it and finished third.

The 1500 metres was won by Jim Van Beek, and again I was third. My time of 4 mins 10 secs was the best I had run after earlier doing a 5000 metres, so I guess my tactics were sound. I had another week of total rest while I was down with the flu, then I travelled to Stawell, but as usual couldn't get near them. Under the circumstances I had no right to expect to. My fine track season was probably due to all the training last year; however, it sure ended with a whimper!

Little did I know that it would also cause the end of my 'prime of life' running career. I just had to keep going to track events while I was performing so well, but it meant that I had not done suitable preparation for the Great Otway Classic. A day after Stawell, I got straight into doing long hard miles in the hills. I went from ten miles to sixty-five miles to ninety-three miles per week. Again, I trained twice a day and when, after a couple of weeks, my left knee became sore from overuse, well, I just ignored it. Early in May with chronic knee pain, I bowed to the inevitable and withdrew from the 1985 Great Otway Classic.

At this time, I received a letter from Alan Batchelor regarding the proposed relay. It gave a rough outline and had been sent to the top eighteen distance runners in the Army. Before mid-year, but probably after I had done well in the Army athletics competition, the commanding officer, Lieutenant Colonel 'Para' Hills gave me an additional task: he had volunteered the unit to host this year's 3MD cross-country championship and I was given the task of organising the event. Officially I was doing it with oversight and wise advice from the unit's psychology officer, Lieutenant Drury. In reality, he knew nothing about athletics and was a necessary figurehead.

Designing the course and organising the competition was pretty full on, as of course it had to be the best one ever held. In addition, it would be nice if the unit had a team compete and win the event. No pressure then! I spent more time on the cross-country than I did on my day job.

I had a couple of months without any running and then cautiously began some light training. I figured that I had to, as no doubt I was expected to perform well in the race I was organising. The course I devised was in and around the property on which the School of Army Health was located. The centrepiece was Summerleigh

Lodge which sat high along the ridgeline. My thought was to make it as hard as hell so it would be a challenge for visiting teams. Of course, our home team runners would suffer also, but at least they knew in advance what they were in for and could train on it.

The course was three laps of 3200 metres and so in entirety it was 9.6 kilometres, or six miles in the 'old money'. My secret weapon was Heartbreak Hill which was right beside the Sergeants' Mess, which makes sense as they would have had a good view from their 'watering hole'. I had never seen anybody run up it, and for good reason – it was almost un-runnable! There was a flat section down along the Sanctuary's fence but the rest was undulating. I did a few laps just to make sure it could be done, which was a bit important. My best training time was just under thirty-seven minutes. An interesting comparison is that back in 1981, while I was still anaemic, I won on the One Tree Hill (Bendigo) course in 33 mins 35 secs. Hmmm!

The pro marathon was held and the results were a surprise to me, with a changing of the guard. John Guerin, whom I was able to beat in last year's Otway, was victorious in an excellent 2 hrs 20 mins 40 secs from Ian Minter (2 hrs 26 mins 12 secs) and Anton Oberscheider (2 hrs 31 mins 30 secs). Of even more interest to me, my Healesville training partner, Brian Simmons, was just behind the placings in 2 hrs 31 mins 36 secs. In all my marathons, only once had I gone faster!

I thought I better get a couple of races in and so the next week we three Healesville boys had our first race together. It was eight kilometres and Brian beat me by more than a minute, with a similar gap back to Wally Butler. My thoughts after that race were that I was very unfit and my left knee still hurt.

At the end of August, I had my first visit to compete in an Army organised event called the Lake Relay. SOAH put a team in to give our cross-country runners an outing. Each team had four runners and they each had to run five laps of Albert Park Lake in South Melbourne, therefore covering in total about a hundred kilometres. My laps were 15 mins 28 secs, 15 mins 39 secs, 16 mins 15 secs, 16 mins 36 secs and 16 mins 28 secs, for 4730 metres. A good day out as I was awarded Fastest Lap and our team of unknowns finished in second place.

The only training I was managing was around thirty miles a week. In mid-September, we had a practice event over the cross-country course and I ran 35 mins 37 secs. Then I had a week of nothing but making sure everything would go smoothly. Our unit draughtswoman had a sense of humour; she made up a bunch of certificates to be awarded to each finisher. Part of the design was a coat of arms with the motto *Nur Nettor*. Might help if you read it backwards!

Chapter 13 To Sydney

It was all a bit of an extravaganza and my old mate from 1969 Medical Orderly course, Wayne 'Shorty' Langford, was Master of Ceremonies. He was very much an extrovert and never short of a word. He even had us down on the parade ground as runners doing laps and pretending to be Formula One cars while he made a video. There were pit stops and all. I am not sure what the visitors thought as they were subjected to it on the big day.

Well, it wouldn't be a story without a happy ending, right? In first place in the 1985 3MD cross-country championship was Greg Wilson (SOAH) in 34 mins 50 secs from Brian Scholes who kept me honest (35 mins 11 secs) and Jeff Rudd (35 mins 50 secs). The winning team – School of Army Health. Job done, I would say! I hope Lieutenant Drury was as proud of his endeavours as the CO was of his unit's achievement.

This tough cross-country was definitely the straw that broke the camel's back. I did no running for the rest of the year and was just thankful that I was able to get up Heartbreak Hill and steal an event I had no right to win on one leg. It was an interesting time to receive another update from Alan Batchelor, stating that relay approval had been given.

So 1985 was a pivotal year for my running and it was the same for my Army career. At the end of the year, the School of Army Health was relocating to the former

Officer Training Centre at Portsea. We were all taken down for a look, with spouses included. The camp was in a lovely setting way down at the tip of the Mornington Peninsula. Portsea was tiny but also the playground of the rich and famous. I was happy enough to continue my career down there, but to my surprise, Sandy was not on board. As she was usually quiet and accommodating, when she was so against the idea, it was time to listen.

I weighed up all the pros and cons. Firstly, I didn't want to force her to Portsea against her will. I could go unaccompanied but that was hardly fair on Sandy and two young children. Truth be known, I would rather work running a Regimental Aid Post (RAP) than a training unit with all its military discipline. Another factor was that I had further correspondence from Alan Batchelor and it seemed that the Around Australia Relay would actually be happening next year. I considered that it would be the experience of a lifetime and I had my doubts the SOAH would release me to participate.

All things considered, I decided that I would request a posting to a RAP anywhere. What I failed to realise was that this decision would eventually lead to the end of my Army career. When I had my interview with my old CSM, Lieutenant Colonel Bob Allen, he strongly advised me to go to Portsea. He added that he had personally chosen me for the TDWO position and pointed out how good it would be for my career. He then asked me how I

Chapter 13 To Sydney

considered my time in the Army; was it a career or just a job? I had served for fourteen years and so I thought the answer was self-evident. Perversely, I said, 'A job,' and that was the end of the conversation.

When my posting came through it, was to RAP District Support Unit (DSU) Sydney at Victoria Barracks in Paddington. After the drive north, we were accommodated in a Rushcutters Bay motel for a few days while awaiting permanent quarters. Unfortunately, we were burgled on day two, so that wasn't a great start. When we were offered a brand-new townhouse in Hurstville South, we jumped at the chance. A bonus was that the other residents were all Army Senior NCOs, so there should be no problem with the neighbours. The only downside was a commute of twenty kilometres through Sydney's traffic.

Victoria Barracks is on a busy road close to Kings Cross, but it was an attractive and historic place to go to work; all sandstone walls, enclosed vast grass parade grounds and grand historic sandstone buildings. It has been a military base since the Rum Corps resided there in the early days of the colony. My staff consisted of a corporal with a serious alcohol problem and a female private who was very efficient. Each morning, a semi-retired doctor would attend for sick parade. Dr Fred Grace was a member of the Bondi Icebergs who ocean-swam throughout the year, rain, hail or shine. One of his swim mates was famous English Channel swimmer Des Renford.

Apart from caring for the sick, we had to order stores, conduct routine medical examinations and immunisation parades. As many of the staff at Victoria Barracks were both senior and sedentary, the medical examinations proved more of a challenge than the sparse sick parades.

I was finally doing the right thing by my body and my only running was a three-kilometre commute each way from the railway station to work. In March, I had a steroid injection into my left knee, but there was no obvious improvement.

Now that I was in Sydney, I was able to be more closely involved in the preparations for the XXXX Army Around Australia Relay. The official launch was in March and coincided with the opening of the Tomkin Gardens in Enfield. In a rehearsal, local members of the team and a few ring-ins were waiting around when a press photographer decided he needed a photo. We were all in our running gear, but he insisted we wear greens and boots, which no one had available. There was also an Army ceremonial guard in attendance. Ten minutes later, the problem was solved as we pretended that we were running around Australia in oversized uniforms and heavy boots. I am not sure of the reaction of any visitor using the public facilities who might have found an Army ceremonial guard shivering in their underwear!

Chapter 13 To Sydney

On the night, we ran in, formed up on an elevated ramp and listened to speeches before being introduced to dignitaries, who included Prime Minister Bob Hawke. Then we had a taste of reality. As the guests tucked into a sumptuous dinner, we were out in the cold rain, freezing in our singlets, as we foraged for some cold meat and salad in the dark!

In April, I started some light training, not due to my knee improving but because I had to: the Around Australia Relay was only three months away! I ran in the 1500 metres at the NSW (2MD) Inter-Service Championship and finished a close second to Corporal Glenn Norris, recording 4 mins 12 secs.

People magazine visited Victoria Barracks to do a story and took shots of Alan Batchelor, Tammy Menzel, Mike Connor and myself. Later, we journeyed out to Ingleburn for a publicity poster shot where six of us were running just in front of a loud and threatening armoured personnel carrier. As few of the initial shortlist were available for the relay, the ANZAC Day Marathon was used as a selection trial. It was also the Services Championship and John McCrystal was our top finisher with a third place overall in 2 hrs 26 mins, another outstanding performance. We also had fifteen finishers home in under the required 2 hrs 50 mins to qualify for the team. Due to my unfit condition, Alan and I decided I could be timekeeper and just work towards being able to perform in June.

CHAPTER 14

The XXXX Army Around Australia Relay Marathon

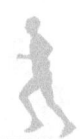

The idea of having a fundraising relay around Australia was hatched between Barbara MacKay-Cruise and Sir Peter Abeles following a family tragedy. It was created to launch and raise funds for an Australian Cancer Research Foundation (ACF). Who would be capable of undertaking such an epic challenge? They decided to enlist the assistance of the Australian Army.

Lieutenant Colonel Alan Batchelor was given responsibility for organising the Army team, which meant a lot of preparation. He was assisted by Major Craig Leggett (Operations), Captain Ed Nicholas (Logistics) and WO2 Lionel Scott (Stores). On the ACF side, Barbara enlisted former Army officer, ultra runner and adventure tour organiser Charlie Lynn. He did a lap of Australia by vehicle, organising the run stages and receptions at population centres all around the country.

Chapter 14 The XXXX Army Around Australia Relay Marathon

In June, team members gathered together for the first time at 2 Training Group, Ingleburn. We spent an evening getting to know each other while receiving an update on preparations. The next day we travelled to Victoria Barracks, Paddington for a general publicity launch.

My own preparations were not going smoothly. I was managing around thirty miles a week and did a couple of low-key races. I went to see a sports medicine specialist, Ken Creighton, who confirmed the diagnosis of chronic patella tendinitis. He referred me to a specialist physiotherapist who devised a set of exercises and sport tape strapping to improve my condition. He also said that if Jenny's physio treatment was unsuccessful, surgery was the next option. His opinion was that I could complete the relay without completely wrecking my knee.

A week before the relay was due to start, I swore off further physio as it was too painful and the after-effects left me unable to run. Members of the team gathered at Bardia Barracks, Ingleburn for a final week of preparations. I departed, knowing I was leaving two young ladies with a big job. Sandy had to care for our young children as a single mother for three months. At work, Michelle had the big job of running the RAP, even though she was the junior rank there.

The runners were divided into five teams of four, with senior ranks nominated as team leaders. Captain

Mark Burgess, Lieutenant Tammy Menzel, WO1 George Russell, WO2 John Kelly and I had a meeting to select our teams. The plan was to have teams with an equal spread of experience and ability. My teammates were Sergeant Ernie Stewart (Broadmeadows, Vic.), Craftsman Rob Combe and Private Vic Perry (Townsville). During the evening we had lectures on administration and operations from key personnel.

The next day we were allotted our team vehicles. Nissan had donated eighteen new vehicles for the duration of the relay. They were white and adorned with relay and sponsorship colours. Our vehicle was an Urvan.

It was going to be an interesting challenge to spend three months living very closely with teammates I hardly knew. There followed more days of preparation which included a night practice session around nearby Oran Park car racing track. This was to ensure that what was planned in theory actually worked in practice.

Apart from our runner vehicle dropping us off to complete our leg, which could be up to four hours long, we were also required to spend a similar time sitting behind another team as their safety vehicle. In dangerous areas, we would be required to spend another long period further behind as an advanced warning vehicle. We would rotate through these tasks until stopping for the night at the next major town. In the outback, we would just keep rotating until we arrived back in civilisation. Apart from the above, we also had fundraising duties and had to drive forward to get some rest and then do it all again.

My relay almost ended right there. As our first runner, I had forgotten to change into the previous team's runner vehicle to be taken forward to warm-up. We called them up and I leaped from the Urvan only to have my feet go out from under me as I tumbled to the ground. It was pitch-black and on the smooth road, I didn't realise we were still moving as I stepped out into space. A learning experience!

On 24 June, our convoy headed off to Canberra and an afternoon tea reception at Government House, where Sir Ninian and Lady Stephen were our hosts. We followed up with a farewell dinner where we got to mingle with the ACF, sponsors and supporters, without whom the relay would not be happening. Barbara MacKay-Cruise was there and she was also to travel the complete route with the team. Then it was a comfortable night in the Park Royal Motel. I really could get used to this!

The next morning, we had a live TV segment on *Good Morning Australia*, outside Old Parliament House. Unfortunately, this involved an hour of standing around in our singlets on a frosty Canberra winter morning. Another downer was losing one of the ACF's key fundraising personnel and our Stores manager just as the relay was about to begin.

Late morning, the support crew formed all our vehicles up in front of Old Parliament House. The runners strode down between them and formed up for speeches and a farewell from Prime Minister Bob Hawke. First leg runner Alan Batchelor and our group followed a police escort through the northern suburbs of Canberra. The XXXX Around Australia Relay Marathon was under way.

*

The first day gave us some insight as to what we were in for. My Team 5 had collection duties in the towns along the highway to Sydney. That night's dinner was a hurried takeaway from the Berrima McDonald's! After dark, we drove forward to where we expected to commence safety duty high on the Great Dividing Range in the Penrose State Forest. I was unable to sleep and spent a frigid few hours reading until we were required.

At 9.15 pm, Team 4 took over runner duties nearby and our job for the next three and a half hours was to sit behind the runner at fifteen kilometres per hour while we illuminated his passage, kept him entertained with music and informed on his progress. At 1 am, we commenced runner duty near Bargo, where we each had to cover twelve kilometres at four minutes per kilometre. This was after sitting in a vehicle for hours and having had no sleep. Our shift took us through to the Campbelltown

Post Office. Where usually we could look forward to a group run-in, a ceremonial welcome and a nice afternoon tea, we arrived at 4am. There was only us and the support crew Urvan, 'Niner,' who had provided our safety while other running teams got some sleep. We drove through the empty streets to 2 Training Group at Ingleburn where we got some well-overdue sleep. The relay would recommence early next morning.

Sydney and other cities were fairly chaotic. As a matter of fact, the whole east coast to Brisbane was the same. There was not much running needed between Ingleburn and Sydney and most of the day was spent on receptions with the Premier, Lord Mayor and sponsors. It was a relief to get to bed, but after three hours of sleep, we were up for our first shift. It was an eerie but relaxed departure from Sydney at 5am, on safety following the runner over a deserted Harbour Bridge at fifteen kilometres per hour.

By late afternoon, we had arrived in Newcastle, but for reasons unknown, we bypassed the city centre. We performed an extra safety for Alan Batchelor when he decided to run across to Mayfield so we could have an unimpeded exit the next morning. We then joined the rest of the team at Stockton, where our 130 Signals Squadron was putting us up for the night.

When every stage was completed, we would have an orders group (O-Group), during which key personnel would discuss issues and how to overcome them. This included detailed plans for the next stage and all members had to wait around until their team leader passed on this vital information. I was surprised to learn that, instead of sleeping on a hard gymnasium floor, Team 5 had been given a night in a motel in the city. High above Newcastle, we were lulled to sleep with the sound of surf crashing on the rocks of a nearby headland.

My first real challenge was on day four, after turning off the highway at Bulahdelah for a reception at Forster. Simultaneously, we received word that there were map-to-road discrepancies and we were now behind schedule. As luck would have it, I had just replaced Ernie in running up one of the biggest hills I have seen. My knee got a big test it didn't really need, but I managed to maintain four minutes per kilometre for nine kilometres and then left it to others to pick up time on the downhill.

The sun was setting over the broad reaches of the Manning River as we did our group run-in to Taree, with our theme song, Dire Straits' *Walk of Life*, blaring from our speakers. The central park was swinging as our kitchen truck provided dinner for all comers, as an O-Group was held under trying conditions. Ready for an early night, we had to drive fourteen kilometres out to Wingham for a function and our accommodation.

We tossed our bags into a room at the ramshackle Wingham Hotel, looked longingly at our beds and set off across the village green for a function at the RSL Club. The town was dead quiet and as we reached our destination, we understood why. The six of us that had made the effort to attend were greeted enthusiastically by a huge crowd, as we were plied with free drinks and hot snacks. A couple of us even got dressed up and participated in the floor show. At closing time, we stumbled off to bed, only too aware of an early start tomorrow.

A bare six hours' sleep and we were up at 5am for a drive to Coopernook for a scheduled breakfast function. It was still dark as we passed through Taree and noticed the first runner setting off. Twenty kilometres further on, we arrived in tiny Coopernook. At the football field, there was a thick blanket of frost and nothing to eat but frozen hay bales. We sat in the van chilled to the bone and awaited developments. Eventually some locals turned up and got things going, but for Team 5, breakfast at Coopernook was a real anticlimax. We were first to arrive and before any food was cooked, we had to leave for our safety duty.

As we progressed up the east coast, the running was the least of our problems. Locating the rendezvous point where we would meet for a group run-in to the stage destination was a continuing problem. Another was ensuring that we all took the same route out of town, as our maps were not that detailed. At various stages, there were so many towns and receptions that we struggled to attend, let alone consume all the offered tea and scones.

At Kempsey and Coffs Harbour, running team members were billeted out with local families. I was fortunate that my host woke up and drove me to the 4 am start for our advanced warning shift. Unfortunately, we had to leave without Rob, as perhaps his family slept in. Eventually he found his way back to us, but that was the end of this form of accommodation.

Adding advanced warning to our duties meant a long day of sitting in the Urvan, so it was a relief to get out for a run. My share was twelve kilometres in 45 mins 45 secs around the Maclean bypass. After ten hours, it was then a pleasure for us to settle down on the banks of the mighty Clarence River and enjoy a picnic lunch. Our reverie was interrupted by an indistinct radio call, informing us that Barbara and her driver Cheryl had taken a wrong turn and were calling for assistance from a ferry in the middle of the Clarence. We may have been overtired, but we were unable to offer assistance as we were too busy rolling around in hysterics! When recovered, we drove on to tiny Woodburn where we had a reception to attend. We had quite a wait, thinking the town deserted, but then I was relieved to see Barbara arrive in one piece. We had a group run into the CWA Hall and there we found all the missing locals gathered to welcome us. The runner arrived and then set off in a hurry to make it to Lismore

Chapter 14   The XXXX Army Around Australia Relay Marathon

before dark. We stayed and had a great time meeting the townsfolk. Their enthusiasm was emphasised by the cheque for $2000 this community of 800 had raised, which per capita was one of the best in the whole relay.

It was after dark when we got to Lismore for a reception and accommodation at the local Army Reserve (ARES) unit, 41 Battalion. Most of the relay team were ushered out early so they could have some dinner, while the team leaders and command element continued entertaining the locals. By the time we got away, there were just cold leftovers for dinner, but we still had an O-Group to attend to. We had four and a half hours of sleep and then nineteen hours of duty before finally getting to bed at 11 pm on a concrete floor. I was tired, irritable and had been suffering from the 'flu' since early in the relay. Canberra, singlet, below freezing – had not been a great start!

After six and a half hours, we were up again, still in the dark for first run. I set myself the challenge of first run up the range on the road towards the coast at Ballina. I attacked the climb in order to keep us on schedule and covered eight kilometres in 31 mins 35 secs. I shouldn't have bothered as my teammates were feeling frisky as the sun rose above the fertile hilly country around Alstonville and we were minutes ahead by handover.

So, a couple of hours in the early morning and job done!? No, there was a bit more to this day. Up the closely settled Tweed coast, we had receptions and obligations every half-hour. Surely there is a limit to how many morning teas you can consume? Through Lennox and Brunswick Heads, it was a hectic, subtropical confusion of activity.

We followed up with a stint of advanced warning on the dangerous section across to Murwillumbah and then had the final safety across the border and up to Surfers Paradise. There was a group run to celebrate crossing the border, but when Ernie and I jumped out of the van, the legs wouldn't work. The rest of the group had dashed off and our safety vehicle followed as Ernie and I were left languishing and fighting the traffic jam our convoy was causing.

Off to a lavish reception at Jupiters Casino and then a trip up to our accommodation at Southport. No sooner had we arrived than we were told to drive back through the length of the Gold Coast to the Twin Towns Services Club at Tweed Heads where we were to attend a floor show by Danny La Rue. Good as he might be, I was exhausted; by half-time I gathered an Urvan full of passengers and headed back up to Southport. It was after midnight when I got to sleep on a concrete office floor, after another eighteen-hour day.

*

Chapter 14   The XXXX Army Around Australia Relay Marathon

I was a bit over cities by now and just wanted to go bush. From the Gold Coast up to Bundaberg, my flu was pretty bad. We were getting little sleep and now I was coughing at night and would have get up so as not to disturb the others.

We arrived in Gympie after dark, and it was very low-key. What I do remember fondly is our accommodation at a forestry camp. Modern timber buildings were set among stately eucalypts and soft, green lawn. The facilities were as nice as the setting. We had dinner in a mess hall and hot showers in a sparkling-clean bathroom, then relaxed in a recreation room in front of television. We had been on the road for thirteen days, and this is what I missed. The only sore point was having to sleep on the floor with forty others when there were stacks of lovely bedrooms.

I must have been feeling good as I breezed through Maryborough with a ten-kilometre speed of 42 mins 20 secs. Included in this was stopping for three minutes at the Town Hall to hand over the scroll and do an interview with a local radio station. (On arrival in population centres, the runner would carry a baton containing a scroll to be signed by civic officials of every town and city we passed through.) I was crook again at Bundaberg and awake most of the night with a headache and incessant coughing. There were no doctor's appointments available. In desperation, I settled for the local chemist's home brew cough mixture.

Some of the best occasions were least expected. We had civic duties at the tiny towns of Bajool and Marmor, where we spent half an hour chatting to enthusiastic primary students, signing autographs and dispensing mementos of our visit. An impromptu fun run at Marmor ended at the highway just as Vic came past as the runner.

On day sixteen, we had our first continuous overnight stage covering the old Bruce Highway 'horror stretch' of 336 kilometres in 22.5 hours. After leaving Marlborough, there was nothing to see except unbroken stretches of dry eucalypt forest. (Well, I did want to get into the bush!) Team 5 left Rockhampton late and drove through for dinner supplied by the support crew at Marlborough. While still eating, we were startled to see the runner speed by. We hurriedly got on the road again as we had next safety just north of town.

In the 160 kilometres covered since leaving 'Rocky', the relay was now thirty minutes in front of schedule. This was bound to cause problems further along as teams were still asleep and suddenly found they were needed earlier. I experimented with the 'Cliffy Shuffle' to see just how slow I could run. I took two extra minutes per kilometre; it was boring, but I got us back to schedule.

When our run leg was completed, we drove on to a sign saying Ilbilbie, though in the dark there was no sign of a town. At the only crossroad, we found the sleeping

Chapter 14 The XXXX Army Around Australia Relay Marathon

convoy and chose a quiet spot near some cane fields to get some sleep. After three and a half hours, it was dawn and we got on with a lethargic morning routine. After a while, I noticed that there were very few people remaining at the camp. On enquiring, I was told the runner had passed through an hour earlier.

I alerted the others as we packed in record time and rushed up the highway, trying to contact Team 4 on the radio. They had very professionally continued up the road performing their own safety and were quite relieved that we eventually turned up for work. Part of the problem was the relay was way in front of schedule again. This was also a problem at the next town of Sarina where they passed through without any locals seeing them.

Just past Sarina, we set Rob off on our first run leg while we returned to town for a morning tea. We told him to just keep running in case we were enjoying ourselves too much. It was too early for tea and we couldn't wait, but while we were there, a relay re-enactment was conducted for the innocent locals.

Alan 'Blue' Ingram ran in with Team 4 performing their own safety (again!) and presented the scroll to the mayor. About this time, I had a pang of guilt about leaving Rob running through the heat of the never-ending cane fields. We hurried off to replace him for the final legs into Mackay.

In addition to being ahead of schedule, we were also

closer to town than expected, so Ernie and I ran the final leg together. Sometimes, especially when approaching a city stage end, some support crew had a sudden desire to run with us. (It never seemed to hit them out in the middle of an overnight stage in the middle of nowhere.) Anyway, Phil Thorne jumped out and joined us, so we kept the pace hot, ensuring he would have to earn his publicity. On the way in, we were interviewed for local TV and had action shots taken for the paper. Then on arrival at the rendezvous, we all had to sit and wait until the correct time to run in.

After five hours' sleep, I roused my teammates at 2.50am for the first run of the day out of Mackay. At that time, I was sluggish but got through nine and a half kilometres in 38 mins 12 secs to have us right on schedule. I shouldn't have bothered as Vic immediately had us three minutes in front. He just couldn't help himself!

We were way ahead of any other relay members to arrive at Bowen. Sunday morning in Bowen had to be seen to be believed – and immediately forgotten! It was dead quiet, but Bowen did turn out to be a relay highlight. After the reception, we walked out along Bowen's long, ancient, wooden pier; moored there was Sir Peter Abeles' $1.5 million cruiser. We had a pleasant evening cruise around the bay and had to hold on to our hats when the skipper put the foot down. When we turned for home, the sun was setting behind the ranges far to the west, and the

Chapter 14 The XXXX Army Around Australia Relay Marathon

hills around Bowen were silhouetted as the sun's dying rays thrust long fingers of gold across the placid water.

On day twenty, we had a late start for the final run into Townsville, which was appropriate as Rob and Vic currently served at Lavarack Barracks. I was pleased to reach the northern city where I had first taken up running sixteen years earlier. I handed over to Vic and Rob and they did the final leg into the Army camp accompanied by TV, reporters and a police escort.

I had a feeling of nostalgia as we crested the range and I saw the familiar panorama of Townsville spread before us. This approach is dominated by the brooding grey mass of Mt Stuart with its sheer face towering over the Army's immense Lavarack Barracks. Ever expanding suburbs had filled in all the flat land between Mt Stuart and Cleveland Bay. On the ocean side, the city centre was similarly dominated by the vivid red and orange hues of Castle Hill's cliffs and rocky slopes.

Our group run-in was an amazing experience as we ran between solid walls of supporters with the whole population of Lavarack Barracks cheering us home. We had a day off and I enjoyed catching up with old friends and in between a Cleveland Bay cruise that took us close to Cape Pallarenda, my first Townsville home. The only low point was the insect screening at the transit lines; I think it was there to keep the mosquitoes inside and I hardly got any sleep at all.

The next night, we spent at the Army's Field Force Battle School, which is set in thick rainforest on the western side of the mountain that looms above Tully, Australia's wettest town. We had the first run out of Tully the next morning through mist and a steady, warm drizzle. I had the rare experience of enjoying a morning run through a tropical downpour surrounded by solid walls of vivid, green rain forest.

We had a dreaded 'split shift', meaning we had to hang around all day to perform the final safety into Cairns, but I knew just the spot to wait! We drove on to near Gordonvale, where the Gillies Highway (also known as the Gillies Range Road) turns off and winds up to the Atherton Tableland. There, we found an oasis on the banks of the Mulgrave River and enjoyed our sandwiches below the spectacular slopes of Walshs Pyramid. Ten years earlier when in peak form, I had won the annual eight-mile Pyramid Race up the 3000 feet of this well-named monolith.

Yawn ... oh, hey, look – there goes the runner! Oops. We were a little late taking over safety, but luckily it was George and Team 4, so they were used to it by now. It happened again the next morning after leaving Cairns, totally my fault. I thought we had time to see the picturesque village of Kuranda and Barron Falls, before safety duty. I had underestimated the slow traffic and the difficult winding single lane, and though we rushed, we were late again. Yes, you guessed it – poor old Team 4 were manfully performing their own safety, and we didn't get to see Port Douglas at all!

We had to rush through some of Australia's most beautiful scenery where, for thirty kilometres, the highway hugs the Coral Sea coast and seems almost devoid of civilisation. A magnificent panorama of placid inlets bordered by pristine white sand beaches and rocky headlands unfolded. Tall palms marching along rock strewn bays contrasted with trickling streams and rainforest on the inland side. This was the first time we had passed over territory I had not seen before, and I was suitably impressed. It whetted my appetite for our imminent turn inland to cross our immense nation.

We were still performing safety as Team 4 ran into the most northern town on our run, Mossman, and returned for an inland diversion up onto the Atherton Tableland. Well, that was the plan, except Mike Connor stayed on the highway heading back south. After admonishing him for not wanting to run up the looming climb, we soon got him on the road to Mareeba. It was hot and the range was long and steep, so the runners were not doing any sightseeing. For us riding behind, there was a great view of tiny Mossman in a sea of sugarcane far below.

We took over running as the climb flattened and we emerged from rainforest into dry scrub with ant hills, so typical of the Aussie bush. The temperature was stiflingly hot as the climb continued from Mareeba to Atherton, cutting through the heart of the Atherton Tableland. Team 1 was working hard as we gazed at some of the nicest country in Australia. Lush green farmland flourished due to red, volcanic soil and it was interspersed with patches of rainforest. But by evening, I was a bit over it. Our reception was in a noisy, smoke-filled RSL, dinner was too little too late and was eaten standing in the dark. Early arrivals had used all the hot water and my knee was aching badly.

The next two days would be a challenge, as it was 600 kilometres along the Kennedy Highway and the Gregory Developmental Road to Charters Towers. In the first 200 kilometres after leaving the Tableland, there was only one turn-off to Karumba, 500 kilometres away on the Gulf of Carpentaria. We left Atherton for first safety early the next morning and I thought, now at last, we are heading into the outback. The runners were Team 4 again, and after yesterday they were cursing their misfortune in again copping the hill. As well as a mountain range up to Herberton, they had a stiff headwind and it started to drizzle.

Poor communication was a problem after we took over running before Ravenshoe. There had been no talk of a reception there and town was one kilometre off the highway. We called Alan who said to go through town, seeing it was so close. Vic ran the scroll in as we joined

Chapter 14 The XXXX Army Around Australia Relay Marathon

the few locals out to greet us. We then all adjourned to the CWA Hall where the ladies had gone to a lot of trouble. All we could round up were a dozen team members; as runner team, we should not have attended at all. We had a few hectic minutes of eating, drinking and talking before we rushed off to relieve Vic. He was unamused to find we had been feeding our faces, and as a fully laden Ernie wobbled off without a warm-up, Vic unkindly labelled him 'Beachball'.

A bit further on, there was a sign stating Innot Hot Springs, so we pulled up to investigate. There was a creek with shallow pools of warm water, just what our weary bodies needed. I waded in to take a photo of some bougainvillea. I stepped on a spot where boiling artesian water was gushing and leapt towards the bank. Unfortunately, my camera didn't make the trip and sunk into the cauldron. I risked more scalds in rescuing it, and then we thought we better see if Rob had finished his leg.

I had the 'glory leg' through to Mt Garnet and through a steady climb, I covered thirteen kilometres in 50 mins 45 secs. It was the only town in 470 kilometres between Ravenshoe and Charters Towers. It seemed closed for Saturday afternoon, with no sign of life. After running, we followed directions to the golf club/racecourse where we found some locals relaxing with footy, races and beers. We enjoyed an hour out of the hot, humid weather before it was on with the show.

We came across the convoy at the dinner point, near the junction of the Gulf Developmental Road. It was located among rock, dead wood, long dry grass and ant hills, so not inviting a long stay. At dark, we headed off for another hundred kilometres south and at 9 pm our headlights picked out a sign stating 'The Lynd Junction' (now Conjuboy). We sat there confused in the pitch-black night. Some sign of civilisation, including a petrol station, would have been nice. We were mulling over the problem when our salvation came via a radio message. All teams were informed that petrol was available at The Lynd Oasis, a cattle station a few kilometres to the west down a corrugated dirt road. It was an oasis of civilisation; a small 'junk food' shop was packed with relay team members. We filled up, ate up and drove back to the junction to grab some sleep before our next safety.

It seemed my head had barely hit the pillow when our tranquil night location became chaotic. I was startled awake by the noise of truck engines, brakes, hundreds of bawling cattle, flashing torches, headlights and a huge cloud of smelly dust. It was 1 am and after two and a half hours of sleep, it was time to prepare for safety again.

From 1.15 am, we took turns at the wheel, trying to stay awake and not knock the runner over, as we crawled along at fifteen kilometres per hour, headlights piercing the darkness, music blaring from our speakers and the infernal blipping of our hazard lights. After two and a

Chapter 14 The XXXX Army Around Australia Relay Marathon

quarter hours of that, the last thing we felt like doing was running. But run we did, from 3.30 am until we reached the Greenvale area at 7.30 am.

With the first faint flush of dawn, I hit the road for my thirteen kilometres. It seemed interminable. Irritable from lack of sleep, I struggled just to keep on schedule, confusing time calls and frustrated from constantly running in pain. As I neared the end of my leg, I passed a solitary Urvan parked near the breakfast camp. There was no one waiting to take over and so I picked up pace, thinking I hadn't reached the runner yet. A kilometre further on, there was another Urvan and upon enquiry, they said they were the new safety. I had had enough of it, and as I plodded back to the camp, I gave a nonchalant John McCrystal a mouthful of advice to hurry him on his way.

My mood worsened when I found the only food remaining was cold leftovers. I was not pleased that after twenty-six hours on the road, runners on easier shifts and support crew had hogged the lion's share. When our sandwiches were ready, I gathered my teammates and headed straight off before I said something I would regret. We drove a course parallel to the upper reaches of the mighty Burdekin River and were closer to Townsville than Charters Towers, still 180 kilometres away. On arrival there, we discovered that it was Sunday and the town was closed!

So far, this has been a description of a typical relay shift in the outback. There were many more as our journey continued, but I shall ignore most of those repetitious kilometres and stick to the highlights. So, westward ho! Hughenden, Richmond, Julia Creek to Cloncurry – pretty much flat, desolate, dry and boring, but it had to be crossed.

At Cloncurry, the terrain changed to rugged hills and dry watercourses flanked by majestic rivers and ghost gums. This was the harsh Gulf Country that Burke and Wills passed through before meeting an untimely end more than 150 years earlier. Thirty days into the relay, we crested a range of rocky hills, and there was an urban panorama spread across the valley below. From a far hill, we could see the buildings and huge chimneys of Mount Isa Mines dominating the landscape. It came as a pleasant surprise to find this dot on the map was actually a city of 30,000 people.

We had a rendezvous for the run-in and then an RSL function, but after another twenty-two-hour day, I was ready for bed and welcoming a rest day. It was one of the good ones, as we had a guided tour of the mine over one kilometre below the surface and in the afternoon a drive south-east through rugged country to do some fossicking for 'Maltese Crosses'. These small stones are believed to be from meteor fragments, and some have the pattern of a Maltese Cross on the surface. One of our access roads was an old mining railway tunnel just wide enough to fit the Nissan Patrol through. A little further on, we dropped into a valley and found a huge crater with impassable walls and a deep lake. The day was completed with a visit to a modern ghost town, the site of the Mary Kathleen uranium mine.

Camooweal was a further 188 kilometres west, our final tiny town in Queensland. It is reached via the Barkly Highway, which continues as the only thin strip of bitumen west to its junction with the Stuart Highway. In the whole 500 kilometres, there seemed to be nothing except a couple of roadhouses, as most of the vast stations were far distant from the highway. So, humble though it was, Camooweal rates a mention.

It was the middle of the dry season and we had just travelled 900 kilometres through terribly drought-affected country. Yet, it was raining steadily when we left 'The Isa' and it never let up all day. There was also a bitterly cold southerly wind that had us reaching for our cold-weather gear. The land of the Barkly Tableland through to central Australia is dead flat and it soon turned into a sea of mud. If we moved our vehicles off the narrow strip of bitumen, the show would be over. It was extremely hazardous to remain on it as the huge road trains stopped for nothing and would not budge an inch.

Except for a rare vehicle, there was no sign of any living creature during the whole day except a solitary dingo. On arrival in Camooweal, there were a pub, primary school, service station and a few houses huddled beneath the low cloud and sodden from the downpour. Our welcoming committee was a kid on the pub verandah, holding a sign which read, 'Camooweal, the town where you make your own fun'.

Some of the team must have taken note as there were a couple of practical jokes played out. We were setting up our bedding in the primary school. Mary Kerwin of the support crew, in particular, had lots of bags and was meticulous in her preparations. When she finally stood back to admire her handiwork, she was given the message to pack up as she had received a billet for the night with some of the locals. One would have to have seen Camooweal school in the middle of a rainstorm to appreciate the enthusiasm Mary displayed in packing up and stumbling out, heavily laden, into the teeth of the gale. Mary sloshed through the sea of red mud and had almost made it across the road to an unsuspecting Aboriginal family before the joker called her back. It says a lot about Mary's temperament that when she arrived back, soaked through and puffing heavily, she just calmly and doggedly set up her gear again.

When the kitchen truck served dinner, I rushed out to get it, but by the time I got back to shelter, I had a plate full of water. A high point was some teachers arriving and putting TVs on with the Commonwealth Games

Chapter 14 The XXXX Army Around Australia Relay Marathon

in full flight. Not so good was the horde of mosquitoes in full flight! Our relaxed evening was shattered when Tammy Menzel let out a piercing scream. On climbing into her sleeping bag, she had come into contact with a cold, slimy object. When a somewhat shaken Tammy investigated, she did indeed find a snake, albeit a small, black and white rubber one. She spent the rest of the evening trying to discover the perpetrator while I was occupied with the horrendous mozzies.

*

Thirteen kilometres from Camooweal, the border with the Northern Territory is marked with a signpost adorned with outback Australia's national emblem, the shotgun blast. A couple of signs were the only features in the entire landscape, man-made or natural, to be above ground level. It was an eerie feeling to be standing in the drizzle, the sky blotted out by mist and low cloud, with the dead flat, treeless tableland extending to the horizon in every direction. We were in the tropics, yet I was shivering while clad in a tracksuit, balaclava, two jackets and gloves. Welcome to the Northern Territory! It would be a furnace in summer.

At our first major road crossing for 500 kilometres, we found Three Ways Roadhouse. As we came from the east, the direction choice was obvious, but the relay did a quick diversion south to Tennant Creek, where I recovered from forty hours with only three hours of sleep since Camooweal, then it was directly north through a big empty Territory to Darwin.

Elliott was a dust bowl as roadworks were under way. This dirt surface suited me fine and a roaring tailwind had me cruising through eleven kilometres in 41 mins 9 secs. After the run, lunch was to be somewhere in Newcastle Waters but we didn't know how to get there. A close inspection revealed a small sign in the middle of nowhere indicating a left turn onto a narrow strip of bitumen, which after five kilometres led to a dilapidated schoolhouse. We turned south towards some barely noticeable buildings on the horizon. Good choice, as a winding track led to an oasis in the middle of the harsh bushland with manicured lawns, hedges and palm trees surrounding a huge single-storey building. The best description is that Newcastle Waters station house was owned by Kerry Packer and valued at $3.5 million.

We navigated our way through a maze of paths and rooms until we found some people. The manager Sally Warriner made us welcome, and we got straight into a shower in the plush guest quarters. We moved to the shaded outdoor pool area and team members had a barbeque with pioneer pastoralists who travelled from as far as 500 kilometres away. It was a delicious meal with interesting conversations, and it was easy to forget for a

Chapter 14   The XXXX Army Around Australia Relay Marathon

while that, out on the highway, runners were pounding their way north and expecting to be relieved soon.

Before leaving, I had a look around and found the historic original station buildings of stone and bush timber. There was all the paraphernalia needed for a working cattle station, including bush vehicles, light aeroplanes, numerous animals and stockmen. One hundred metres from green, manicured lawns, the land instantly transformed into a harsh bush landscape.

Further north, late in the afternoon, we did another left-turn diversion to check out the Daly Waters pub. We discovered an historic wood and iron building redolent with outback Australian charm. The publican was pleased to see us but said a big occasion had been organised and then cancelled at the last minute when it became obvious the relay was going straight on by. It sure would have been a nicer dinner spot than the dust bowl of road trains at Dunmurra where we had dined earlier.

Following another 'graveyard shift', we drove on to Mataranka, found the convoy and grabbed a few hours' sleep. After breakfast we took a ten-kilometre diversion to the east to visit Mataranka Springs. On arrival, we found a massive caravan park and a pleasant, forested area. A one-kilometre walk on a path that wound its way through luxuriant tropical foliage brought us to the springs. A stream seeping through the foliage was dammed to create a crystal clear and delightfully warm swimming pool. This was set among palms, tall gums and lush undergrowth, a remarkable sight set in the harsh, dry Territory scrub.

Another safety and runner shift brought us to Katherine, the Northern Territory's second-largest population centre. We visited it twice, going north and returning, and never saw much at all. We did the run-in, which was low-key as most of the relay members were out cruising Katherine Gorge. After five minutes at the reception, we snuck out and drove flat out for twenty kilometres east to catch the final cruise for the day. On arrival, we ran through the tourists and flung ourselves down, panting, just as the skipper was casting off. Now to try to relax and enjoy it!

It was scenic and peaceful cruising this large river with its blue-green hues walled in between towering cliffs of orange sandstone. All too soon, it was back to the showgrounds for dinner in the dark and then on the road again for night shift. Our second session as runner brought us to the outskirts of Darwin where we received an unusual donation: grateful but scratching our heads, we mounted a huge set of water buffalo horns on our front bull bar and continued on our way. I ran the baton down The Mall of an enthusiastic and busy central Darwin. My only previous visit had been on return from South Vietnam in 1972, and all I saw then was the airport.

Darwin is a nice place to visit, and the evening

Chapter 14 The XXXX Army Around Australia Relay Marathon

reception was a crowded affair. I joined Alan and Barbara for the scroll signing and a wonderful donation of $20,000, while all dined on spit-roasted buffalo. I enjoyed a relaxed rest day in Darwin and then during the evening at Larrakeyah Barracks, we also had TV with Rob de Castella, Lisa Martin and Steve Moneghetti excelling in the Commonwealth Games Marathon. At 10 pm, I had to leave Lisa to the final kilometres as we had to leave at 3.15 am for a 343-kilometre haul back south to Katherine.

Team 5 seemed a bit subdued; perhaps it was the early start, leaving the bright lights of Darwin or that we were retracing our steps. More likely it was the realisation that our next capital city was Perth, more than 4000 kilometres away. We arrived in Katherine well after dark, purchased petrol and went straight to the showgrounds for dinner. At the O-Group, we were informed that we were first safety, with another 3.15am start. We had certainly not recovered from the Darwin trip and were about to set off on the most difficult leg yet undertaken. Our next night stopover was at Wyndham in the Western Australian Kimberley region, 613 kilometres away.

This was the outback, a single lane, bumpy strip of bitumen called the Victoria Highway leading us to the Kimberley. It was rugged, isolated and empty. After our run, we drove 150 kilometres west, and there were very limited places to stop for a break. We passed one road junction, a dirt one signposted 'Wave Hill, 300 kilometres'.

In the end, we just drove off into the bush and located a couple of trees to give some scant shade for the Urvan. The flies, termites and heat were annoying as we read, slept or walked around to pass the time until our next safety.

Afternoon safety brought us through to the Victoria River where there was a roadhouse, and the support crew had set up a dinner camp. Most of the convoy had spent a relaxed afternoon enjoying this large river and the spectacular mountain scenery. Not for us though, as we ran past, across the bridge and along the Victoria River valley. There was no twilight in the valley and when I had finished my eight kilometres in 32 mins 12 secs, it was pitch-black. Dinner was delivered out to us, and I was beyond disappointed to see salad and half-cooked chicken when my body was crying out for carbohydrates.

On we drove until we refuelled at tiny Timber Creek, probably the most isolated town on coastal Australia. Its nearest neighbours, Katherine and Kununurra, were about 300 kilometres away. We pushed on until we pulled over near our next duty point and had four hours of sleep until 1 am. After another graveyard shift, we located the convoy camped at the Baines River and halted for a couple of hours until breakfast.

It was always an eerie feeling to have spent the night on safety and runner duties and arrive at a camp of sleeping teammates. We had done plenty of night

Chapter 14 The XXXX Army Around Australia Relay Marathon

stages but this one had a difference, in that there had been a dramatic change of scenery. The breakfast camp was dominated by a semicircle of brooding cliffs and in general the terrain had the rugged grandeur I associate with the Kimberley. It had been a long haul, and we had a decision to make: were we dedicated relay professionals or tourists?

*

On we drove across the border into Western Australia for a hundred kilometres to have a look at the Ord River Dam. Not far from the border, a well-constructed road took us south for thirty kilometres to Lake Argyle. Cresting a ridge, we were greeted by a vast panorama of blue bays and inlets enclosed by walls of red rock. We enjoyed a brief stay at the original Argyle homestead of the Durack family that had been relocated from the floor of the lake. A very windy lookout gave a brief but rewarding view of this huge lake that stretched to the horizon. We saw the massive rock fill dam wall that holds it all back and a powerful jet of water from near its base which feeds the Ord downstream.

Time was on the wing and we rushed back just in time for a group run across the border. Then it was straight into safety and a run through the Ord River valley near Kununurra. It was near sunset when we arrived at

Western Australia's most northern town of Wyndham. We passed a settlement named 6 Mile, drove on through 3 Mile and then the road ended at Port Wyndham. There was no room for expansion at the port as most of the narrow peninsula is taken up by the brooding bulk of the Bastion Range. The town then spread along the narrow strip between it and Cambridge Gulf.

The port area was very old and tired but, just for Vic, there was a crocodile viewing platform. We walked through low green bushes to a small concrete platform which was open to the nearby mangroves. There were no crocodiles, and as the sun had set far over the rugged ranges behind Cambridge Gulf, we suddenly became aware that we could be 'main course'. We beat a hasty retreat and drove back to the football field at 3 Mile. We were at a loose end as there were still a couple of hours until the reception. Alan Batchelor was getting some shut-eye on his sleeping bag, so I followed suit.

At 8 pm, I awoke to a deserted camp. It had all happened and we slept through, as no one thought to rouse us. I arrived with my team at the Sportsman's Club light-headed, hungry and decidedly antisocial. When encouraged to socialise by Barbara and the support crew, I did not respond too well. Food and sleep were my only priorities. The manager had some steak and leftover salad prepared.

Alan mentioned that he was getting the support crew to do some running through the Kimberley to

Chapter 14   The XXXX Army Around Australia Relay Marathon

ease the burden on the runners. When I conveyed this information to the other team leaders, they were equally dismayed and we trooped into the back room to discuss Alan's decision with him. Our determination to continue with all running duties unless injured and a few facts regarding the support crew caused a re-think. The Commanding Officer, Alan, had every right to have his order obeyed without question, but kudos to the runner in him that he was willing to have us continue. I later worked out why we were so down. In three days, we had run from Darwin to Wyndham a total of over 900 kilometres. In our sixty-five hours on the road, we had managed only nine hours of sleep in three sessions, and it was finally getting on top of us.

There's not a lot to say about the next couple of thousand kilometres, with the exception of Broome. The highway is largely a semicircle as it loops around the top of the Great Sandy Desert. After Halls Creek we passed through featureless and flat country, over which a road crew were laying a final section of bitumen. So, George Russell and Mike Connor became the last people to run on an unsealed portion of Highway no.1. Another 900 kilometres and four days later, we ran into Broome.

It was after dark when our group strode a spot-lit path between walls of Broome residents and mounted a semi-trailer stage. We were individually introduced and welcoming speeches were made with genuine enthusiasm.

Team members were presented with Broome mementos and a giant cheque for $8500. This was our best reception of the relay; full plaudits to local dynamo Sally 'Big Sal' Aston and the town for their interest and effort.

Once down from the stage, we mingled with the locals at the Mardi Gras before the party continued at the nearby Roebuck Hotel. Most walked there and I only followed when I realised the Urvan keys were there – somewhere! It was bedlam: packed to the rafters, earsplitting music and jostling bodies. After rescuing the keys, I quickly left them to it and settled for an early night in my tent at the caravan park. Ahh! A full night of sleep and a rest day in Broome. Where better to recharge the batteries?

Broome is set on a low peninsula which separates Roebuck Bay from the Indian Ocean, with jetties where the pearling fleet harbour. There is a modern shopping centre but I was particularly attracted to the old shopping strip, which was all historic shops and quiet streets with an oriental flavour. The shop of the pioneering Streeter and Male Company was like something I had seen only in old movies. There were also a couple of pearling luggers up on blocks for tourists to experience.

The afternoon was spent at Cable Beach. It has a magnificent stretch of pure white sand which is soft underfoot, not overcrowded and devoid of rubbish and pollution. The turquoise vastness of the Indian Ocean merging with the horizon and the cloudless azure sky

Chapter 14 The XXXX Army Around Australia Relay Marathon

completed an unforgettable picture. The only downside was that it was very hot, and we had an emergency evacuation from the surf when a deadly sea snake was spotted.

The rest of the west coast gets skipped over and if you need to ask why, then you haven't been there. It is hot, harsh and empty! Keep in mind that the Dutch and William Dampier were in Australia long before James Cook and decided no one would want to live here. You can guess which section they discovered.

In a 500-kilometre-long trip south-west, with the ocean on one side and the Great Sandy Desert on the other, the only civilisation was the Sandfire Roadhouse. Port Hedland at the other end was everything that Broome wasn't. It only rates a mention because we stayed at an Army Reserve (ARES) depot and had a party to celebrate reaching the halfway point of our epic journey.

From Karratha, we took the 'scenic route', meaning it was another 1000 kilometres down to Carnarvon, with plenty more open spaces. There was a planned diversion to Onslow which was on the coast some eighty kilometres west; however, some map-to-ground errors had been made. The arrived-at solution was for the convoy to make the trip to the coast while two teams waited at the turn-off to Mt Minne for six hours before resuming our trip south. I have no idea what Onslow was like as I spent a hot afternoon at an isolated picnic shelter. What we saw was a relentless sun in a cloudless sky beating down on a parched landscape. Red sand and rough, rocky plains were covered with scrubby bushes and spinifex. The far distant hills were majestic with contrasting hues of red rock and pastel green foliage.

After four hours of alternating safety and runner shifts with Team 2, 160 kilometres south of our isolated junction, we stopped for a sleep just short of another isolated junction. Alan Batchelor came past on Team 1's final leg, during which he turned west onto a very wide and very bumpy dirt road. After three hours' sleep, we were up for another graveyard shift of safety and runner. I would usually enjoy the dirt, but this was a different challenge in the wee small hours. There were corrugations, sand patches, small stones, concealed rock and a vicious camber, all the more difficult to see when the safety vehicle was bouncing around as much as I was.

It was eighty kilometres across and the same distance back north to a very isolated Exmouth. This small town exists to serve the military base at North West Cape. No doubt this explains our visit and their interest, as demonstrated by an amazing $8500 donation to the ACF. We were last into Exmouth on safety and left soon after on our run, so I didn't even get to see the place after all the effort to get there. At least, we were heading south again.

After our long haul from Broome, we crossed the Gascoyne River bridge, and on entering Carnarvon, the

Chapter 14 The XXXX Army Around Australia Relay Marathon

landscape changed immediately. The town of 8000 had cultivated farmland and outlying settled areas, making it more like a 'normal' town we see in the east. Our arrival coincided with a bikie group's Sandhurst Run and their outdoor rock concert. We were introduced on the back of the usual semi-trailer stage, but two more disparate groups you could not find. There were drugs, drinks, heat, dust, aggression and arguments. I was soon out of there and slept for thirteen hours; since leaving Port Hedland four days ago, we had totalled only eighteen hours of sleep.

We enjoyed a well-earned rest day, although it did rain at night. Some tents that hadn't been tested failed, while those sleeping in the open sought shelter – except our Vic, who was still out there fast asleep with sleeping bag and contents thoroughly soaked. He wasn't even aware it had rained.

Halfway to Geraldton, about 500 kilometres south, we grabbed five hours' sleep on the roadside. At this stage, we were inland of Shark Bay, Australia's most westerly point. One of my run legs was through the historic village of Northampton, which was all sandstone buildings set in green, fertile farming land. After what we had passed through since leaving the east coast, we could have just stayed put. In fact, that's exactly what Ernie's running shoes did, as he left them airing out on a post.

Geraldton, with a population of 26,000, was the largest place we had passed through since Darwin. It was attractive, with many imposing historic buildings, surf crashing on a sea wall and large port facilities. Our accommodation at the football clubrooms was modern and clean, and when I saw carpeted floor, even I spent a luxurious eight hours asleep there.

Early on day fifty-eight, we prepared to enter our first capital city since leaving Darwin, 4221 kilometres and nineteen days ago. From Midland, it was a slow drive in as we encountered wet roads and traffic. Our rendezvous at the city end of a bridge over the Swan River was a scene of chaos, with police and television crews adding to our own preparations for the run-in. The runner's arrival coincided with a torrential downpour and a gale force headwind, a soggy but memorable entry into Perth.

The next morning when Vic set off as first runner, the rain was absolutely bucketing down again. Our course was south-west towards a corner of Australia I had long wanted to see. Robert Holmes à Court's magnificent Heytesbury Stud was a delight to the eye after our long trip through the outback. Thoroughbred horses were grazing on lush, green grass and there were many kilometres of white painted fences. The highway was about sixteen kilometres from the coast, with a range of hills along the eastern side enclosing fertile farmland.

Our evening arrival in the large port city of Bunbury coincided with the grand opening of the Lord Forrest Hotel. We jogged into the foyer and lined up in an atrium formed

Chapter 14 The XXXX Army Around Australia Relay Marathon

by the base of the cylindrical multi-storey building. It was magnificent as all rooms had internal balconies overlooking pools, gardens, waterfalls, fountains and hanging gardens. Many speeches were made, but as we were right next to the waterfall, I have no idea what they were about.

A rumour had gone around earlier that our accommodation for the night was the Lord Forrest, but alas, it was ill-founded. The reality was a sleeping bag on the floor of a draughty office in the local ARES depot. The next day, I was last runner into Manjimup and it was rather low-key. With no one around, I climbed into the van and it was off to the footy field for a sleep.

While we slept, the next day commenced at 1 am in appalling conditions. It was raining heavily and the temperature was down to six degrees. I don't think we had acclimatised yet! When we woke, everybody was gone except the XXXX representative, David Park. We shared our muesli with him and then headed off to Pemberton to find the Gloucester Tree. This huge kauri has a viewing platform at a height of sixty-one metres, accessed via a staircase consisting of steel pegs driven into the trunk and a wire rope to hold on to. Rob was straight up it, but the rest of us had second thoughts. It was wet, slippery, I was wearing my Ugg Boots and had badly injured my thumb the previous day; however, I couldn't leave without climbing it! It was worth it for the 360-degree uninterrupted view of the forest.

We drove on through superb forests of kauri and jarrah, and when we reached the coast near Walpole, we boiled the billy in the pouring rain. After a long day on the road, we had the final run into Albany. The highway crests a saddle between two hills and runs in a straight line down to the Southern Ocean. There are many imposing historic buildings and a large port facility.

The next morning, we drove to a rocky bluff where the lookout there had a huge memorial to local ANZAC volunteers. It had unforgettable views of Albany's historic buildings in their hilly green setting and the vast waterways of Princess Royal Harbour and King George Sound. We had left our usual safety margin to get to work on time, but the runner was so far ahead of schedule that we still managed to be late.

During safety, we were able to enjoy a wildflower display in the Stirling Range National Park. Then the only town I remember in the long haul to Ravensthorpe was Jerramungup, and that's only due to its name. As the relay was passing through Ravensthorpe in the middle of the night, we were tasked with civic duties to fly the flag while the little town was still awake. We enjoyed doing the rounds of the hotel and hospital, and chatting with the locals, whose enthusiasm was evident. The 300 residents had raised $1300. If that wasn't enough, we were invited to a free dinner and accommodation at the Palace Hotel. We had to be up again by 1 am but this was

Chapter 14   The XXXX Army Around Australia Relay Marathon

too good an offer to refuse over such a technicality. The beds were not wasted as when Team 1 arrived, we guided them in and handed them over 'pre-warmed'. We were at it all night, with three and a half hours of safety followed by our runs, which took us past the breakfast camp at Munglinup. I had to run straight on by for a steady uphill twelve kilometres before returning for leftovers. It was dawn and our day's work was done, except for a hundred-kilometre drive through to stage end at Esperance.

Esperance was a disappointment as they had done no fundraising at all. It was a touristy place, but apart from a Pink Lake and an impressive Bay of Islands, I couldn't see why. Norseman was 200 kilometres north and exactly the opposite. It was a mining town, and we were back in the Aussie outback. There were huge tailings dumps, mine works and lots of old buildings, with many closed. During a night spent at the football ground, a southerly buster blew in and I awoke to a bitterly cold morning for us to begin our return across the Nullarbor.

Norseman, Balladonia, Caiguna, 372 kilometres. Caiguna, Cocklebiddy, Madura, Mundrabilla, 373 kilometres. Mundrabilla, Eucla, Nullarbor, Nundroo, 409 kilometres. Nundroo, Penong, Ceduna, 152 kilometres. There it is, four days and all done – nothing to see here! Well, just a bit, then. Each run leg was twelve kilometres and that meant three and a half hours as runner and three and a half hours as safety, followed by ten and a half hours to eat, rest, drive to next duty point and sleep. Repeat, repeat, repeat. It was long and tiring but without towns and civic duties, it was less complicated and almost seemed easier. There were roadhouses at regular intervals, and we seldom missed calling in.

On night one, in the middle of nowhere, we found a water tank with a large section of roof that had the sole purpose of catching lifesaving water in this parched landscape. We found another use for it, as a splendid sleeping shelter. We found the next dinner camp at Madura where the terrain had a dramatic variation. From undulating, scrubby forest, the highway dropped down the escarpment onto a flat, almost treeless plain that stretched to the horizon and beyond. In the middle of a cool, rainy night, we had the final runs before reaching the border with South Australia.

While on safety, we saw a group of team vehicles off to the right, parked at a lookout. Mark Burgess came up on the radio and said it was worth a look. What's more, he offered to fill in as safety while we did so. Who could knock back an offer to be relieved of the tedium of safety?

I was unprepared for the sight that awaited us when we drove over. The grey-green saltbush gave way to a rock surface worn smooth by millions of years of erosion, and a few tourists no doubt! Then at our feet – nothing! The ground fell sheer, and in some places overhanging. Far below, the powerful surf of the Southern Ocean

Chapter 14 The XXXX Army Around Australia Relay Marathon

broke on rocks or crashed onto the cliff. The huge swell marched in unbroken ranks from the far south where turquoise waters and the blue sky seemed to merge. The combination of flat treeless plain halting without notice and falling sheer to another empty expanse of blue water was truly majestic. When combined with a cliff face which receded in a series of headlands of consistent height to the limit of ones' vision, it became the view of a lifetime. It was an eerie feeling, though, to stand on the edge of this abyss without any safety rail between a slip and certain death. I still had relay duties to complete so I stayed a respectful distance from the edge.

*

Our next feature was that there were no features, except a sign stating we were crossing the Nullarbor Plain. Absolutely flat with no water, no shade, and the only vegetation looked and felt harsher than the rocky soil that somehow sustained it. I enjoyed my run on this traffic-free, dead-flat, straight bitumen. However, I got a stiff neck from looking over my left shoulder at the spectacular sunset. As the sun's red orb sunk below the distant horizon, a pink tinge spread across the plain, highlighting a million tiny bumps that were a carpet of stunted saltbush.

I'll skip Ceduna and the large diversion down to Port

Lincoln and back up to Whyalla. Yes, we did it and the only highlight for me was the little town of Streaky Bay. A couple of days later, we had a despised split shift on entry into Adelaide. I did a solid eleven and a half kilometres around Port Wakefield, running into the strongest headwind of the relay. This only gets a mention as a resulting photo is now my Facebook cover photo.

We had the final safety, and as the runner was a little late in arriving, the bunch was pretty toey. Away they went as our vehicle halted to let Rob and me out for the run-in. It was difficult to run at 3 mins 30 secs per kilometre after being cramped up in an Urvan for over three hours. In a repeat of Tweed Heads, we were just left in the dust to fend for ourselves. But wait! All was not lost, as the baton carrier was support crew member Ian Bromeyer, and he wasn't a runner. He couldn't hold the pace, forcing the pack to slow, so eventually Rob and I made contact as we entered the Adelaide Showgrounds at Wayville. After all that rushing, we had to wait for a gate to be opened and then walk through the Adelaide Show Day crowd. We jogged a lap of the trotting track and were welcomed by South Australia's marathon-running Premier, John Bannon.

After a rest day, we had first safety, which was better than having to run up Mt Lofty. It did mean we were too busy with navigation, and then our run, to enjoy the lovely towns and countryside of the Adelaide Hills. At sunset, we ran down along the Coorong, with the sun's dying rays reflecting off the silver mirror of water. We had a few hours' sleep at Kingston SE and were up before dawn for the morning shift. It was just as well the road was quiet when a farming couple came out with tea and toast. We stopped to enjoy it and a chat while Tony Kleiner dutifully kept on down the long straight until he was a dot on the horizon.

At Mt Gambier, we had a look at the famous lakes and then a brief sleep at the ARES depot. Have you really slept at a place if you have to get up at 2 am?

*

Safety had us across another state border to Victoria and then we ran ten and a half kilometres through bush and farmland towards Portland. As indicated by the name, this large town is set on a fine harbour and was the site of the first white settlement in Victoria. We rocked up to the modern Shire Offices, set on a hill with a great view of the ocean and requested use of their showers. Freshly cleaned up, we enjoyed a view of large pine trees set in manicured lawns with the original bluestone buildings retained to give a sense of the town's history. I was outside admiring the surroundings as Paul Van Leur ran the scroll in to the reception. The public servants then went back to their paperwork while we continued around Australia.

Warrnambool was memorable mainly due to the rain and a bitter southerly blowing in from Bass Strait. Then it was on through fertile, green farmland to Colac, famed as the home of ultramarathoner Cliff Young (actually nearby Beech Forest). We got some photos of our Cliffy lookalike, Mike Connor, with the folk legend himself and then it was on to the day's end at Queenscliff.

For me, it was a couple of days with friends at Healesville, while a reduced team made its casual way into Melbourne. When I next saw them, it was at the top end of Elizabeth Street where I was handed the baton and led the group into Melbourne. The city folk could not ignore our arrival as I was right behind an armoured personnel carrier that made a lot of noise on the bitumen. On arrival at Town Hall the first person I encountered was my old pro athletics friend Jock Logan. We had a chat and handshakes and then I belatedly remembered I had the baton and perhaps the gathered dignitaries could do with my attention.

*

On day eighty-two, we flew to Tasmania and from the flight over and the drive into Hobart, I knew I would enjoy our lap of the island. We drove to our accommodation at historic Anglesea Barracks, located on a hill between the city and casino, all vivid white

Chapter 14   The XXXX Army Around Australia Relay Marathon

painted sandstone with areas of lawn and a majestic avenue of pines. Nice though it was, we headed straight up Mt Wellington to take in the panorama in case it was our only chance. Thick fog blanketed the peak and it was bitterly cold and windswept. We kept warm with a snowball fight and built a snowman, complete with XXXX gear. After five minutes, it was back in the van with the heater on full.

The east coast was all up and down, with names like Bust Me Gall Hill and Elephant Pass. After lots of forest country, it was a real contrast to arrive in St Helens and see boats on Georges Bay. We arrived in the dark and by accident, I parked between the kitchen truck and the dining tables, so a sleep-in was not an option.

We were soon on the road again, winding up Weldborough Pass in lush rainforest and dropping into the old tin mining town of Derby. We spotted a bloke carrying a tea urn to a house and made some enquiries. The house turned out to be the Shire Offices and we had to reassure him that we were just an advance party, so not to panic. We socialised as George Russell ran the baton in, before it was back on the road again.

For me, northern Tasmania was 'Reunion Central' as I kept meeting up with runners I had competed against in Victorian professional events in recent years. This began at Scottsdale and continued across to Burnie. This part of Tassie was like the Central Coast of NSW in that towns and receptions were so close together it was difficult to get to them all on time. Too many choices of entry and exit roads added to the problems.

We had time for brief sleeps at Launceston and Burnie before setting off at 4am for a couple of tough days down the wild, west coast and the south-western wilderness. I had first run leg, and it was raining heavily as I set off, winding up a hill. When the sun did finally come up, we had left farmlands behind and entered rainforest and then rocky plateau country. As we had the final safety into Queenstown, we drove on to Rosebury where we had civic duties. Around the Hillyer Gorge, we encountered mirror image lakes, gushing mountain streams and steep hills thick with vivid green rainforest. We passed another barren plateau and stopped for a look at Lake Mackintosh through the misty rain. Once over the highest point of the Murchison Highway, we dropped down into Rosebury (population: 3000). As we had four hours before the runner arrived, we were pleased to get an invitation to the local RSL Club. Getting an early start on tea and snacks in front of a roaring log fire sure beat sitting in the van awaiting the runner. Then it was on through rugged mining country past Renison Bell and winding through forest to Zeehan. It was raining still, so we enjoyed a look at the mining museum while we awaited the change-over and our safety into Queenstown.

The isolated grandeur of the road to Queenstown

reminded me of its namesake in New Zealand. Approaching town, the road wound steeply down into a valley so deep the sun had already cast shadows over its depths. By the time the runner arrived at the RSL for a reception, it was cold and dark, so we were quickly whisked inside the RSL where dinner was scheduled. I was tired and irritable as our split shift had meant a long day on the road. After a long wait in a crowded, noisy and smoky room, my meal arrived. I had to interrupt eating it, so I could obtain petrol prior to the station closing. My main regret with Queenstown, though, is that I did not see it, as we were last in and first out.

After a two-hour catnap, I awoke feeling pretty seedy, and woke the others before jogging to the start point for a warm-up. At 10.30 pm, I galloped past the safety vehicle and set off into the wilderness. Gormanston Hill climbs directly out of Queenstown and winds through 100 bends in just four and a half kilometres. I ran as hard as I could through the pouring rain, with only my strained breathing and the whining of the safety vehicles' engine interrupting the stillness of the night. The van's headlights didn't light up the road in front due to the constant bends and steep climb. My spectacles fogged up, so I removed them, put my head down and just plugged on up. Towards the end of my leg, the road crested a ridge and dropped steeply down the other side. For only the third time during the relay, I had run flat out and my leg muscles were like jelly as my feet slapped the wet pavement down towards where Ernie was waiting to relieve me. I hoped he would be waiting, as there had been a junction at the hilltop and in the pitch-black night, I had taken a guess at the correct route. With much relief, I handed over and retired to the comfort of the van. When I checked my time for the six kilometres, I was satisfied to see 23 mins 40 secs, proving to myself that I could maintain the schedule no matter what the conditions.

We drove on into the wilderness through rain and fog, with intense concentration required to keep on the narrow, winding road up to King William Saddle. At 2am, we parked near Derwent Bridge for three hours of sleep before our next safety, through until dawn. Alan Batchelor had a tough leg down a steep gorge to cross the Nive River and was fairly distressed when he handed over to me near the top of the matching climb. I warmed up near Tarraleah, overlooking the hydro-electric station far below.

With daylight, we were done with the wilderness and entered the green pastures of the Derwent Valley. On reaching historic New Norfolk, we popped into the Colonial Inn for a look. It is 151 years old and is symbolic of Tasmania's links with England as a former penal colony. My great-great-grandfather, Richard Tonks, was a convict and later publican in Hobart and surrounding area. We enjoyed a guided tour and a complimentary

Chapter 14   The XXXX Army Around Australia Relay Marathon

Devonshire tea. The perfect way to finish our jam-packed four-day lap of Tassie!

*

On day ninety, we set off from Melbourne with just a week of the Princes Highway between us and the end of the relay in Sydney. There was confusion through the outer south-eastern suburbs as a busload of team members from Watsonia Barracks tried to meet up with the locals who had enjoyed a day away from the convoy. To add to the mess, our vehicles with support crew were yet to locate their owners following a ferry trip across Bass Strait.

Once reunited with our vehicles, we had a couple of routine days through to East Gippsland. All the preparatory work we runners took for granted when we arrived at a new town seemed to come apart at Bairnsdale. We arrived in town an hour early and the locals seemed confused about the timing and the route to be taken. With none of the decision makers around, the running teams in town took the initiative to ensure it went smoothly.

We had a group run-in with an APC and police escort, and ran a loop through the back streets to meet the schoolkids, before arriving on schedule at the main street reception. Our senior member, Captain Mark Burgess of Team 3, lined us up and made a good fist of his impromptu speech debut. Team 5 were on safety through to Lakes Entrance, but Ernie and I stayed behind to bolster the numbers at the reception. After some photos of us draped over the RSL cannon, we got a lift up the road to rejoin our mates.

My run was through undulating eucalypt forest near Nowa Nowa and the delightful spring day had me running well. I tore through eight and a half kilometres in 29 mins 36 secs without apparent effort. The town itself did slow me when I realised that students from the tiny primary school were out to cheer us on. I hurriedly put a team singlet on and we 'disappeared' the bawdy songs from Kevin 'Bloody' Wilson that were blaring from the speakers.

A sportsman's night at Orbost caused much anguish among the decision makers as sport sponsorship politics reared its head. Charlie Lynn, in his old hometown, had organised for Cliff Young to be at the same function we were to appear at. Conflicting sponsor parties were not happy! We were not to go if Cliff was there, and as the cook had been told no need to prepare a meal, it looked like we would go hungry.

Ed 'Captain Zero' Nicholas had us off to the local pub, but then Craig Leggett overruled and we were off to the function after all. A compromise was reached: running teams heading off at midnight would leave in small shifts for dinner at the pub where our cooks had been given a free rein! On a full tummy, we were back to the footy

Chapter 14 The XXXX Army Around Australia Relay Marathon

ground for one and a half hours of sleep before a midnight start to another long day.

How much can change in one day! Dawn had arrived as I tried to coax some speed from my sluggish body, and I guess lack of sleep would do that. I then realised that I had been going uphill when the road suddenly became really steep. There were sharp bends and I passed a sign denoting Mt Drummer, from where I had glimpses of the icy waters, where Bass Strait meets the Tasman Sea.

Just after cresting the top of the range, it nearly ended for me. A heavily laden log truck came speeding down from behind us and went straight around the safety vehicle on a blind corner. He immediately cut back in to avoid an oncoming car and I ended up in the deep gutter beside the road. No injuries, but after the run, the safety crew assured me that it had been a close call.

Rather shaken, I continued through the tree fern gullies and spectacular mountain views. While Tammy cruised down the range, we located the kitchen truck in a parking bay by a small stream cascading over the rocks. We joined Team 1 in a leisurely breakfast, while the rest of the relay had gone ahead, and the support crew were making sandwiches and trying to pack up around us.

After tiny Genoa, we stopped for a few photos of our final border crossing and drove north into NSW.

*

All beautiful country, and towns like Eden, Bega, Cobargo and Batemans Bay were duly visited and enjoyed over the next day. The end was getting very close, and with a couple of short days to finish off, not all runners were required. I got a lift up to Nowra where I enjoyed getting to meet my family again. Then we continued up the highway where I had the luxury of a day off at home, as only half the team were used on days ninety-five and ninety-six.

On Sunday, 28 September 1986, all I had to do was drive a few kilometres south from Hurstville to Sylvania and locate Paul Arthur before he completed his leg. All went smoothly as I cruised down the gentle slope, across Tom Uglys Bridge and up the winding concrete highway until at Kogarah, I handed over to another local in Glenn Norris. I had covered my final eight kilometres in 30 mins 50 secs – job done!

We drove into Victoria Barracks for the final rendezvous and awaited Alan Batchelor's arrival on the last relay leg. We walked to the adjacent showgrounds and upon Alan's arrival, we were unleashed on 50,000 fans who were enjoying the rugby league grand final half-time break. On completion of our lap of honour, we lined up on a stage and were individually introduced to the crowd. Handshakes and congratulations came from dignitaries including the Prime Minister, Lieutenant General Peter Gration and Sir Peter Abeles.

Chapter 14 The XXXX Army Around Australia Relay Marathon

Our final run was back off the Sydney Cricket Ground, and the XXXX Army Around Australia Relay Marathon was over.

CHAPTER 15
Orienteering in Norway

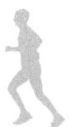

What do you do after being in career-best running form, getting injured and then running around Australia? It's like having two different worlds and you return to the comfortable, non-challenging one. At Hurstville, I returned to being a husband and father to two young children. At Victoria Barracks, I marvelled at the job Michelle had done in keeping the RAP running and settled back into Army Medical Corps work.

As a result of the relay, we all received a Chief of General Staff Commendation for exemplary service. Later in the year, I saw the pecking order for promotion courses, and I had fallen off the perch. It seems my not pursuing the Portsea position far outweighed anything the CGS thought of my abilities. From that point, I decided to position myself for retirement from the Army when I reached twenty years of service. It is worth commenting that I retired five years later at my current rank of

Chapter 15 Orienteering in Norway

Staff Sergeant. Private Michelle Mirfield was by now Corporal M. Wyatt and eight years later was deservedly the highest-ranking enlisted nurse in the Army, as Regimental Sergeant Major of the Royal Australian Army Nursing Corps.

In May 1987, I did a month's training, hoping to be selected in the Great Otway Classic. I was kidding myself and did not get chosen. Late that month, I ran in the NSW Novice Cross-Country Championship over ten kilometres. I have no idea how they choose what a novice is, but I am not sure what amazed me more, running 32 mins 41 secs or only coming fifteenth!

In June, I competed in the ACT/NSW Services Orienteering Championship and finally had a win over a star Engineering Major.

- 1: Greg Wilson, 56 mins 16 secs
- 2: Alan Clarke, 57 mins 18 secs
- 3: Peter Rose, 59 mins 12 secs.

I was training only thirty miles a week when a top Victorian pro runner, Mark Boucher, stayed with us while up to run the City to Surf of fourteen kilometres. Eight years after my first City to Surf, I ran only slightly slower, but this time 47 mins 30 secs only placed me one hundred and twenty-fifth. Mark had a bad day and at halfway, he took his number off and just jogged to the finish. I ran flat out all the way and was amazed to catch him as we approached the finish line.

After that, I ceased all running again and took up riding my road bike forty kilometres a day for the commute to work. My knee must have been bad because riding in Sydney traffic is not for the faint-hearted! Even so, I did two weeks of training and then competed in the NSW (2MD) Inter-Service Championships. Rick Bromley (RAN) ran 16 mins 38 secs, defeating my 16 mins 54 secs in the 5000 metres. In the Masters 1500 metres, I had a win in 4 mins 30 secs.

'Blue' Ingram a teammate from the XXXX Army Around Australia Relay convinced me try to have a go at a triathlon. I told him I was a terrible swimmer but he promised me I would not be last out of the water. I gradually built up my swimming distances until I could cover over a kilometre in the pool. The HMAS *Penguin* Tuff Triathlon was held in May at Ku-ring-gai National Park, on Sydney's northern outskirts. It consisted of 1.2 kilometres of open water swimming, fifty kilometres cycling and ten kilometres running. My swim took 41 mins 54 secs and I was third-last out of the water. I couldn't see without my glasses and zigzagged the whole course as I adjusted my direction. Cycling for 1 hr 51 mins 11 secs saw me pick up eighteen places and I did the fastest run leg of 37 mins 55 secs, passing another eight. Overall, I was twenty-seventh of fifty-three. I never volunteered for another!

At the start of 1989, I received a posting as Wardmaster

Chapter 15 Orienteering in Norway

at the Medical Centre, District Support Unit (DSU) Watsonia in suburban Melbourne. My idea was to be in Victoria so I could plan my future beyond the Army. We were shown a married quarter in the eastern suburb of Scoresby. It was so nice we decided to live there and I would endure the long commute. The only running event I recorded for the whole year was a Melbourne marathon in October. I did two months of light training and managed 2 hrs 48 mins 47 secs. So after sixteen years of running, it seemed I was back at the marathon level I started at in 1973.

We looked around Sandy's hometown of Healesville with a view to building a new home for post-Army life. On a trip up the range to the tiny town of Toolangi, we saw an acre bush block for less than the small town blocks down in the Yarra Valley. We sold our poorly designed Badger Creek house and purchased the Toolangi property. A lot of time was spent up there clearing the block and deciding what we were going to build on it.

A Mornington Peninsula builder had a design we liked, but before we signed up, they said, 'Oh, Toolangi! It will cost much more to build there'. A local builder lived just down the hill from our block. We showed him the plans and asked if he could build it. 'No worries, but ... have you ever considered building in mudbrick?' We looked at a couple he had built, loved them and signed up with Overend Constructions.

In February 1990, during one of my regular weekends up in Toolangi, I ran in the Healesville Fun Run over ten kilometres. The visiting stars of previous editions were absent and it was fought out by the locals. Brian Simmons, who had finished well back in my latest attempt in 1985, was now a fully developed runner. He won a good battle with 33 mins 21 secs to my 33 mins 28 secs.

Three months later, I attended the Australian Services Orienteering Championships (ASOC), my first for a number of years. I had done only three orienteering events in the past three years, had done no training and had a chronic hip injury. Fair to say that I went to Cooma as a member of the 3MD team with low expectations. Yes, it was won by another Engineering major! Where do they keep getting them from?

- 1: Ross Coyle, 2 hrs 22 mins 14 secs
- 2: Bevan Hill (RAN), 2 hrs 45 mins 7 secs
- 3: Greg Wilson, 2 hrs 51 mins 5 secs.

Apart from my surprise third placing, our Victorian (3MD) team won the team event. On the final day, I combined with Bill Gradden, Jeff Rudd and Penny Knott to claim victory in the relay.

Eighteen years earlier when I had my first try at orienteering in the jungle below Mt Stuart in Townsville, I had told Graham Moon, 'Never again'. Now at age thirty-nine and half-fit, I had just won a spot in a team to represent the Australian Defence Force (ADF) at the

World Military Orienteering Championships (CISM). This was the first team to travel overseas since 1975 and I would have been on that trip, except I had decided to get out of the Army. Ironic that I was soon to retire again, but this time I would go out in style – the event would be in northern Norway!

I had taken six months' long service leave on half-pay so I could be involved in assisting with the house build. I returned to full duties so I could participate, with the deal being that team members found their own way over in mid-June and the ADF would arrange our return trip.

The cheapest flight I could find was with Philippines Airlines, and I understood why. On the positive side, I ended up with a trip around the world; on the downside, I saw nothing but airport lounges. Melbourne to Sydney and on to Manila, where we had a long night of stopover in a lounge with broken air-conditioning and limited supplies. Then it was on to Bangkok where I went for a long walk but never got to the end of the huge terminal building. When we landed in Karachi, the plane was surrounded by armed soldiers to prevent anyone from setting foot on the tarmac. On we went to Frankfurt and finally arrived in London. My former Ingleburn Joggers training partner, Glyn Cox, had a cousin in West Dulwich and I had enjoyed a week seeing the sights with Wayne and Frankie.

I was shown around all the inner-city places that tourists travel to see. I also had a day at Sandown races and saw Wimbledon on the way, but it was the wrong time of year for play. One day, I ran west through parkland and saw a bunch of squirrels before having a look at Crystal Palace. Down on the track, champion British track sprinter Linford Christie was being filmed in an advertisement for milk.

The adventure continued with an Air Europe flight from London to Oslo, Norway. We landed alongside Oslo Fjord in cool weather with a steady drizzle from a leaden, cloud-filled sky. Summer in Norway – huh! I decided that I had seen enough cities after a week in London, and besides, it wasn't ideal tourist weather.

While waiting for an 11 pm train departure, I ran into my teammates, Dave Gratwick and Mick Hodge, at Sentralstasjon, Oslo's main railway station. They were burdened with huge packs and passed on some harrowing stories of backpacking around Europe for the last few weeks. Although it was good to catch up with them, I stuck to my original plan while they headed off to Sweden.

The night train from Oslo to Trondheim took nine hours, leaving me with a bare ten minutes to catch my northern connection. Though the outside sky was almost dark, I saw plenty of good, if steep, orienteering country – railway stations, waterfalls, wall-to-wall mountains fjords and tiny mountain villages.

The train almost went on without me when it stopped at Hell – I just had to get a photo! The large port city of

Chapter 15 Orienteering in Norway

Trondheim was asleep, and then it was another ten hours north to where the train line terminated. I stopped for the night at a little town called Fauske where all I noticed was a kilometre hike with my bags to the youth hostel for some badly needed sleep. I saw my first Norwegian TV show; the movie they had on was *A Town Like Alice* with Norwegian subtitles!

The next morning, I boarded a bus for another eight hours north to Narvik, the site of some decisive WWII battles. There was more great scenery during a journey which involved ferry crossings and tunnels a few kilometres long. The weather up north was excellent with clear days of bright sunshine.

Narvik was very scenic, being set on a fjord and surrounded by tall mountains. Winding through them was the city's lifeline, an iron ore train line and terminal for ore shipped from Sweden. All too soon, it was back on the bus for two more hours further north to Bardu in Tromsø Province. During the trip, it was fascinating to see a sign denoting the Arctic Circle.

My destination was one of three military bases which comprise Setemoen and use nearby Bardu township for support and amenities. I had arrived early and stayed at the Bardu Motor Inn for a few days. The town is in a broad valley on a gushing river of the same name and a major road junction. Even in midsummer, it was surrounded by snowcapped peaks. As Bardu is inland, it was only settled in the past 200 years, unlike the ancient coastal settlements frequented by the Vikings.

Once I had settled in, I headed off on a forty-minute run to do some sightseeing. When I was out getting some dinner, I met a group of soldiers who turned out to be liaisons for the visiting orienteering teams. Drawn from the lower, national service ranks of the Army, they all seemed enthusiastic and spoke excellent English. We shared some pizza and chatted for hours in a very noisy disco, which seemed the only night life venue for hundreds of young Norwegian soldiers.

When I headed off to the forest trails for another run, the weather had turned cool and cloudy. Later our team liaison Trond Hermansen collected me for an afternoon drive to Narvik to pick up Dave and Mick. An uneventful drive brought us to a bustling and tourist-infested Narvik, and the train from Sweden duly arrived with my teammates. It seems strange that this city is connected to Sweden by rail, but not to the rest of Norway.

Our team was accommodated at the 10th Heavy Artillery Battalion who had as their unit emblem a wolverine. The reason was that in winter it was one of the few creatures that endured the freezing conditions with them. We settled into our barrack block accommodation and enjoyed the first of many similar dinners: fish and boiled vegetables, with no bread, hot drinks or sweets! After dinner Lieutenant Commander Adrian Wotton

(RAN) and Lieutenant Zoe Read (RAN) arrived after a tour of Scotland and a flight via Bergen and Bardufoss. As the organisers were unaware of any female competitors, Zoe decided to stay at the Bardu Motor Inn in preference to sharing with three males.

As competition time neared, teams from all over Europe and further afield arrived. The Norwegian meal timetable and diet took a bit of adapting to. They enjoyed a huge breakfast of foods we didn't usually partake of at that time of day – fish dishes, salad and brown goat's cheese – but which I soon came to terms with. Somehow, they didn't do lunch, so dinner was eagerly anticipated. I joined many others in sneaking a snack pack out to ensure I made it through to dinner time.

A practice course was set on a map adjacent to the town and we headed out there at midday. The map was titled Leirvassfjellet after the major feature, which was depicted as a multitude of very intricate contour lines. Thankfully, the course was set on the lower slopes and included some areas of green and tracks.

Lulled into a false sense of security by this, I stepped into the bush and was immediately chest-deep in vegetation, climbing on my hands and knees. The course seemed simple but I had problems with every control I attempted. I failed to locate number six and ended up on a large rocky outcrop overlooking a vast forest. At that stage, I decided to abandon and run straight back to the finish to ensure I met our self-imposed two-hour-finish deadline.

Half an hour of solid running had me back in time and I tried to gauge the others' reaction to the area. Although some were loathe to admit it, all had suffered similar disorientation. A major problem had been several new trails and rides that were not marked on the map. Our prospects did not appear to be bright if things continued in this vein. The one consolation was that the forest was lovely and very soft. Dense silver birch, denser ferns and soft soil enveloped one (and the controls also!) but eased the pain of falls from concealed logs and rocks.

Dinner was a Midsummer Day treat of a traditional meal. My anticipation faded as I gazed at a table with thin wafer bread, oily sliced meat and a porridge made from curds. After attempting the traditional fare, I filled up on the only other available food – watermelon and cordial. Roll on, breakfast! The only thing keeping my morale up was Trond's promise that a special menu was in store from tomorrow when the other teams arrived.

Soon after a vehicle arrived and Trond took us on a fifty-minute drive northwards through the forest. We were off to join the locals in their Midsummer Night celebrations, whatever that entailed. After escaping the car park which was full of tourists, we located a nearby table overlooking a waterfall on the Målselva River (Målselvfossen). The evening was spent sampling the local beer, eating grilled laks (salmon) and watching the sun sink towards the horizon. Later, we joined a group of Norwegians in the valley beside the raging rapids and sat around a bonfire singing Beatles ballads.

While we chatted, sang and drank, nearby salmon fishermen were trying to catch breakfast as the sun scooted sideways to the right before beginning to rise again. At 1.30am, we decided to call it a night and headed home. On leaving, our driver noticed a police vehicle and swerved all over the road while attempting to get his seat belt on. After commenting that it was nice he managed to finally get his belt on, the police then breath-tested him. With all that swerving, they must have thought they were on a certainty. Alas, he was all clear and we continued in high spirits back to the barracks and bed at 3.30 am.

We had a late breakfast in an area set aside for the orienteering teams and met the Irish team who had arrived last night. There was a real international feel about the place now most international teams had arrived. At midday, we drove to the Heinvassfjellet map, where we joined the Irish in becoming more familiar with the local terrain. It was very warm and sunny as I covered the course cautiously in reverse order, deliberately avoiding the early controls of yesterday. We had no time limit after deciding we could be out there for a long time completing the fifteen-control course.

I navigated from fifteen to six with very little trouble and then jogged to the finish with Dave Gratwick. We had spent two hours on course, and I didn't want to get too tired. From overheard comments, it seems the Irish team had a lot of trouble with the early controls. Oops! We forgot to tell them about the unmarked track and power lines.

On our arrival back at the unit, we were greeted by Captain Arnold Simpson, Lieutenant Bill Gradden, Major Alan Clarke and our Chief of Delegation, Major John Suominen. They distributed team orienteering suits, leggings and northern hemisphere compasses and then went for a practice run while the rest of us relaxed in the now open CISM Club, formerly the Officers' Mess! I did the right thing and called it a night at 10 pm but then lay awake for three hours. Lack of sleep could pose a problem as the event wore on.

There was an early breakfast next morning and all teams travelled by bus to Svartvatnet which was another local map. No wonder the Scandinavians can orienteer when they only have to walk out the door onto their local maps. Svartvatnet was a large lake and most of the controls were set in a circle around it. Some others were located on a very steep and detailed mountainside. Strictly for the adventurous!

The event was largely a matter of doing your own thing, so I set off through slow, tough terrain, completing seven and a half kilometres and twelve controls in 1 hr

57 mins. I encountered some minor navigation problems and fell, hurting my back; however, my sore knee ligament held together and I was generally happy leading into the first day of competition. The team from the United Arab Emirates seemed to wander around in a confused huddle, so we became confident of defeating them at least. They were overheard asking if there were any trees on the competition map area!

We spent the fine, sunny afternoon resting in preparation for the evening opening ceremony at Barduhallen. The venue consisted of a large hall with an adjacent sporting oval. The various countries were an impressive sight in their respective uniforms as they formed up behind their national flags.

With Trond holding an 'Australia' sign and Arnold nominated as flag-bearer, we marched on and paraded, while speeches, music, dancing and flag raising ceremonies were performed. After some hang-gliders made the descent from the snow-covered summit of nearby Big Alla, we adjourned to the hall for eats and drinks. There was no alcohol which I found commendable, but it led to an early night. When it wound up, I spent some time at the CISM Club before retiring at midnight. Outside the sky was cloudy with an ominous look about it.

*

Day One, 26 June 1990.

I awoke at 6 am to a cool day and pouring rain. A bus trip of one and a quarter hours brought us to the competition area east of Bardufoss, a map titled Råvatn. The rain kept streaming down, so I grabbed a hat, put anti-fog on my glasses and lost all confidence.

On 'Go', I grabbed my map and flew a hundred metres on into a cleared strip. I immediately halted to look at my map and realised I had rushed ninety degrees off course down the wrong clearing. I ran to the right and up a gully, expecting to locate the first control, but it was nowhere to be seen! I searched, then over into the next gully for more searching.

Okay! Run back to the ride to start over again, but still no good. There were others running around looking for it, then suddenly I was out of the gullies and on a steep slope. No one around, no features I could recognise – lost. What a frustrating start to the first day of an event on the other side of the world!

In despair, I went downhill trying to find the start point but I couldn't locate it. Eight hundred metres on, I came out on the main road near the assembly area. Very subdued, I went back into the bush and trudged carefully uphill; once in the control area, I was led to it by teammate Flight Lieutenant Adrian Rowland.

If it had been any other event, I would have gone home.

Chapter 15 Orienteering in Norway

As it was, I faced the daunting task of covering a further nine kilometres and locating twelve controls. I followed Adrian for a couple of controls, letting him do the bulk of the thinking while I tried to recover my composure. I veered right to a parallel error at control four and lost another fifteen minutes while Adrian disappeared.

I managed to navigate solo to the next few controls and caught Adrian Wotton near control eight. After indicating my distressed state to him, I accompanied him on the 1600-metre leg to control nine. On reaching the area, he decided to go to a nearby track to relocate his position. Incapable of making a decision, I just stood in the rain while he disappeared from view.

Sometime later, I did the same thing, and attacking from the track, I found Bill Gradden instead of the control. Bill was also having a few problems and we decided on togetherness for the final few controls. I am not sure how we got to the finish as it was a case of the blind leading the blind! Eventually, we came out beside an elevated bank and on deciding to climb it, we found the finish area.

We had to run back along the bank in full view of the crowded finish area and across the rifle range to get to the final control. We then plugged to the finish. While taking 3 hrs 32 mins 55 secs for nine and a half kilometres was disgraceful, I was too exhausted to care. My only thought was relief at having finished. Later on, seeing the results, I was amazed to see I had still managed to beat three competitors, not counting the Emirates who all failed to finish. In fact, our unofficial competitor, being the lone female Lieutenant Zoe Read, was very popular after finding five of them in a stationary bunch and leading them to the finish.

*

Day Two, 27 June 1990.

Arnold Simpson flew the Australian flag in A Klasse while the rest of us happily settled for the shorter and easier B Klasse. Determined to go slowly and carefully to the first control, I still had problems. I located control two first and retraced my steps back to control one, but at least I had taken only fifteen minutes to retain my title of slowest first leg. The next few controls went carefully to plan before a parallel error at control five had me visiting an A Klasse control and losing twenty minutes.

I ran hard and fast with a Dutchman, passing Adrian Wotton on the long leg to control seven. From there, it went fine as I only lost a couple of minutes on the last seven controls. I was very pleased to have finished off so strongly, but two costly errors were the difference between fifteenth placing and my thirty-sixth of forty-two starters.

Chapter 15 Orienteering in Norway

Adrian Rowland was sixth, only five minutes behind the winner, in 58 mins 30 secs, with Bill Gradden improving to twenty-sixth in 1 hr 13 mins 31 secs. The rest of our team finished in a bunch from thirty-fourth through to thirty-seventh. On day one, we had pledged to never follow any orienteer from Luxemburg, a sound decision as they finished in a block behind us. The United Arab Emirates were sent out in two non-competitive groups for a walk in the forest!

Meanwhile the Scandinavians and Swiss were dominating A Klasse. Arnold Simpson finished an admirable forty-third position. While he was not satisfied with his performance, the rest of us thought he did well just finishing the difficult twelve-kilometre course.

Just in case we were not exhausted, we completed the day with a two-hour bus trip to Senja Island, not far south of the provincial capital of Tromsø. It was cold and windy, with sleety rain detracting from any sightseeing enjoyment. The island is joined to the mainland by a two-kilometre bridge. Our route took us over a steep snow-covered pass, through a two-kilometre tunnel onto a winding road alongside isolated fjords. Eventually we halted at a tiny remote fishing village where we enjoyed an evening of feasting. There was plenty of singing and dancing with the few local residents. The highlight of the trip was intended to be watching the midsummer sun almost set; however, that was thwarted by heavy cloud cover. I was too tired to enjoy the festivities and was happy to crawl into bed back at the barracks at 3.30am.

We enjoyed a rest day, and that's exactly what I did, except for a sight-seeing flight in a Piper Bear Cub. The pilot threw in a few light aerobatics, which had me asking to be taken back slow and steady and be placed on *terra firma*.

*

Day Three, 29 June 1990.

It was time for the relays and one last chance to pull out a satisfying result. Australia had an A team of Captain Arnold Simpson, Flight Lieutenant Adrian Rowland and Major Alan Clarke. The B team consisted of Lieutenant Bill Gradden, Lieutenant Commander Adrian Wotton and Staff Sergeant Greg Wilson. Our standing in the competition was emphasised by the fact that the winning Finnish team had already crossed the line for victory before the final runner of our A team set off. That being said, they still managed eighteenth place of twenty-nine teams.

- Leg 1: Adrian Rowland, 1 hr 9 mins 54 secs
- Leg 2: Alan Clarke, 1 hr 25 mins 53 secs
- Leg 3: Arnold Simpson, 1 hr 1 mins 25 secs.

Shortly before my start time, Mick Hodge settled any

Chapter 15 Orienteering in Norway

nerves by informing me that our RAAF plane for the flight home had blown an engine and was stranded in Washington. This, combined with the fact that I was last runner to set out (by twenty-six minutes), did little to create enthusiasm.

I ran solidly to the first control, knowing there was a track to pull me up. When I missed the control, I searched left instead of right and lost a couple of minutes. (I seem to have this thing about first controls.)

With number one out of the way, I settled into solid running and (for me) accurate navigation. I lost another minute or two but imagine my surprise when at control eleven, I caught up with another competitor. He was from Luxembourg, of course, and now I had a race on my hands. He left the control just ahead of me and ran directly through the scrub. I took a punt and detoured twice as far around through a cleared ride. I ran hard and was pleased to see him still approaching as I left control twelve.

There was one control to go. Running flat out, I stumbled into a lake. Too disoriented to look at my map and detour around it, I waded on through and reached the control just as my opponent was punching his card. With 300 metres to go, I sprinted for home, but nearly fell on the final tight bend and failed to catch him by two seconds. I felt I had done a good job of holding last place of the teams that completed the course.

The time I recorded saw me finish as the third-fastest Australian behind Arnold and Adrian. I was pleased to finally achieve a worthwhile result, but Bill Gradden was wandering around mumbling about 'blokes that can only perform well in relays'. I think he could recall me doing something similar at our last ASOC (Military Championships). The French and Dutch no.1 teams, and of course the United Arab Emirates, failed to finish after punching wrong controls.

The competition spirit was epitomised by the last two placegetters sprinting flat out, only two seconds apart. We didn't care that the winning team had finished more than two hours earlier, as we held each other up celebrating our rearward placings.

- Leg 1: Bill Gradden, 1 hr 33 mins 8 secs
- Leg 2: Adrian Wotton: 1 hr 43 mins 33 secs
- Leg 3: Greg Wilson: 1 hr 20 mins 16 secs.

There was a formal dinner on our final night and the main course was three servings of *finnbiff*. This turned out to be delicious, but it was three courses of Bambi!

*

We received word that we had to get back to London urgently to catch the next RAAF 'milk run'. The British came to our aid and gave us a lift in an RAF Andover to their base in Hanover, Germany. There we were accommodated overnight while being warned not to go out on the town. In view of recent IRA terrorism, they were concerned we may be mistaken for British servicemen and come to some harm. The locals were not paying much attention as Germany were playing in a football World Cup semi-final that evening.

The next morning, we had a spin down the autobahn on a bus to coastal Hamburg, from where we flew to England, landing in the village of Brize Norton. We stayed the night, and I enjoyed my first stroll around a pretty English village. The next morning, it was back through London and south to Gatwick airport where we finally boarded our RAAF flight back to Australia. I did mention earlier a trip around the world!

As the RAAF use the same crew for the complete trip, they have to have stopovers and make duty calls along the way. Our first leg took us across the Atlantic and when we landed at Washington, we were told to amuse ourselves for a couple of days.

One of the others had a hire car and was heading north, so I got a lift up to Gettysburg, Pennsylvania. There I had a great time catching up with a couple of our close friends from the mid-1970s in Townsville. Jim and Patsy Hartnett had both been American exchange teachers and had returned to settle in Gettysburg. It was great to catch up and meet their teenage children. On the first day, Jim took me to a small local fun run at Waynesboro and I had a win. Jim was now a cyclist and had a training ride arranged for the next day, which happened to be 4 July. He told me about another fun run and having given me directions, threw me his car keys and said, 'Stay on the correct side of the road!'

I managed to travel interstate, leaving Pennsylvania and passing through the Blue Ridge Mountains to Fort Ritchie in Maryland. The event was held from a military base, and being Independence Day, there was plenty going on. They were surprised to have an Aussie soldier competing and I came away with the first veteran (over thirty-five, that is) trophy.

All too soon, it was goodbye to this lovely green part of the east coast and back on our plane odyssey. The next leg was right across the US to San Francisco, where there was a good view of the Golden Gate Bridge as we landed to refuel. On we went and, oh, bother, we had to overnight again – in Hawaii. I got to have a look around the world's largest shopping centre, lazed around Waikiki Beach and went out for a close-up of the volcano. Another long haul over the Pacific and we touched down at Richmond, to the west of Sydney.

CHAPTER 16
Ultramarathons

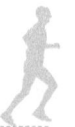

Following this delightful interlude, I resumed my leave and spent a lot of time camping out in the new home in Toolangi. Chris Overend had constructed a lovely three-level mudbrick home which stepped down the sloping block. Unlike our first house, this one was correctly oriented to take full advantage of the sun and the view. It also had a lot of timber on the deck and a wraparound solar pergola. Much of my time in the latter half of 1990 was spent painting the house.

We moved in the next year, as the house was livable but with a number of finishing-off tasks still required. We had it built to lock-up stage plus plastering and carpets, but the rest was up to us. Sandy and the kids moved there in time for them to begin the new school year, just down the hill at tiny Toolangi Primary School. Sandy obtained a shop assistant position at the only shop in town, the Toolangi General Store.

It should have been simple for me also – resume full-time duty at Watsonia for nine months and then take my discharge from the Army, having served for twenty years. However, there was a twist in the tale as they decided to re-post me to the RAP at Broadmeadows. This was just a bit further than I was happy to commute to on a daily basis. I opted to live in at Broadmeadows Sergeants' Mess during the week and then spend weekends at home.

In January, I decided to start back with a bit of running training. Week one was thirty-one miles and week two was seventy-two miles. Then after a week off tired and sore, I, for some unknown reason, decided to run in my first ultramarathon. I suspect that star veteran athlete Dot Browne may have mentioned it at a mid-week Croydon Veterans' Athletics Club meeting, as she was a prime mover in Victorian ultra running at that time. The event was the first edition of the Mansfield to Mt Buller 50 kilometres. As you may deduce from the name, there is a hill in the latter stages.

I was well aware that I wasn't fit for the event, so when the leaders tore off at a frantic pace, I took it cautiously. I didn't see the placegetters again and after the finish, I realised the reason. First over the line was an English star called Carl Barker (3 hr 53 mins), who set a race record that would stand for years. Second was Bruce Cook from Queensland (3 hr 59 mins), an Australian ultra record holder. Anton Oberscheider from Victoria (4 hr 7 mins) at third was, like myself, a sub-2:30 marathoner. So my fourth placing (4 hr 14 mins) was against some stiff competition.

The ascent from Mirimbah to the peak is steep and around sixteen kilometres long, with a kilometre scramble over rocks to a cairn before running back down to the village. As I neared the top, a spectator called out, 'Well done, second place. Only one has been up here before you!' Make of that what you will. It was an interesting debut, to say the least.

A month later, I took it to the other extreme and joined Brian Simmons on a trip to Canberra for my first Australian Veterans' Athletics Championship. It was poor timing as I was right at the top of my M35 age group. My results were: 1500 metres, sixth in 4 mins 29 secs; 5000 metres, sixth in 16 mins 25 secs. On the way back, we called in at Nowa Nowa and I came third in their fourteen-kilometre King of the Mountains (54 mins 30 secs).

A couple of months later, I made my final trip to the Australian Defence Force Orienteering Championships. They were held at Camp Cable in the hinterland of Queensland's Gold Coast. Four years earlier, I had become lost trying to locate the venue, so just competing would be an improvement. I had competed in these events on five occasions for three minor placings, and every time they were won by an Engineering major.

My orienteering experience, that began twenty years

earlier in the jungle below Mt Stuart on a course set by Major Graham Moon RAE, ended in the jungle of Camp Cable with the event won by Major Ross Coyle RAE. The minor placings went to John Bizjak (RAN) and Adrian Rowland (RAAF). I was pleased to finish at age thirty-nine with fourth place. Need I say that I did better still in the relay. In a fitting finale, I was a member of the victorious team representing the Army and managed second-fastest time for the course.

As I was commuting and spending time at Broadmeadows as well as finalising the house build, there was little running. I did have a reunion with some Around Australia Relay mates when I combined with Rob Combe, Ernie Stewart, 'Blue' Ingram and Pat Thomas in the Lake Relay.

Toolangi Primary School wanted to hold a fun run and I volunteered to design a local course for them. There was a four-kilometre race straight up past my home, looping down to finish off along Messmate Forest Walk. The ten-kilometre race had a larger initial loop and a steep climb before descending and returning along the same forest path. In what would become a tradition, one of my running friends would come up and win it. On this first occasion, it was Captain Rolf Zimmerman who relegated me to runner-up.

In September, I retired from the Army and enquired about becoming an ambulance officer. I could hardly

Chapter 16   Ultramarathons

believe it when they said that I was too old and they would have to completely retrain me. Rather than argue the point, I took on board that it would mean working down in the suburbs, and this wasn't why we had moved to Toolangi.

The local strawberry co-op was run by George Weda who just happened to have been one of the Army patients I cared for back in my first posting at 4 Camp Hospital, Townsville. On enquiring about employment, I don't think he even got back to me. I walked down the road two kilometres from home to the Alex Demby Timber Company and said, 'Give me a job.' The owner-manager Gary Demby said, 'Okay, start Monday.'

It was far from my ideal job, but it did have some advantages. It was so close to home I could go home for lunch and the work was physically demanding which no doubt kept me a bit fit. They started me on the 'green chain', one of the heaviest jobs at the sawmill. For the first few years, that was okay; I had to stack 'house lots' of timber, which kept the brain working as well.

I must have managed enough training because on Australia Day in 1992, I was back on the start line at Mansfield, preparing for a second attempt at the fifty kilometres up Mt Buller. Keith Fisher took it out solidly, but with consistent twenty-one to twenty-two-minute 5 kms, I had reeled him in by the start of the climb at Mirimbah. I reached the thirty-kilometre mark ten minutes ahead of my debut last year. A strong run up the mountain saw me clear out to win by twenty-five minutes from Graham Alford and Keith Fisher. My time of 3 hrs 57 mins 25 secs was an improvement of 17 minutes and made me one of an elite group to have broken four hours on this course.

Now that we had settled in as Toolangi residents, I resumed running training, but it was a balancing act. The main difference was that I now recorded kilometres in my training log, as it made it appear that I was doing more than when using miles. After working physically hard all day, it was often an effort to drag my protesting body out for more exercise. There were also continuing problems, particularly with my left knee, if I did too much.

A month later, I ran my first Coburg 24-Hour track event. There was a top field of twenty-nine, with a third of them from interstate and Neville Mercer from New Zealand. The number two-ranked Australian, David Standeven, and champion female Helen Stanger headed the field, but all the media had turned up to see Cliffy. Cliff Young had just turned seventy and was attempting to break the M70 world age best of 173 kilometres.

It was very hot, with the temperature on the black rubber/bitumen surface recorded at fifty-five degrees. After the first four hours, I was in unknown territory for the next twenty hours. In the first twelve hours, I covered 122 kilometres and strained my groin. The second half was pretty much a walk as I added another fifty-nine kilometres. I went from second place at halfway to finish sixth, having run 181.419 kilometres – but I did finish!

Due to the conditions, there was an adverse effect on performances and several withdrawals during the event. David Standeven won from Peter Gray, and Helen Stanger put in a remarkable effort for fourth. Cliffy was unable to do it on the day and achieved 153 kilometres.

How things have changed since 1971 when Trevor Newton was a Queensland hero for running a hundred miles in twenty-four hours. Twenty years later, I run a hundred miles in 19 hrs 43 mins 18 secs, and it is my worst ultra performance.

I did a full season of professional cross-country with the VCCL and was running well again – for a forty-year-old. By September, the regular racing had me in contention and I ran my best eight kilometres for sixteen years (26 mins 35 secs). A week later, I ran my best half-marathon for thirteen years (74 mins 19 secs).

Another week on and the conditions were perfect for me at Jells Park where my training partner Brian Simmons had sponsored the race. It was hilly, cold and raining, and that combined to slow the faster runners enough for me to have a handicap win over eight kilometres (26 mins 55 secs). Mid-week, I journeyed down to join Brian in an RACV team competing in the Lake Relay, which was now open to civilian corporate teams. It was now a full five kilometres and teams of five runners each had to do three laps. Mine were 16:38, 16:58 and 16:55 and we finished in second place, beaten by three minutes by National Mutual.

I was managing 200 to 300 kilometres per month and in October, my results were satisfying. My fastest six and a half kilometres for the season (21 mins 33 secs) was followed a day later by my second marathon since 1984. In the People's Marathon, I finished twelfth in 2 hrs 48 mins 16 secs. A fortnight later, it was time for the local derby, the Toolangi Fun Run.

Back in the late '70s in Sydney, I ran well in a tough 33.4-kilometre race at Warragamba, where way back was a teenager named Bruce Graham. He went on to become one of Australia's top orienteers and a fine runner. On my hilly Toolangi course of bitumen, dirt and trails, Bruce ran a superb 32 mins 25 secs for a hollow victory. I played to my strengths and did the seventh kilometre up a really steep hill in 3 mins 46 secs which allowed me to get a break on Brian, which I held for second place. My Veteran record of 34 mins 5 secs was a minute faster than I had done on flat courses with the pros and a rare victory over Brian by ten seconds.

I followed up with another attempt at a track ultra, the Australian Ultra Runners' Association (AURA) Six-Hour Track Race. There were twenty-two starters which included the event record holder, Jeff Smith (77.083

kilometres). Opting for a conservative start, my thirty-three laps in the first hour had me back in sixth position. I moved through to fourth at the halfway mark and although well in front, the leading trio were no longer increasing their lead. During the fourth hour, Ian Clarke collapsed on the infield with cramps in both calves. The other leaders were slowing and for the first time, I was pulling them back.

With one and a half hours to go, I hit the front as Jeff Smith dropped off the pace and Tony Dietachmayer had to take longer walking breaks. When six hours had elapsed, I had totalled 78.426 kilometres and set an event record. For a few short days, it was thought to be an Australian record but no sooner had they claimed that when a few other performances came out of left field. Apparently, Trevor Jacobs of Canberra had run further and then Yiannis Kouros put up his hand. He had also run faster and then gone on to run at that pace for a full twenty-four hours. Game, set and match to Yiannis!

Well, that did it for the year and most of 1993 as well. My left knee was a crunching mess again and rest was the only option. In March, I ran in the Healesville fun run and on no training came second (35 mins 21 secs) while also scooping up first local and first over-40. In May, I managed second in the M40-44 division of the Victorian Veterans ten-kilometre Championship (37 mins 34 secs). A bit of training saw an improvement when I was narrowly beaten by Ross Martin for first Veteran (35 mins 40 secs). They were not my best runs; they were the only ones, as I had to stop again with pain in both knees and my left big toe.

During the winter, Brian and Christine Simmons combined with Sandy, myself and a couple of others to form a team for the Toolangi Tennis Club. Sandy is the local star tennis player and Brian is talented at whatever sport he attempts. Christine was capable and I, well, I filled up my corner of the court. Like orienteering, I was fast but erratic. Anyway, we had fun and ended up winning the grand final.

So in September, we won at tennis and Essendon won the Aussie Rules Grand Final. Inspired by this and a week off work, I decided to attempt some training again. I managed four weeks of about a hundred kilometres while trying to ignore pain in both knees. On this background, I again fronted up for the AURA Six-Hour Track Race. For some strange reason, I also entered the Australian Six-Day Race later in the year at Colac.

The Six-Hour seemed pretty good at the start, as Keith Alexander led the first hour at record pace with fourteen kilometres, from Brian Simmons who was making his ultra running debut. Superstar Lavinia Petrie was in third from myself, being a bit conservative due to my lack of preparation. During the second hour, the dark clouds came over and rain belted down, flooding the track.

Chapter 16 Ultramarathons

By the halfway point, Brian had moved into the lead and that's when the 'cyclone' hit. Storm force winds and driving rain flattened tents, destroyed the leader board and sent sandy grit over everybody. Runners were blown out into lane three on entering the straight and reduced to an angled walk, trying to make headway against the wind. Lane one was now two inches deep with water as runners sloshed through it. The worst conditions I have ever experienced by far!

While all this was happening, Lavinia still managed somehow to break the Australian record for thirty miles by 1 min 13 secs and promptly retired from the event. An hour later, the track was steaming in bright sunshine as helpers tried to coax floodwaters off the track. At the four-hour mark, Keith Alexander started to fade and I moved into second place behind Brian. Apparently, Dot was supplying a feast of pancakes, honey, strawberry jam and ice cream, with some competitors stopping to partake.

Not for Brian and me, though, as we pushed our depleted bodies through another two hours of suffering. The latter stages were tough with the pair of us staging a run-walk-cramp battle to the finish. In the end, I got it done, perhaps due to my more cautious pace in the early stages. It was nowhere near last year's distance but probably a better performance in the terrible conditions.

- 1: Greg Wilson, 74.19 kilometres
- 2: Brian Simmons, 72.29 kilometres

- 3: Keith Alexander, 70.28 kilometres.

Brian had surpassed my times in all distances from 800 metres through to the marathon, where he ran sub-2.30 and represented Australia. He chose a very tough day for his first ultramarathon.

I cannot explain why I entered the Australian Six-Day Race at Colac, when I knew I was unfit for it. Anyway, in November I went and I am glad I was able to participate in this historic event and soak up the atmosphere of that park in the centre of Colac. I ran 150 kilometres in twenty-one hours; then while having a shower break, I had a think about whether I would be able to run the next day. The answer was no, and if that was the case, I may as well be back at work. To my regret, that was it for my multi-day ultra career.

Two weeks later, I had recovered well enough to place third in the Toolangi Fun Run in 36 mins 36 secs. Meanwhile, two stars were having a great battle out front. Bruce Graham (34 mins 29 secs) won again after a close battle with Brian Simmons (34 mins 56 secs).

I was having trouble with right-side sciatica and it was only when I commenced Christmas leave that I started training again. From a fifty-eight-kilometre week at the end of December, I went straight to over a hundred kilometres for a couple of weeks. Then just after I recommenced work in early 1995 and was feeling flat and tired on a Friday evening, I received a phone call. It

Chapter 16 Ultramarathons

was a bloke called Tony Collins ringing from New South Wales wanting to know if I would like to enter his twelve-hour ultramarathon which started on Saturday evening. After a year of inadequate training and fresh off pulling out of the Six-Day at Colac, the last thing I felt like doing was driving interstate for an ultramarathon.

I explained this to Tony, but he insisted I would be fine and mentioned that he had a novel incentive scheme. The winner would receive a prize of $3 per kilometre, second $2 per kilometre and third $1 per kilometre. I finished up saying I would think about it and hung up. The trouble was that it was due to start in less than twenty-four hours at Wyong, north of Sydney, and I was in my lounge at Toolangi. There was not much time left for thinking!

An hour later, I set off in my old work car and drove nine hours up to Ingleburn. There I handed over driving to my old Ingleburn jogger friend Bob McMurdo, who was happy to crew for me. A couple of hours later, we found the venue, a deserted football field at a dot on the map called Tacoma, near Tuggerah Lake. I hadn't given any thought to the fact that I had driven all night and was now going to have to stay up and run all night. I flopped down on a sleeping bag and awaited developments while hoping to recharge my batteries.

As afternoon rolled into evening, runners and officials began to arrive. I had no idea of the field, as no doubt

Tony hadn't wanted to dissuade me from making the trip. Australia's best home-grown male runner Bryan Smith (world rank third, 1993) and champion female Helen Stanger were a handy pair to start with!

Trans-American athlete Pat Farmer led the field at an ambitious pace and after four hours, the early leaders started to fade. Bryan Smith took the lead, and I followed through into second place. I led the field briefly during the night but with three hours remaining, I was three laps behind Bryan. The rest of the field was quite a way back, so I decided on 'death or glory' and went into attack mode.

In a short time, I had taken back a lap and headed off to pull back another. However, the title champion is not lightly bestowed and Bryan saw to it that I got no closer. I did pay for my aggression by losing a few more laps before the finish, but you never know unless you try.

- 1: Bryan Smith, 131.111 kilometres
- 2: Greg Wilson, 128.858 kilometres
- 3: Bob Channells, 120.946 kilometres
- 4: Helen Stanger, (117.069 kilometres), first female by twenty-three kilometres!

Cliff Young beat half the field, recording 88.429 kilometres.

During the long drive home, I had plenty of time to reflect on what might have been if I had more notice to prepare. I don't think a long drive and no sleep contributed to a top performance. I also had to accept that my dramatic acceleration and then not being able to sustain it may have cost me a 130-kilometre total. In any case, I regard this defeat as my best ultramarathon performance, and it ranked among the best that had been done by an Australian.

With my lack of training, you can imagine how my legs felt during the following week. Five days later, I managed a four-kilometre hobble around the Messmate loop. Then at 4.30 am on Sunday, I made the ridiculous decision to drive to Mansfield for the annual challenge of Mt Buller. To compound matters, I only just made it to the start in time.

Kelvin Marshall set a strong early pace. When I got the legs warmed up, I moved to within a couple of minutes after twenty kilometres. Ian Clarke and Keith Alexander lost contact when I made a move to be with Kelvin at the base of the climb. At Mirimbah, I went past and hoped my hill climb skills would see me through. It was a near thing as Ian Clarke closed to 150 metres but then faded. On the way back down from the cairn, I could see my nearest pursuer and knew I was safe.

My winning time of 4 hrs 7 mins 37 secs was ten minutes slower than in 1992, but how can you measure the merit of a win a week after a twelve-hour race? I had still not been passed by anyone up the mountain. Bob Harlow (4 hrs 12 mins 49 secs) came through the field from well back for second, with Ian Clarke third (4 hrs 16 mins 25 secs). I was surprised and pleased to get away with that one.

I had a month off to recover and then in March 1996 after three weeks of a hundred kilometres, I travelled to Wollongong for my second attempt at a 24-hour. My reasonable assumption was that I should be able to achieve 200 kilometres, but again it was not to be. In an action repeat of Coburg, I cruised through the first twelve hours amassing 119 kilometres but my second half was only seventy kilometres. This time, my blood sugar went awry and I couldn't run in a straight line. My hands and lower legs swelled with oedema. After some advice from Helen Stanger, I took a few hours' rest and ate some carbohydrates that enabled me to plod on to the finish. My total of 188.9 kilometres for sixth was an improvement, but I knew I should be capable of more.

There were some great results, with visiting Russian Gennady Groshev (229.617 kilometres) defeating Bryan Smith (222.294 kilometres). A fantastic run by Helen Stanger saw her third overall and, in the process, set four female ultramarathon records: 100 kilometres in 9 hrs 6 mins 40 secs; 200 kilometres in 22 hrs 16 mins 35 secs; 125.16 kilometres in twelve hours and 213.494 kilometres in twenty-four hours.

I had plenty of time for thinking as we continued north for a visit with old Townsville friends, the Clitheroes, who now resided on the Gold Coast. I felt the oedema would be due to either heart or kidney problems, because of the stress I was putting my body under. I knew I should be up there near Helen Stanger, but it wasn't worth dying for. I decided that in future I would stick to what I knew was safe and achievable at lesser distances.

I had just narrowly surpassed my largest monthly running total with 526 kilometres, but perhaps it is cheating to do 190 kilometres in one run. I did very little up at Ray and Judy's Burleigh Waters home except lie around and complain about how much my legs hurt. After a week, we returned via Newcastle and Ingleburn where we visited the Cox and McMurdo families. After about ten days, I was able to gingerly hobble a few kilometres.

Continuing south, I turned off the Hume Highway and headed to Canberra. Sandy wondered if I had discovered one of my renowned shortcuts, but no, I sheepishly admitted that there was a race to attend. The Australian 50km Championship would be my first race of that length that didn't have Mt Buller awaiting at the end of it. The course was a complete Canberra Marathon and then keep going out and back for the extra eight kilometres.

There were plenty of highlights to report. It was the first time that the visiting Russians had tasted defeat in Australia. In his defence, Gennady Groshev was leading clearly at the forty-six kilometre point but was unable to read in English the 'Turn Around' sign and just kept on running. By the time he realised his error, Kent Williams, using his local knowledge, had taken the lead.

- 1: Kent Williams (ACT), 3 hrs 16 mins 45 secs
- 2: Gennady Groshev (Russia), 3 hrs 19 mins, 11 secs
- 3: Peter Fitzpatrick (NSW) 3 hrs 24 mins 4 secs.

Bob Harlow, who had been behind me up Mt Buller, came fourth (3 hrs 25 mins 41 secs) and was placed in the Australian Championship. Four minutes back, a close battle played out as Igor Streltzov (Russia) at 3 hrs 29 mins 31 secs held me off (3 hrs 29 mins 47 secs). This was the only flat road fifty-kilometre race I ran while fit and remains a career PB. I can't help but wonder what it may have been had I not destroyed myself in a 24-hour so recently.

The other huge story was the performance of Lavinia Petrie, at age fifty, finishing tenth, first female by almost nine minutes. As she passed through the marathon in 3 hrs 8 mins 3 secs, Lavinia won the Australian Veterans Marathon Championship and set a W50 Australian record. By continuing on to fifty kilometres in 3 hrs 41 mins 56 secs, she smashed the female course record by 12 mins 17 secs and set an Australian road fifty-kilometre record. Lavinia also broke the world best time for a female over fifty by an amazing 30 mins 4 secs.

Needless to say, I was a cot case afterwards, with a very painful left knee and thigh. Still, after a week off, I fronted up at Coburg 24-Hour and hobbled

Chapter 16   Ultramarathons

twenty-two kilometres in two hours before retiring hurt. Igor Streltzov won the event with 221 kilometres. I pretty much retired from training and racing, unless something of special interest came up.

Six months later, after a month of thirty kilometres per week, I ran in the Toolangi Fun Run 10 Kilometre and managed 36 mins 14 secs on the hilly course (fourth, and first over-40). I played some poor tennis for Toolangi and joined the Army Reserve (ARES) as a paid replacement activity. At this stage, I was down to twenty kilometres per week, if I felt like it, and they decided to hold the Victorian Mountain Running Championship up nearby Mt St Leonard. It was only eight kilometres away from home, so what the hell, may as well run in it! The event involved running thirteen kilometres from Healesville to the top of Mt St Leonard, an ascent of 1000 metres.

- 1: Robin Rishworth, 59 hrs 40 secs
- 2: Greg Mandile, time unknown
- 3: Nigel Aylott, time unknown
- 4: Greg Wilson, 72 hrs 30 mins, first Veteran.

A few months went by when, out of the blue, my phone rang. Geoff Hook, President of Australian Ultra Runners Association (AURA), was holding something called the AURA Dam Trail 50 Kilometres. It was in three weeks and would happen in my backyard, the Great Dividing Range above Healesville, 'so it would be nice if you ran'.

Training: week one, fifty kilometres; week two, seventy

kilometres; week three, ninety kilometres; week four, nil (injured). The day before, I did my four-kilometre loop pain-free and so I fronted the start line at Fernshaw with nine others. To quote Kevin Cassidy, who quoted American President Franklin D. Roosevelt after the Pearl Harbor attack, this was 'a day that will live in infamy'. Make what you like of the results as they were of little relevance.

The course was incorrectly marked, causing us to run extra kilometres along a trail called the Maroondah Highway before we reached the twenty-kilometre aid station at Dom Dom Saddle. Had we known what was in store, we might well have remained there. Everyone except the leader, Safet Badic, was directed on to an incorrect route.

Brian Simmons and Kelvin Marshall had raced away in pursuit of Safet, except he was running up to Mt Monda and they were running back down to the start. Clive Davies and I both realised after a kilometre downhill that we should be going *up* Mt Monda. We ran into the pursuing Ian Clarke and advised him to about turn. Then to our surprise, we ran smack into Safet Badic who had been correct until he asked a park ranger how to get to Maroondah Dam. We turned him around again and that is the last we saw of him until the finish.

Just over halfway, I was reduced to a walk in second place, although in hindsight it was up Mt Monda. Clive Davies ran past strongly and Ian Clarke passed me in my

Chapter 16 Ultramarathons

wife's car, as he had given it up as a bad joke. Halfway up Mt St Leonard, Geoff Hook was there asking if anybody had seen Safet, as he had not been seen at course checkpoints. Over the top with no one in sight, I spotted Clive on his way down. Thinking I might be in front, I ran past Clive and headed for the finish. There was a big hill from Donnellys Weir back up to the dam wall, and it was there my lack of fitness told.

Mine was the first time logged at the top of St Leonard, so perhaps Clive skirted the top, and who knows what Safet did! It was alleged that he was seen in a car out on Myers Creek Road, heading for the finish. There was a presentation and soon after, exhausted and confused, I jumped in the car and headed home back up the same road. Halfway up, who should I spot running down towards me but Kelvin Marshall who had been three minutes in front of me after twenty kilometres and was now an hour behind. I offered him a lift to the finish but he was determined to get there on foot, even going the long way on the bitumen.

I record all this detail because this was the first Dam Trail 50 Kilometre and now, over twenty-five years later, it has grown into a major trail race, the Maroondah Trail 50 Kilometre and attracts a large field. Although Kelvin may have run an extra fifteen kilometres or so, it was important he finished, as he is the only person to have completed all of them until recently!

1: Safet Badic, 4 hrs 42 mins 40 secs
2: Clive Davies, 5 hrs 3 mins 30 secs
3: Greg Wilson, 5 hrs 5 mins 12 secs
4: Brian Simmons and Kevin Cassidy, 6 hrs 40 mins 40 secs.

Brian and Kevin had been thirty minutes apart at twenty kilometres with me in between. I never saw them again, and they somehow finished together. We didn't ask them where and how because they had no idea. Kelvin was a minute behind them after his road trip. What a marvellous experience!

After I recovered, I trained on for a couple of weeks, but it petered out when I became injured again. Out of the blue, Leigh Privett from Albury rang wanting accommodation for the touring Russian ultra runners for the night before the Coburg 24-Hour. So Gennardy and Igor stayed with us and I went down to the event with them. I had no intention of finishing but did one hundred kilometres in 10 hrs 30 mins and then pulled up stumps and went home. I mention this event only because it is the day that world ultra champion, Yiannis Kouros, broke the Australasian record with 282.981 kilometres.

Five months later on minimal training, I placed third (36 mins 24 secs) in the Toolangi Fun Run behind two top runners, perennial winner Bruce Graham (32 mins 30 mins) and my workmate Brian Simmons (35 mins 46 secs). I could get away with ten kilometres, but when

World Rogaining Champion Nigel Aylott rang wanting a partner for an event the next week, I should have said no. I told him how unfit I was, but it was in the Murrindindi State Forest, just up the hill from home and he wouldn't take no for an answer. Oh, did I mention it was a twelve-hour rogaine, running flat out all night trying to navigate through the bush? Nigel did all the navigation and as a team must finish together, I slowed him down in the second half, but, yes, we came first.

In twelve months from August 1995 to August 1996, I trained a total of 180 kilometres, most of it in two weeks of the latter month in response to another phone call from Geoff Hook. The result was left knee pain again. After a week off and a couple of jogs, I ran in the Victorian Veterans 10 Kilometre Road Championship.

1: Brian Simmons, 33 hrs 41 mins
2: Russell Johnson, 35 hrs, 18 mins
3: Greg Wilson, 35 hrs 32 mins.

The upshot was a strain to the right hamstring to balance out the knee pain.

This mini comeback was due to Geoff wanting a full Victorian team of three finishers for the first Athletics Australia 100 Kilometre Championship at Shepparton in Victoria. He had Yiannis Kouros and Safet Badic, which was a great start, and so I and Michael Grayling registered to make up the numbers. The big problem for me was that in September, coming off almost nothing,

I managed eight training runs, with the longest being twenty-two kilometres. I was going to have to be very careful to make it to the finish.

For some reason I decided I could run each five-kilometre lap in 25 mins 30 secs and be sure of completing the course. That was my plan, based on nothing, and I stuck to it all the way, even though it meant putting ego aside and being back beyond midfield early. Way out in front, Yiannis had a close battle with teammate Safet Badic, until the latter quit the race at halfway. Our team's winning chances suddenly dropped immeasurably as there were three Queenslanders in front of Michael and I. One of the Queensland team was Tony Kleiner, a fellow member of the XXXX Army Around Australia Relay, ten years earlier.

After halfway, Yiannis just kept lapping at an amazing 19 mins 30 secs per five kilometres and was soon a lap in front of the field. Peter Spehr and Mick Francis came through strongly as two of the Queensland team paid the price for their early heroics. When Yiannis breasted the finish line, he had run a world class 6 hrs 56 mins 46 secs and was fifty minutes clear of Peter Spehr. Mick Francis was next over the line but was ineligible for a championship place as he had not registered with Athletics Australia.

I was between the Queenslanders, and we were all in before nine hours had elapsed. The Team Gold medal was now all on the shoulders of Michael Grayling, who gamely battled on to finish fifty-six minutes after the last Queenslander. The calculators came out and the Australian Championship result was:

Teams:
1: Victoria, 25 hrs 2 mins 31 secs
2: Queensland, 25 hrs 38 mins 5 secs
3: New South Wales, 27 hrs 19 mins 25 secs.

Individual:
1: Yiannis Kouros (Vic), 6 hrs 56 mins 46 secs
2: Peter Spehr (NSW), 7 hrs 36 mins 14 secs
3: Mick Francis (WA), 7 hrs 52 mins 56 secs, was ineligible
3: Asim Mesalic (Qld), 7 hrs 57 mins 31 secs.

My fourth place in 8 hrs 17 mins 34 secs is an achievement I am proud of, and as I did no other 100-kilometre events, it remains my career PB. The reason for the pride is not that it was in any way an outstanding result. I understood how limited I was by lack of training, so I planned and ran accordingly and achieved the aim without any distress. Yes, I could have gone faster, but the risk of having to pull out was overriding.

It's ironic that twenty-three years after turning professional, as I was not up to national class in the amateurs, I had won an Athletics Australia Championship Gold Medal (Team). It was a joy to share a team victory with the greatest ultramarathon athlete the world has seen and I am sure Michael Grayling feels the same. That was a fitting end to my ultramarathon career.

At one of my regular low-key Tuesday evening meetings with Croydon Veterans, one of the faster runners asked why I was wasting my time doing ultras when I still had so much speed. When that was combined with how much I was hurting myself in trying to go so far on insufficient training, I eased out over the next few years.

CHAPTER 17
Easing into the next millennium

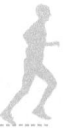

Toolangi is a special place, more a farming community than a town. There are only 500 residents in the area. It is located in a fold of Victoria's Great Dividing Range along the headwaters of the Yea River. Depending on what part of town you live in, the rain, which is abundant, eventually reaches the Murray River in the north, or cascades into the Yarra Valley and the Yarra River to Melbourne. The soil is a rich, red volcanic loam and much land has been dedicated to horticulture. The remainder is a mix of tree ferns and messmate forest, even in the centre of Toolangi. North to the top of the range, there are magnificent stands of mountain ash, while in the opposite direction there are outstanding views over the Yarra Valley. The spectacular peak of Mt St Leonard is only ten kilometres away and is often snow-clad in winter.

Toolangi is a great location in which to be a runner, as it has a network of hilly, dirt roads which are almost traffic-free. The air is clear, the climate bracing and the scenery outstanding. I have no doubt that my local environment is what kept me running after my time in the Army.

Two events occurred in the 1960s which had a big effect on Toolangi. Firstly, electricity finally made its way up the escarpment from Healesville, making life much more comfortable. Secondly, the 'Dips Me Lid' Hotel, located at the junction of Chum Creek and Myers Creek Roads, burned to the ground. In earlier days, the poet CJ Dennis had a second home in the town and enjoyed a beer or two there, hence the name.

There was a general store but most supplies were at the end of a steep, winding road to Healesville, or further to the outer suburbs of Melbourne. The Singing Garden of Arden was a tearoom located where CJ used to reside, and the main employers were the Strawberry Runner Grower's Co-op and Alex Demby Timber Company. The local tennis club battled on, but apart from a couple of stalwarts, most of the members were from the Matthews and Wilson families.

Sandy was fortunate to obtain a shop assistant position at the general store and I worked at the timber mill, as previously stated. Daniel and Kimberley attended tiny Toolangi Primary School and then Healesville High School. Dan was a talented tennis player and excelled academically, which made him a hard act for a little sister

Chapter 17 Easing into the next millennium

to follow. Kim was artistic rather than sports-minded and had difficulties in her secondary schooling.

By the mid 1990s, Kim was refusing to attend school and had to do remote learning. It was thought she had chronic fatigue and she became a recluse in her room. Dan was very close to his mum and Kim often argued with them both. I tended to support her to give her a friend and keep the fragile peace. In their late teens, both left home and lived in separate shared accommodation with friends.

A week after the Australian 100 kilometre Championship in 1996, I made one of my annual trips into Melbourne to compete in the Lake Relay. My teammates included Rolf Zimmerman, who had won the first Toolangi Fun Run, and Ernie Stewart, my teammate from the XXXX Army Around Australia Relay. My times for the short five kilometres were 16 mins 18 secs, 16 mins 23 secs and 16 mins 29 secs, which helped our team to third place.

A month later, I gave up trying to win my own fun run and dropped back to the shorter four-kilometre event. In the easier company, I managed to win in 13 mins 38 secs, taking a minute off the Over 40 record.

In December, I gave my local trail ultra another go. Perhaps a year off had been enough time to forget the debacle that was the first AURA Dam Trail 50 Kilometre. Morley Walking Track along the Watts River from

Fernshaw was very overgrown, and combined with the steep goat track, it took leader Tony Dietachmayer an hour for the first ten kilometres. On our second visit to Dom Dom Saddle, I was one minute in arrears but lost ground when forced to walk on the climb to Mt Monda. Peter LeBusque breezed past and then Peter Hoskinson caught me, but then dropped back as we caught the early leader. At the gate leading to the steep climb up Mt St. Leonard, Peter had a two-minute lead, but I was encouraged seeing him struggling on the steep track above. I made up gradual ground over the peak, and with ten kilometres to go, I went by into the lead which I was able to hold to the finish.

1: Greg Wilson, 4 hrs 35 mins 19 secs
2: Peter LeBusque, 4 hrs 37 mins 48 secs
3: Tony Dietachmayer, 4 hrs 42 mins 12 secs.

A close race which is what happens when most of the field follow the correct course. Apparently, Kelvin Marshall went astray again and Geoff Hook spent most of the race time searching for him. My time was a forty-minute improvement on the first time and just four minutes outside Safet Badic's course record. Very surprised on no training worth noting down!

In September 1997, I returned to the Lake Relay and joined a team of old military runners and one useful ring-in from the fire brigade. Peter Hunt was a handy addition as one of the best Over 40s in Victoria. Also in

Chapter 17   Easing into the next millennium

the team were old mates Ernie Stewart, David Holland and Frank Kresse from the Navy. We came second overall and broke the Over 40 record by twenty-one minutes.

In January 1998, I did three weeks training and returned to the Mansfield to Mt Buller 50 kilometre after a four-year break. I had lost a lot during that period, or I just had a bad day, needing lots of toilet breaks.

1: George Berger, 4 hrs 15 mins
2: Bert Pelgrim, 4 hrs 20 mins
3: Kelvin Marshall, 4 hrs 22 secs.

I came fourth another fifteen minutes back, with a similar distance to Lavinia. It was a very disappointing result because I was thirty minutes slower than I had run just after a 24 Hour race. Kelvin was in front of me for the first time, and while my record climbing the mountain was intact, Lavinia had come close to catching me. Champion that she is, the fact remained that a female eleven years older was getting too close.

A week later, I ran in a slightly shorter event with Bert and Lavinia, but this time we were on the same team. Croydon Veterans had a talented group of distance runners and top 800-metre runner Colin Paige was the other in our team for the Andy Salter Relay, where each member had a 3,200-metre loop to complete. The rules stated that a team's cumulative age had to reach a certain total and contain at least one female to compete. Having a fifty-four-year-old who could outrun most other females was a huge advantage. Basically, whatever team had Lavinia should have won.

- 1: Croydon 42 mins 22 secs, with Colin Paige (10 mins 1 secs), Greg Wilson (10 mins 10 secs), Lavinia Petrie (11 mins 57 secs) and Bert Pelgrim (10 mins 14 secs).
- 2: Springvale (42 mins 59 secs).

However, it was very close, as three of us were coming off an ascent of Mt Buller. Springvale's outstanding fifty-seven-year-old Theresia Baird was fifteen seconds quicker than Lavinia and each of our men held about the same margin on our opponents.

Two days later, I was off to Wodonga to compete in the 3MD Army 5 Kilometre Championship. It was ten years since I had run in this event, and I had slowed down by thirty-three seconds. So I guess that is a pass. My 17 mins 10 secs saw me in fifth place overall and at age forty-five, I was easily first O/35 Master.

I had three weeks off completely and commenced training in March with a week of seventy-four kilometres. Then the wheels fell off as I had as many days injured as training leading up to the AURA Dam Trail 50 Kilometre. This time, I wasn't disappointed as I had no right to expect a better result.

- 1: Bert Pelgrim, 4 hrs 27 mins 38 secs
- 2: Peter Mitchell 4 hrs 33 mins 26 secs
- 3: Greg Wilson, 4 hrs 44 mins 22 secs.

Chapter 17 Easing into the next millennium

I did no training at all and then went to Glengarry in Gippsland where the Australian 100-kilometre Championships was on. This time, I was sensible and chose to run the fifty-kilometre event instead. The big event was won by Yiannis again (7 hrs 14 mins) from my rogaining mate Nigel Aylott (8 hrs 9 mins) and Kelvin Marshall. I completed the 50 kilometre in 3 hrs 48 mins and was second to Daryl Cross (3 hr 26 mins).

My ultra career was almost over, and I knew it. Ironically, in this penultimate event, they took a photo of me and I was on the cover of the monthly *AURA Ultramag*. I say 'ironic' as it ranks as one of my worst short ultra performances.

The next month, I made the switch and commenced only my second professional season with the Victorian Cross-Country League (VCCL) since I injured my knee training for the Great Otway Classic thirteen years earlier. For May 1998, I trained twenty kilometres per week for two weeks and then spent the same time recovering from a right calf strain. Straight off that, I ran a ten-kilometre race (unplaced at 34 hrs 59 mins) that was my fastest for six years.

A month later, Brian and I travelled all the way to Warrnambool for that country club's big event a five-kilometre race around the city centre. The handicapper stuffed up and I was with Brian, even further back than usual. The race was three laps around the streets and the leader was well into her second lap before we'd even started. We never got near them, but I clung on to finish six seconds behind Brian in 16 mins 41 secs. This was my best five kilometres for five years, but it was a long drive back home.

Through winter, I finally managed to string some training days together and it paid dividends. The Country Championship was held over ten kilometres at Gellibrand Park. It was wet and windy, and the course was hilly, meaning perfect conditions for me. I finished fourth (35 mins 23 secs) which was a big improvement. Graeme Watkins and Gary Rice beat me for the over-40 prize, but I took Brian's scalp, which was a rare occurrence nowadays.

A fortnight later, we trekked up to Murchison for Doug Tuhan's flat, fast ten kilometres. Tenth was as close as I could get in the handicap, but in running 33 mins 58 secs, I was fourth-fastest and the fastest over-40. I ran my fastest ten kilometres since my injury-enforced retirement fourteen years earlier. A thirty-nine-year-old veterinarian from Wangaratta was in front of me and he told the officials he was a 'vet'; without checking, they awarded the prize to him! He didn't lie but it was hardly ethical.

Perhaps you have noticed that I only manage to win races when the conditions are so adverse it slows faster runners down. In August, the VCCL held a King of the

Chapter 17 Easing into the next millennium

Mountains, a very hilly two laps over eight kilometres at Cardinia Reservoir. The sponsor offered to double the prize money if the winner was able to beat the previous year's winning time of 26 mins 56 secs.

I was off a tough handicap with Mark Tomsett and he burnt me off on the downhill sections. In chasing him, we passed Bert Pelgrim early, then up the hill, I left him and got past Peter LeBusque. Over the top, I got past the Petries and down to the boardwalk. After a lap, I knew I was close to the lead. After another solid climb, I could see the two limit marker leaders and was close enough to pull them in. I just had to be able to hold off the top-quality back markers who would come with a rush in the concluding stages.

Down on to the flat, still narrowly behind, but I waited until the final straight and kicked past Aaron McKenzie to win clearly. The first six runners all ran faster than last year and my winning time of 26 mins 20 secs smashed it to rake in the bonus cash. This was my first professional victory since 1991 as they are very rare from a tough handicap, particularly as you get older. If only they held more races on a course that suited me! The reality was that I would be re-handicapped and be uncompetitive on easier courses.

A week later, I drove to Adelaide for their marathon as it also incorporated the Australian Defence Force Championship. I had not run an official marathon for many years, although I did have a time of 2 hrs 54 mins 38 secs from Canberra when I competed in the 50 kilometres in 1994. I ran a controlled race with an easy start and was then not passed by anyone. My time of 2 hrs 50 mins 53 secs placed me twelfth overall, but I was pleased with my ADF result. I was the first Army finisher and third in the ADF. At age forty-six, I was also first ADF Master (over-35).

That was enough for me, and I pretty much had the rest of the year off. In January 1999, I had my annual holidays and jumped straight into a couple of weeks of more than a hundred kilometres. Of course, I started to get sore and had to then ease off. This brief burst of training was somehow supposed to get me fit enough for another crack at the Mansfield to Mt Buller fifty-Kilometre Ultra.

At the base of the climb, I was in second place behind Safet Badic. As soon as I hit the wall at Mirimbah, I, err, hit the wall. Up the mountain, I had to walk a lot and for the first time, I was passed on the climb. Kelvin Marshall and top female Sandra Timmer-Arends came past and I just waved them goodbye. I was the third male to finish and improved by ten minutes on last year with 4 hrs 37 mins. I was not satisfied at all with that performance, although what did I expect on three weeks of training? I resolved then to never run it again unless I was properly fit. A contributing factor was the lack of a support crew,

Chapter 17 Easing into the next millennium

as it was difficult to do ultras without one. Eight years after I first tried an ultramarathon in this very event, my career as an ultramarathoner was finished. Mansfield to Mt Buller was a fitting way to 'bookend' my career.

I am proud of my ultra achievements, and not because they were outstanding. It is that I could achieve the results I did on very inadequate training. I have enjoyed running with some of our legends, met many interesting people and the whole experience has enriched my life. I feel that working physically hard at the timber mill during this period detracted from the training I could manage, but it made me capable of enduring the runs that I did. In eight years, from 1991 until 1999, I competed in sixteen ultramarathons. I won five and finished worse than fourth only on the four occasions that I ventured to 24 hours or beyond. I also managed to win my age category in every event under 24 hours. There is a message there for me if I should wish to heed it!

I went directly back into retirement mode as far as training went. A week later, I did front up for the Andy Salter Relay as Croydon always put in a top team. The fastest runner over the 3200-metre course was Ewan Wilson with 9 mins 44 secs, but our solid team effort (and Lavinia) saw us prevail. Croydon won in 41 mins 44 secs, with Colin Paige (9 mins 59 secs), Lavinia Petrie (11 mins 35 secs), Greg Wilson (10 mins 15 secs) and Bert Pelgrim (9 mins 55 secs). We had improved on last year by thirty-nine seconds, which was mainly due to improvements by Lavinia and son-in-law Bert.

My only other run of note was a fortnight later when I attended the ADF 5-Kilometre Championship at Wodonga. I was ninth overall in 17 mins 28 secs but was again first Master. Other than that, I played tennis, attended Army Reserve and ran a few VCCL events very poorly. When I heard about the Torch Relay being conducted as a prelude to the Sydney Olympics, I threw in a nomination. There was only one person more surprised than me when I got to do a leg carrying the Olympic flame past some cow paddocks up near Mooroopna and that was Lavinia Petrie. Upon hearing of it, she said, 'What did *you* do to get on the Torch Relay?'

A year later in November 2000, I did my only event for that year in the ADF Track Championships. I had only done two weeks of training, so my result was as expected: second in the 1500 metres Masters (4 mins 42 secs) behind Geoff Brewster, a visiting English serviceman.

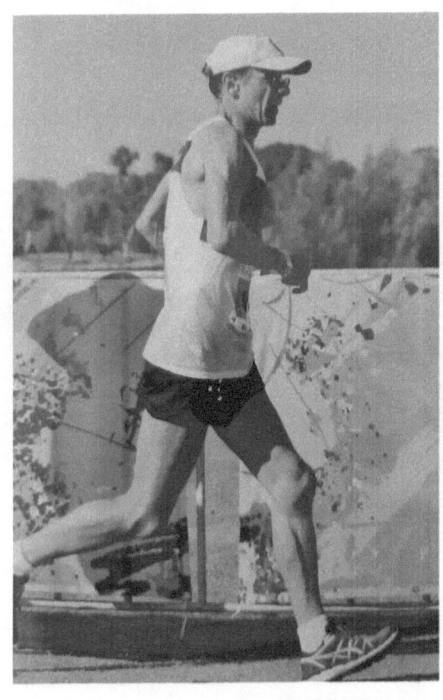

November 2016 World Masters Marathon Championship, Perth WA. Greg in the finishing straight for sixth M60 and a member of the Australian gold medal team.

April 2017 ANZAC Parade, Melbourne, Vic. The two youngest members of the Australian Army Training Team – Vietnam, catch up 45 years after serving together at Van Kiep, Baria South Vietnam. L Don Targett, R Greg Wilson.

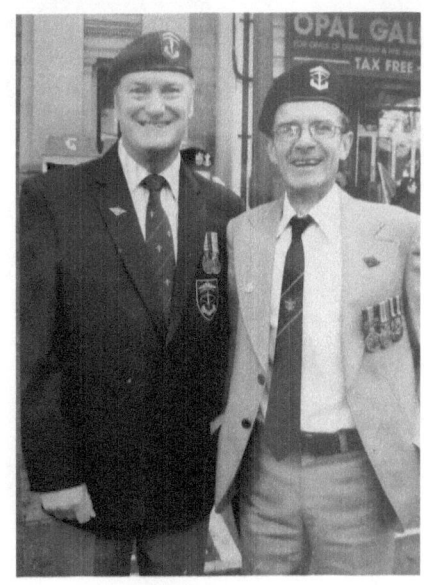

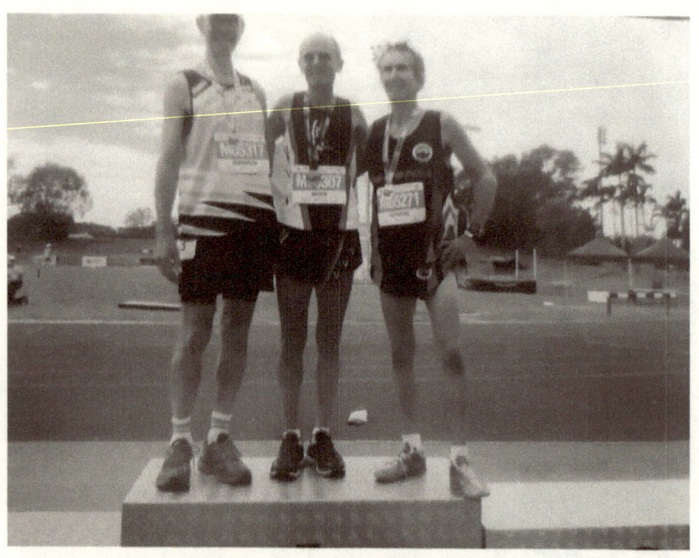

June 2017 Australian Masters 10 Kilometre Championship, Darwin NT. Greg's only victory in this event and on his 65th birthday. Podium L to R Ralph Henderson, Greg Wilson, Ron Schwebel.

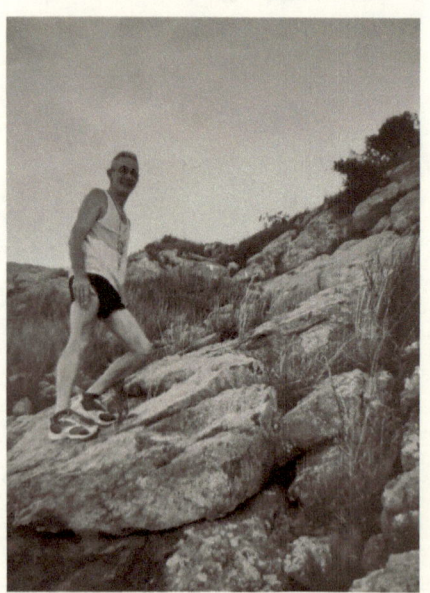

August 2017 Castle Hill Townsville, Nth Qld. Townsville Marathon Club foundation member and Townsville Road Runners legend Peter Lahiff leading the way up the old Goat Track route used during early King Of The Castle events.

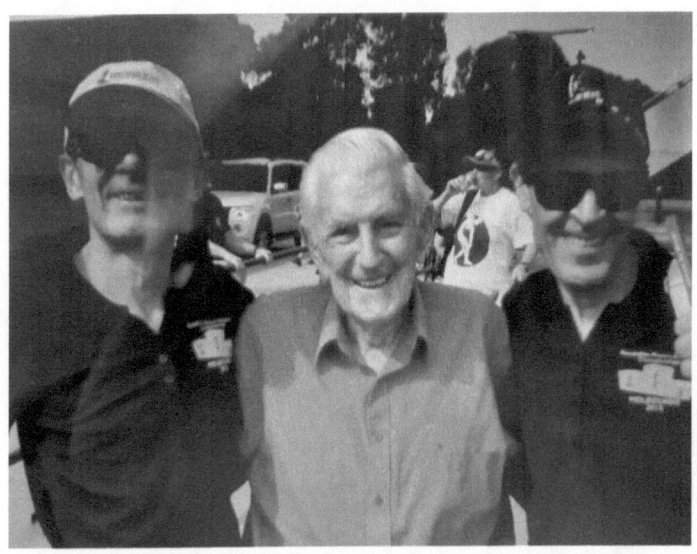

Apr 2018 Australian Masters Athletic Championships, Perth WA. L to R Greg Wilson, John Gilmour, Yassine Belaabed. Our first meeting with a "legend" and just in time as age caught up with John.

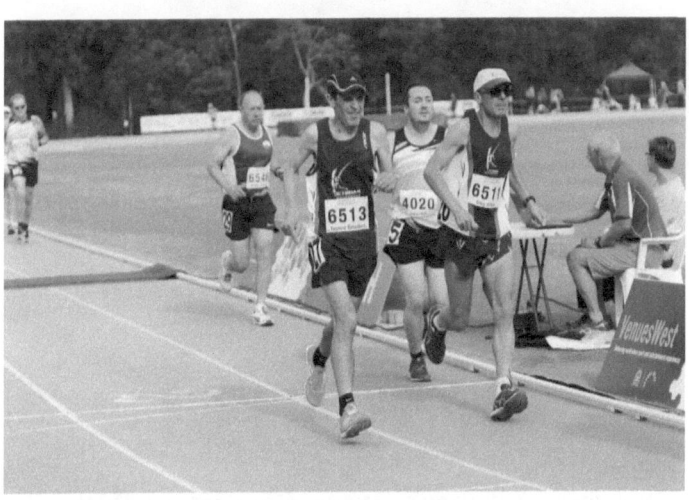

Apr 2018 Australian Masters 10Km Track Championship M65. Perth WA. 1st Yassine Belaabed (L) and 2nd Greg Wilson (R) passing lapped runners.

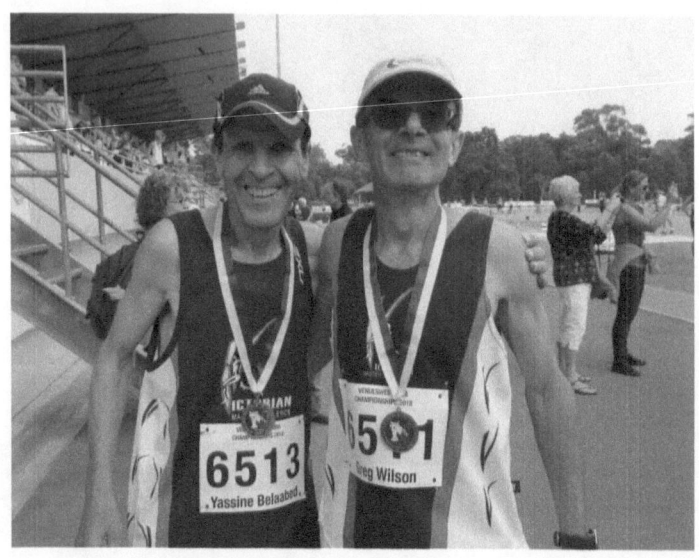

Apr 2018 Australian Masters Championship 10 Km, Perth WA. L to R Yassine Belaabed 1st and Greg Wilson 2nd Post race

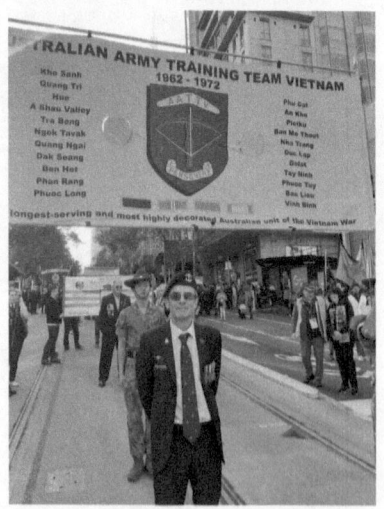

April 2019 ANZAC Parade, Melbourne. Greg marching as the sole member of the Australian Army Training Team Vietnam. The passing of years and closing of AATTV Vic. Branch has thinned the ranks dramatically.

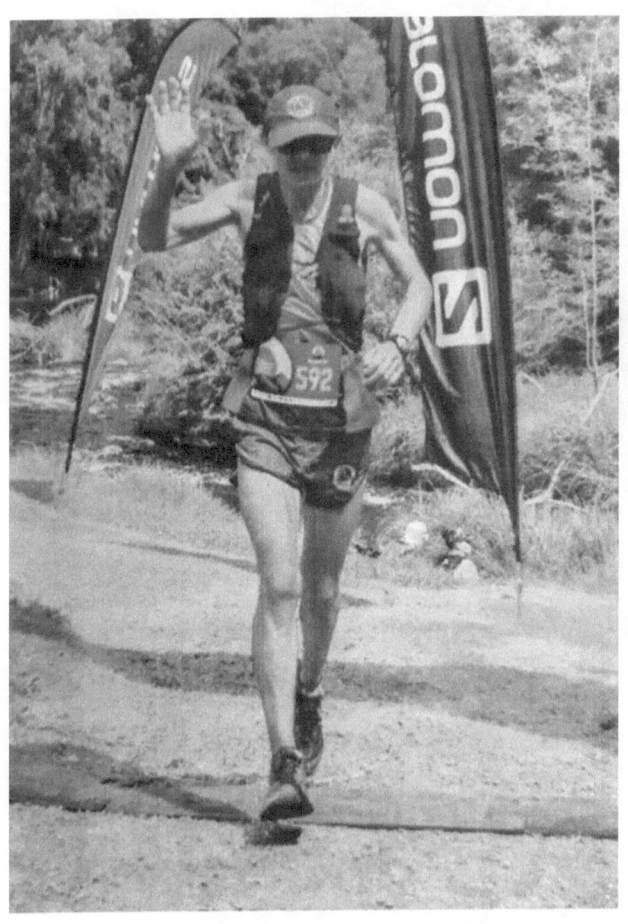

Mar 2020 Lumberjack 50 Kilometre Trail Event, Warburton, Vic. The final event prior to Covid lockdown and Greg waves farewell to Trail races. Almost 30 minutes improvement on 2019 for 18th of 98. Time to find out if this is any good and chase measured age records ... when Covid eventually allowed!

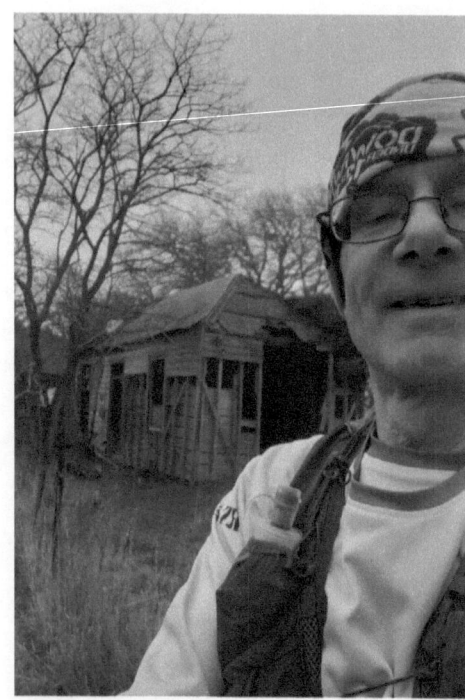

May 2021 Training run from former Calder Hwy. Woodend North, Vic. A revisit to the first house I remember living in, back in 1956.

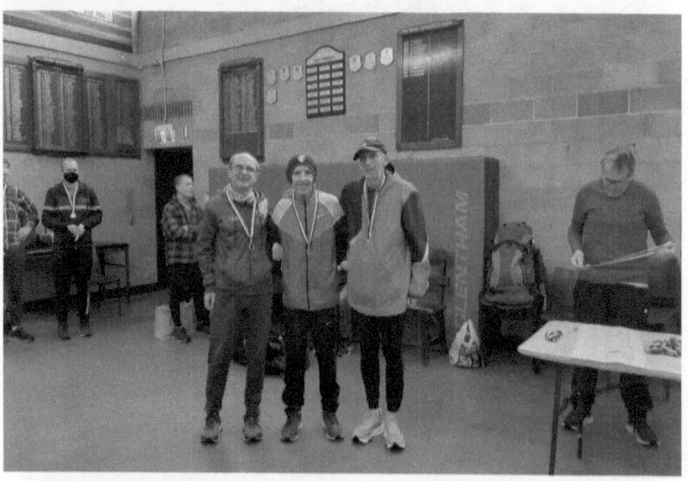

July 2021 Victorian Masters 8 km Cross Country Championship, Yarra Bend, Fairfield Vic. "The Three Amigos" reunited on the M65 podium during a brief respite from Covid Lockdown. L to R Greg Wilson, Yassine Belaabed, Les Williams.

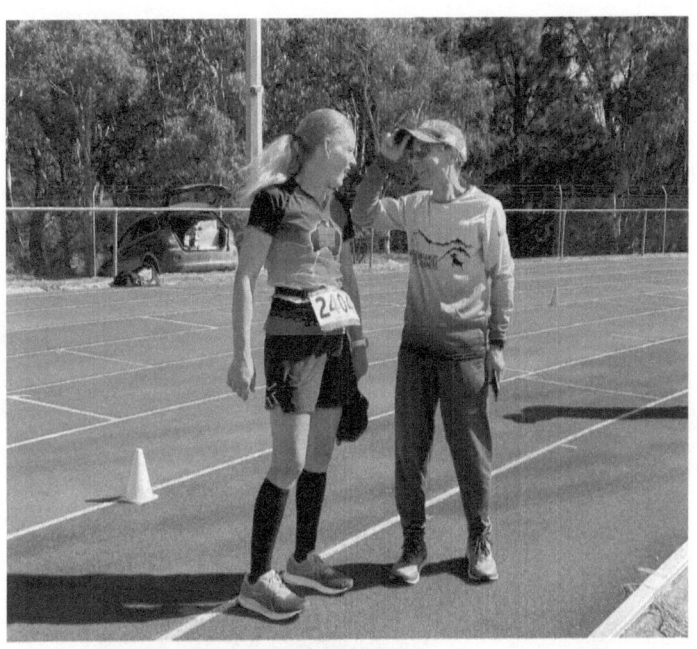

Apr 2022 Victorian 24 Hour Championship, Coburg Vic. Christy Lambert congratulated by Greg Wilson just after a successful completion of her first 24 Hour ultra.

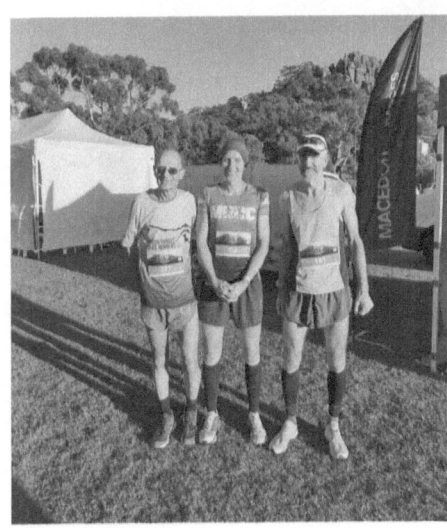

Apr 2022 "Run The Rock 22 Km, Hanging Rock Vic. A trio of local stars in their "local derby". L to R Greg Wilson, Christy Lambert, Steven Williams.

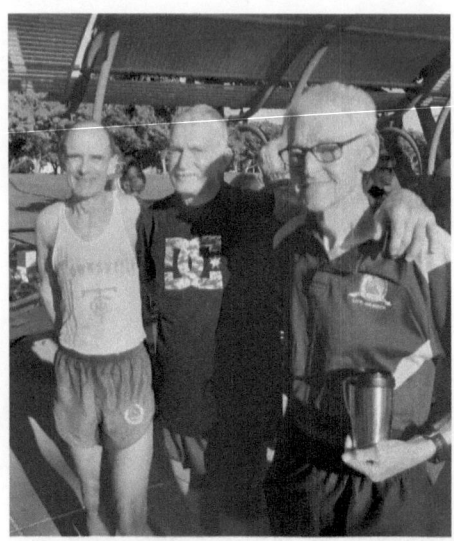

May 2022 Townsville Road Runners 50th Reunion, The Strand Townsville Nth Qld. Three former stars of TRR meet again, 20 years since they were all medalists at the World Masters Games in Melbourne. L to R Greg Wilson, John Herridge, Joe Scott

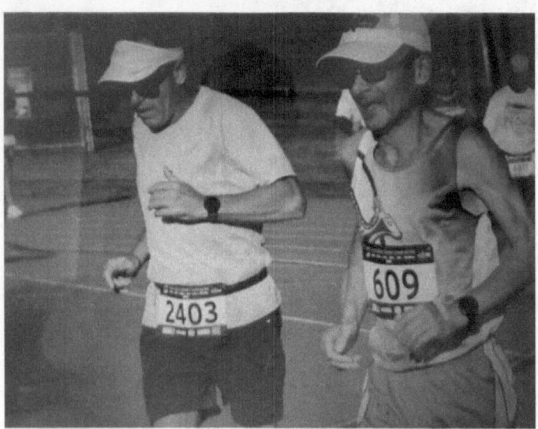

May 2022 Southern Sydney 24 Hour, Barden Park, NSW. What odds about two runners who held the same Army appointment 35 years apart, both excelling in the same ultra marathon. My 6 Hour pace was fairly even with what Kevin Muller did for 24 hours.

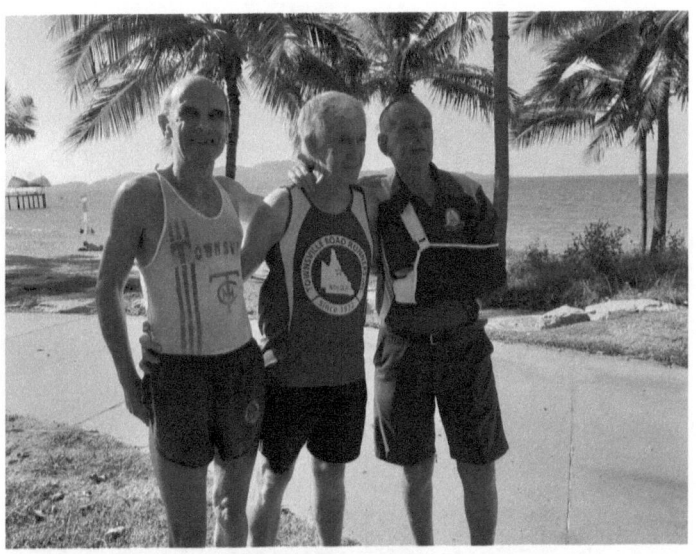

June 2022 50th Anniversary Reunion of Townsville Road Runners (formerly TMC), The Strand Townsville Nth Qld. Foundation members of Townsville Marathon Club L to R Greg Wilson, David Wharton, Bob Down

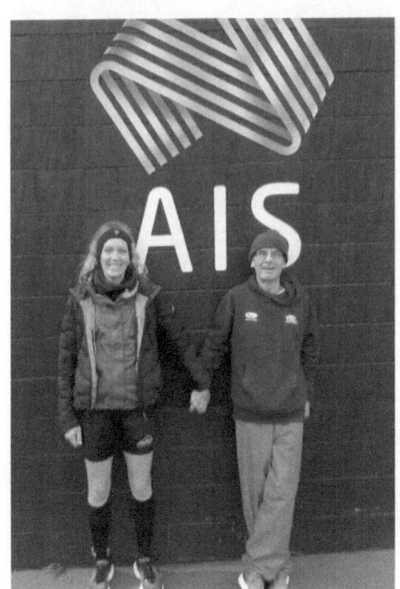

July 2022 Australian 24 Hour Invitational (Open), Bruce ACT. Pre-race Christy Lambert and Greg Wilson. About 25 years since Christy last competed there as a 400 metre hurdler and the same period since Greg had run a 24 Hour.

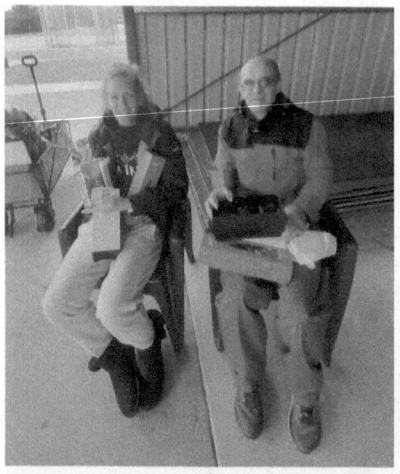

July 2022 Australian 24 Hour Invitational (Open), Bruce ACT. Rugged up against the freezing conditions, but having good reason to be pleased at presentation. L Christy Lambert (1st female and undefeated at 24 hour events), R Greg Wilson (6 x Australian M70 Age Group records).

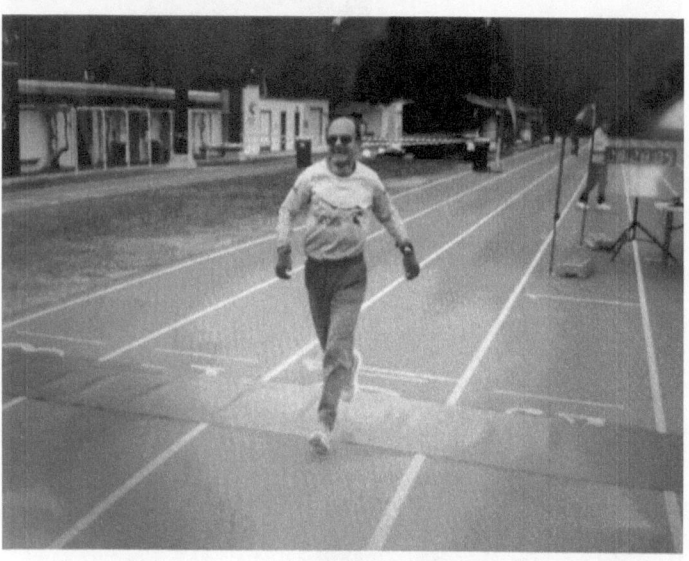

July 2022 Australian 24 Hour Invitational (Open), Bruce ACT. Greg wearing a few layers to ward off the freezing conditions, but running hard to break the M70 record for 50 miles, which Harry Davis held for eight years.

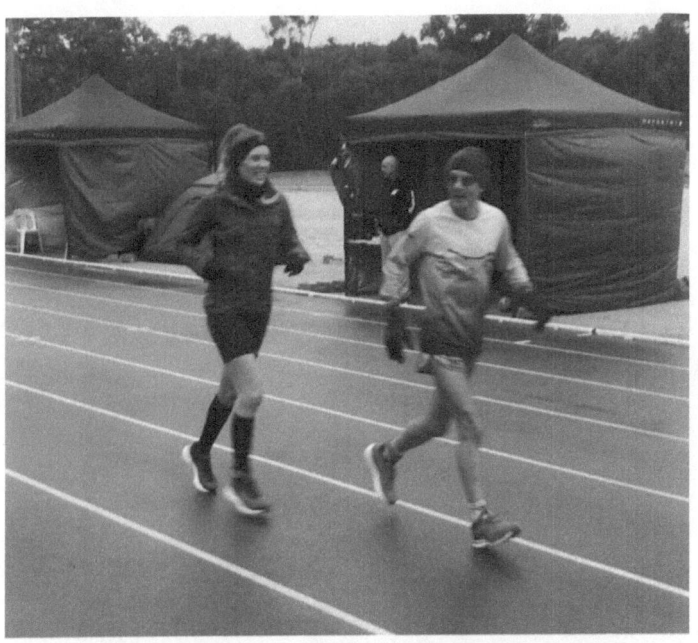

Jul 2022 Australian 24 Hour Invitational, Bruce ACT. Christy Lambert and Greg Wilson during a successful first long track ultra together: female winner and PB and 6 AURA Australian M70 Age Group Records respectively.

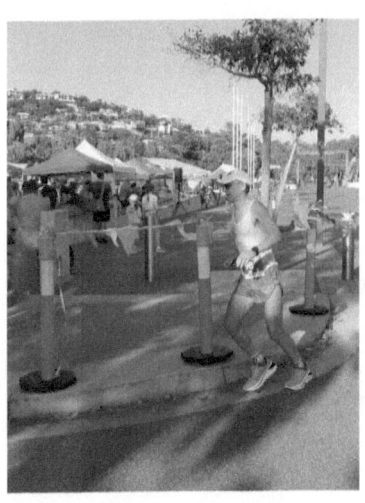

August 2022 Townsville Marathon, Nth Qld. Greg surging for the finish line after a fine run in hot conditions. It turned out to be a qualifying time for the WANDA World Marathon Age Group Championship, Chicago 2023.

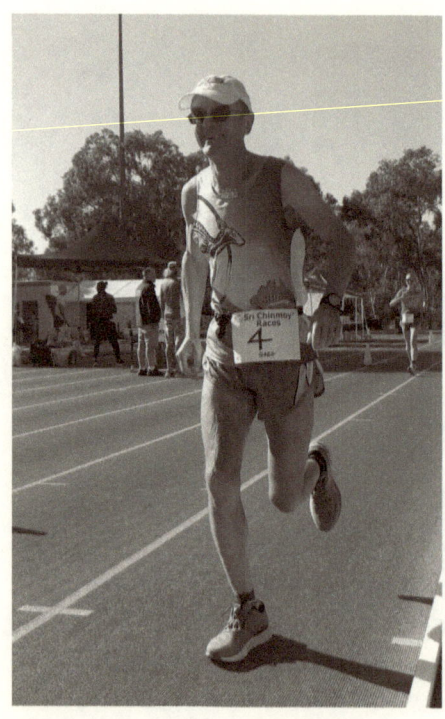

March 2023 Sri Chinmoy Australian 48 Hour Championship, Bruce ACT. Greg pursued by great multi day runner Annabel Hepworth.

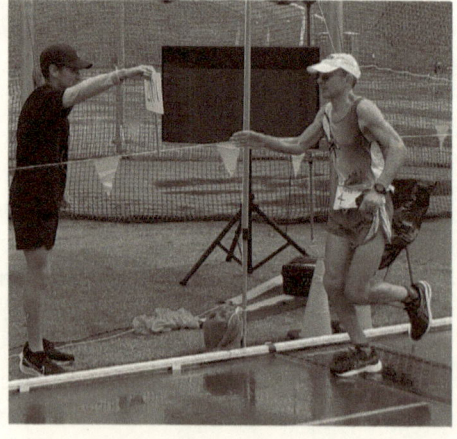

Mar 2023 Sri Chinmoy Australian 48 Hour Championship, Bruce ACT. Greg about to accept a sign denoting his attaining the M70 AURA Australian Age Group Record for 200 kilometres. Very satisfying to break a record by 6 hrs and 36 mins!

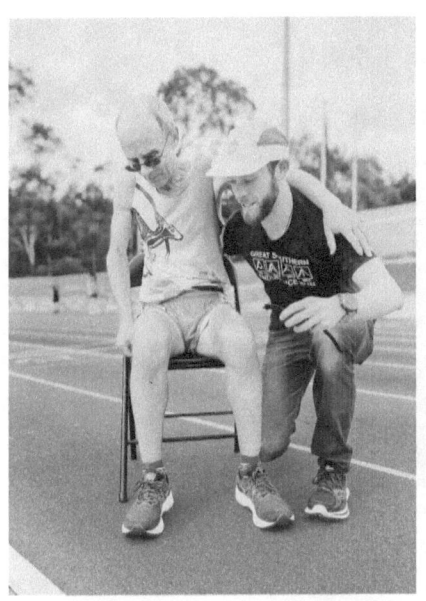

March 2023 Sri Chinmoy Australian 48 Hour Championship, Bruce ACT. Twice as far as Greg's previous longest event, so no wonder "super crew" Justin Hiatt's assistance was needed to sit after finishing. New Australian M70 records for 200 kilometres and 48 hours achieved.

March 2023 Sri Chinmoy Australian 48 Hour Championship. Camille Herron was about 150 kilometres in front, but for almost all the final three hours, after breaking their respective records Greg and Camille maintained a similar pace.

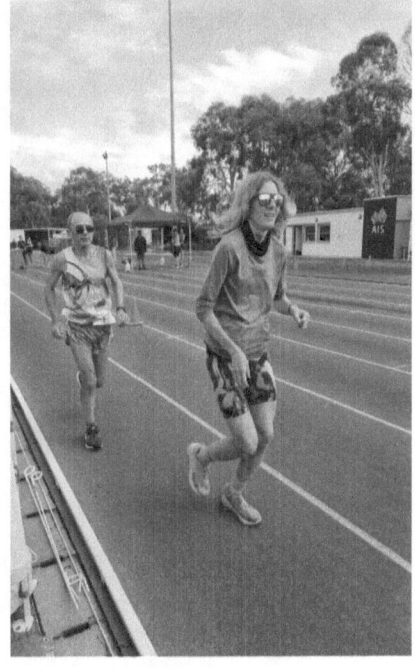

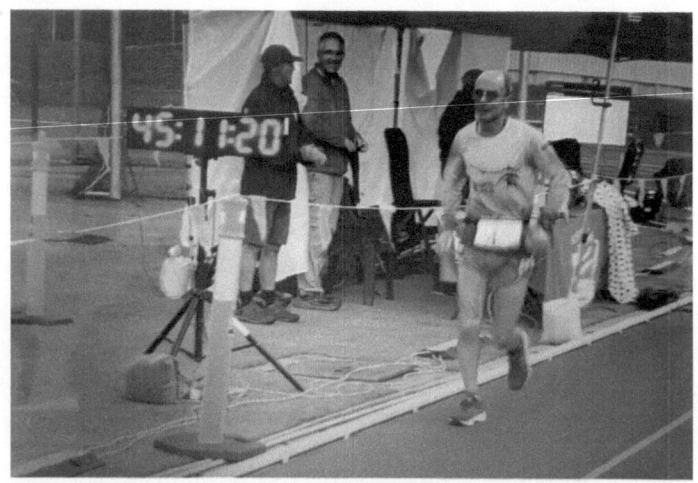

March 2023 Sri Chinmoy Australian 48 Hour Championship, Bruce ACT. The clock says it all as with 45 hrs 11 mins and 20 secs elapsed, Greg has overtaken the distance that Cliff Young ran in setting the longstanding M70 Age Group record for 48 hours.

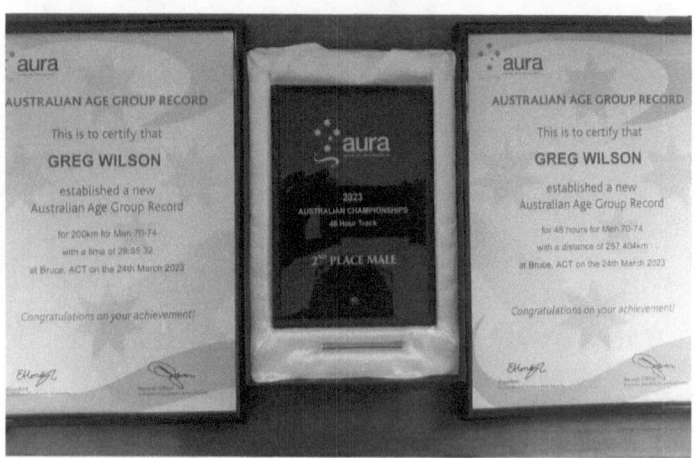

March 2023 Sri Chinmoy Australian 48 Hour Championship, Bruce ACT. The rewards for a step into the unknown of running/walking for double Greg's previous longest race. At age 70 to place second in an Australian Championship, take 6hrs 36 mins off the 200Kilometre record and surpass Cliff Young at 48 hours by over 22 Kilometres. Phew!

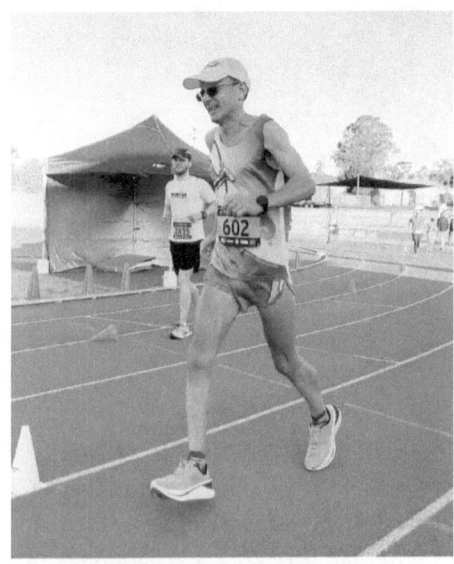

June 2023 Southern Sydney 6 Hour, Leumeah, NSW. Greg Wilson with 200 metres to cover to attain an M70 World Best Performance of 63.800 kilometres.

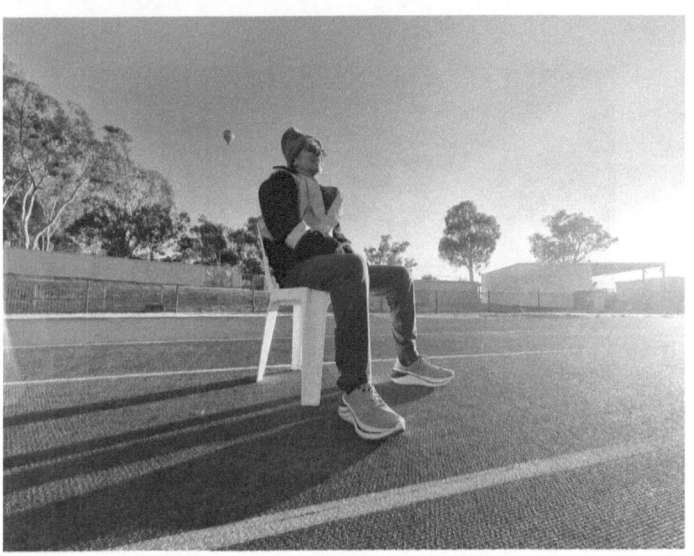

July 2023 Australian 24 Hour Invitational, Bruce ACT. On a freezing morning, Greg awaiting distance measurement after setting new M70 Australian Age Group Records for 100 Miles and 24 Hours.

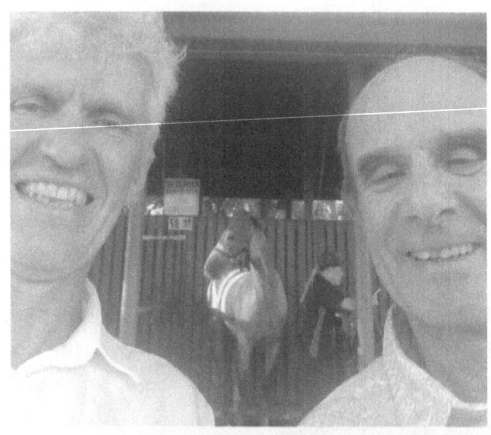

May 2023 Sunshine Coast Turf Club, Qld. Three handy grey runners. Townsville running mate Gerry Maguire joined Greg in part ownership of this former Mt. Macedon trained galloper. L to R Gerry Maguire, Hillcrest Avenue, Greg Wilson. A Saturday city meeting and sixth, beaten less than one length.

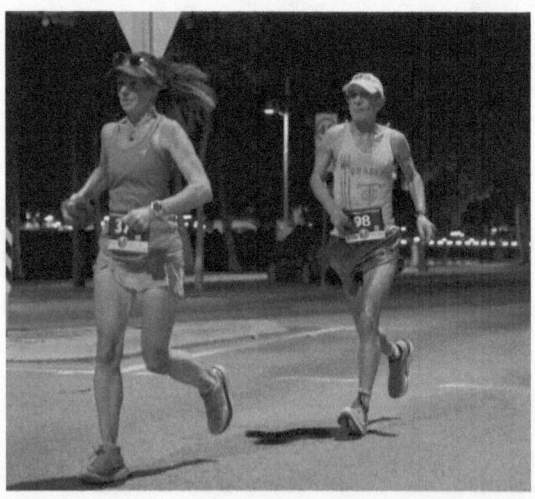

Aug 2023 Townsville Marathon. A small world when you go from being guest speakers, to running together for 25 kilometres. L Karin Thorburn completing marathon number 400 and Greg Wilson best time for seven years (1st M70 by 2 hours)

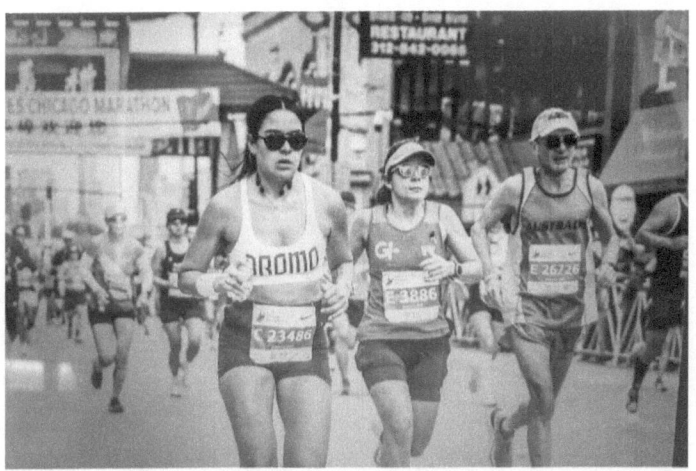

Oct 2023 Chicago Marathon, USA. Early on I spotted a Brazilian female Gislene Calligaris, wearing similar colours. We had a great run as we paced each other and passed thousands of earlier starters.

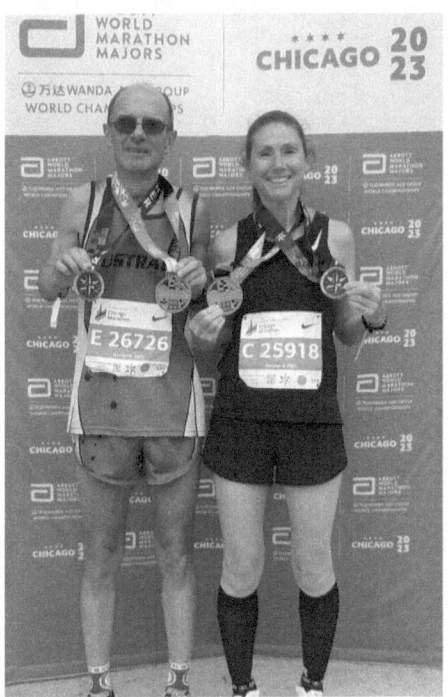

Oct 2023 Chicago Marathon USA. Post-race for a finisher medals shot with friend and fine W50 runner Liz Maguire from Townsville, Nth Qld. In a coincidence we both finished eleventh in the world in our respective age groups.

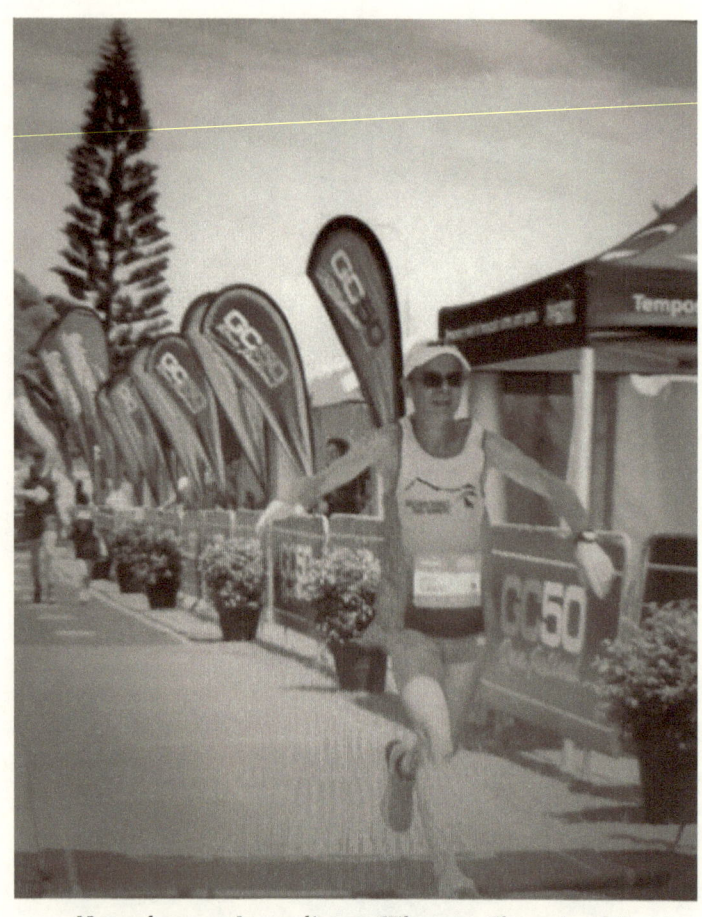

November 2023 Australian 50 Kilometre Championship, Gold Coast, Qld. Sometimes an ill judged early pace in hot conditions can bring even experienced runners undone. That experience though is what enables you to arrive in style for the finish line photo.

CHAPTER 18
Paradise lost

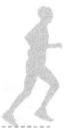

There had been a few changes in Toolangi leading up to the end of the millennium. Dan had long been working and living down in Melbourne, doing data entry at Computershare. When living at home, Kim had pretty much developed into a recluse. She couldn't cope with any noise and we ended up constructing an insulated false wall between the kitchen and her bedroom to keep the peace. When she did come out of her room, it was usually to argue with Sandy and Dan and expect me to take her side.

I am not sure who she was diagnosed by, but she was convinced she was suffering from chronic fatigue syndrome. She spent some years receiving treatment from a local kinesiologist, Lyn McCall, who just happened to be Sandy's boss at the Toolangi Store. I had no faith in that at all but kept silent in order to not rock the boat. You can imagine how much of Sandy's pay remained after kinesiology bills.

Eventually the McCalls closed the store and moved away, so the town lost its local social gathering place. All services were now at the end of a winding sixteen-kilometre road. It was some time before John and Michelle Marshall purchased the site and re-opened the store as a temporary measure. They were only too pleased to re-hire Sandy, and we all became firm friends. Long-term, they planned to augment the General Store business and construct a Toolangi Tavern to replace the long-lost pub.

Brian Simmons had developed 'young man's arthritis' and was easing out of athletics. He and Christine took up playing golf at Marysville and Sandy, who had been struggling with injury on the tennis court, joined them. I gave it a try but the best I can say about golf is that it was in a beautiful setting at Marysville. I saw a lot of the course as I zigzagged around and soon gave up in frustration.

The tennis club folded due to lack of numbers and its fundraising arm, the Toolangi Fun Run, went the same way. At work, I had finally escaped from the green chain when they ceased supplying house lots and began cutting slabs for stacking and kiln drying. I preferred a position where I could use my brain and be further from the noise and drudgery. I was quite content grading, sawing and stacking packs of kiln-dried hardwood, but there were ominous rumblings that it would not last. The boss was just waiting for the political pressure to become too great and cause the forest to be locked away from timber harvesting.

Running in the new millennium began for me with the news that the World Veterans Athletics Championships were coming to Brisbane. I decided that would be a good motivation for a temporary comeback after my years off. My training commenced well with 200 kilometres in January. The next month was a wipeout with hot weather and pain in my left hip. In March, I got back into it before a calf strain and a fall resulted in a painful rib injury. During May, I averaged eighty-five kilometres per week, and as a result, I started to see some reasonable performances in races.

I travelled up to Bankstown in Sydney to compete in my second Australian Veterans Championships. In the ten-kilometre track race, I ran fourth in 36 mins 39.84 secs (age grade performance 80.66 per cent), some distance behind Bruce Cameron from NSW with 33 mins 58.63 secs. I followed up with third in the ten-kilometre cross-country in 39 mins 49 secs (age grade 74.27 per cent) and about the same margin behind Bruce again.

I even managed a win on a fairly flat course with the VCCL in the Bob Cook Memorial ten-kilometre at Heidelberg. It was a desperately close finish as the back marker lunged on the line but fell two seconds short. The champion I had just held off was Sean Quilty, a Commonwealth Games bronze medallist in the marathon.

I received a long handicap start on Sean, but what a nice scalp to take! My winning time was 36 mins 39 secs, exactly what I had run on the track at Bankstown.

In April, the Victorian Veterans' Athletic Club held a warm-up meeting at Box Hill so runners could gauge how their World Veterans Championship preparation was going. For me, it was an outstanding result, as at almost forty-nine years of age I was giving away many years and finished fourth. I was blown away by my time of 16 mins 35 secs, as I had not run that fast for sixteen years. It seemed I was in fine form to attend my first World Veterans Championship – except that when I cooled down, I discovered that I had strained my calf muscle.

In May, the Victorian Veterans held their half-marathon along the Maribynong River in Melbourne. My new-found fitness saw me up in a leading bunch of six, which included my Around Australia Relay teammate, Ernie Stewart. In the concluding stages, national class walker Colin Heywood and I singled out for an enthralling battle to the line.

1: Colin Heywood, M45, 1 hr 21 mins 41 secs
2: Greg Wilson, M45, 1hr 21 mins 58 secs
3: Ernie Stewart, M50, 1 hr 22 mins 36 secs
4: Barry Brooks, M60, 1 hr 23 mins 24 secs.

The main problem with waiting for a World Veterans Championship to come to Australia is that you don't have a choice in what age group you will be in. I was only eleven months from moving up out of the M45 age group, and giving away four years was a big disadvantage. Once I strained my calf and also had a bout of influenza, I stopped training with a view to being able to attend, albeit not being as fit as I would have liked.

We drove up to the Gold Coast where we stayed with Ray and Judy Clitheroe at Burleigh Waters. It was the fourteenth World Veterans Championships and had attracted 9000 competitors from seventy-five countries. It was my first time in an international event of high standing and so it was with some anticipation that I headed off to Brisbane, where I had events on during the fortnight of the championships.

In the eight-kilometre cross-country, I felt flat and tired throughout. I was never near the frontrunners, but these were the best of my age in the world.

1: M. Krempel (Slovenia), 27 mins 27 secs
2: Grenville Wood (Australia), 27 mins 32 secs
3: Ron Peters (Australia), 27 mins 51 secs
22: Greg Wilson (Australia), 30 mins 36 secs.

I wasn't disappointed as I had run the best I could on the day and had no previous idea of where I fitted in at an international level. An idea of the quality is that second-placed Grenville Wood had won the Olympic Marathon trial back in 1984, when I had finished twenty-eighth in a personal best time.

The M45 field for the 5000 metres was so large that

they held three heats, with the winner decided on times during qualifying. There were not many big names in my heat, and I set off at 16 mins 30 secs pace in a leading pack of four. This was trimmed to two as I sat on the shoulder of A. Cerra (Argentina) for lap after lap. Then my hamstring tore! I thought of stopping, which would have been sensible, but I was the leading Australian and decided to stay out there. At a much reduced pace, I hobbled to the finish in second place.

Heat result:

1: A. Cerra (Argentina), 16 mins 41 secs
2: Greg Wilson (Australia), 17 mins 2 secs
3: Robert Herd (Australia), 17 mins 21 secs.

Final result:

1: Ron Peters (Australia), 15 mins 36 secs
2: P. Froucher (France), 15 mins 38 secs
3: M. Krempl (Slovenia), 15 mins 41 secs.
25: G. Wilson (Australia).

My big aim had been the marathon, still five days away. The sensible decision would have been to have gone home, but I had trained for four months and travelled 2000 kilometres! I scratched from the ten-kilometre event and sat in Ray's lounge with an ice pack on my thigh for days. Two days before the marathon, I managed a half-hour, pain-free run and decided to compete.

There was a large and colourful group of competitors and spectators gathered on the South Bank of the Brisbane

River for the marathon. I was there to run at my top and gave no consideration to my interrupted preparation or my injury. I set out at 2 hrs 45 mins pace but as I was near the first female, I decided to hang on and get sucked along by her vocal crowd of supporters. This increased my pace, but who knew if there would be a price to pay.

I was in twenty-fifth place and the ninth Australian when I hit the wall at the twenty-five-kilometre mark. This had never happened to me so early in an event. I was completely out of carbohydrate fuel and my body would now burn fat. If I wanted to finish, I would have to slow down. The idea of surviving another eighteen kilometres was rather daunting.

Many people I had left behind now came streaming past. I just had to ignore them and plod on in ultramarathon survival mode. Over the final five kilometres, it was a delicate balancing act between a brain saying, 'Drive for the finish' and legs saying, 'I am going to cramp if you don't stop now'. I had to stop half a dozen times and then totter cautiously off again. The support from the sidelines was amazing, as I was an Australian and still well up in the large field.

A spectator yelled to keep going as I could still break three hours. In sight of the finish line, I tried to raise a gallop but immediately cramped up. It was hard to believe that amid this painful personal disaster, I crossed the line in 2 hrs 59 mins 48 secs in overall fifty-sixth position.

M45-49 result:
1: Ron Peters (Australia), 2 hrs 32 mins
2: Ivan Golab (Slovakia), 2 hrs 34 mins 20 secs
3: Gavin Stevens (New Zealand), 2 hrs 36 mins 6 secs
10: Gene Sanderson (New Zealand), 2 hrs 54 mins 16 secs
16: Greg Wilson (Australia), 2 hrs 59 mins 48 secs.

The reason for mentioning Gene is that he finished behind me in the cross-country and his position indicates where I belonged if uninjured. I was the sixth Australian M45 to complete the course.

I had only come back to experience a World Veterans Championship and now I was injured again, flat and tired. I went straight back into retirement and this time it was eight months before I pulled the runners on again. It was a long haul back, made more difficult by repeated right calf injuries and a chronic left hip problem. My incentive and long-term goal was another international event, the World Masters Games coming to Melbourne. The big advantage I had this time was that it was on my home ground and I had turned fifty.

Mid-year, I received a phone call from somebody in Townsville. The Townsville Road Runners were having a reunion to celebrate the formation of the Townsville Marathon Club thirty years earlier. Someone had tracked down my contact details and as a foundation member, I was invited to attend. Life gets in the way, and I had not given much thought to my early days up north. It was

Chapter 18   Paradise lost

twenty-six years since I had left Townsville and I decided that seeing they had bothered to locate me, the least I could do was attend.

Before going to Townsville, I had a run with the VCCL. Here I was about to turn fifty and there were only five runners behind me on handicap. The rest I had to give a start, and in most cases, a lot of age. This caused me to wonder why I was bothering with professional running.

I was billeted with Bert and Jennie Part in my favourite spot, North Ward. We had a couple of runs in that area and functions where it was great to catch up with many old friends. Dave Scully, Dave Wharton, Bob Down, Peter Lahiff, Alan Stanbrook, Joe Scott, Rowan Carr and the Gilboys were some of the 1970s crew and I made some new friends among the northern running community as well. On 9 June, I celebrated my fiftieth birthday as well as the club's thirtieth. In my enthusiasm, I aggravated a right calf strain, and this was a problem that reduced my training over the next few months.

A week after returning, I competed in the Victorian Veterans ten-kilometre. I was first M50 in 37 mins 55 secs, which was okay considering my lack of training. If I had looked over my shoulder, former World Veterans champion Bronwen Cardy was close behind and she was in my age group!

After a month recovering, I tried again, this time an Athletics Victoria 16-kilometre cross-country at

Brimbank Park. With a large field of strong runners, my lack of fitness was obvious. The M50 winner was Geoff Clarke in sixty-four minutes and I was back in fifth, about three minutes behind. A week later, I had more luck in the VCCL M50 8-kilometre Championship, managing to win in 28 mins 48 secs. In third behind me was the multiple Australian pro marathon champion Ted Paulin, who had been my nemesis during my early pro years. It just shows that if you are patient enough, your time will come. This time, I pulled up with a sore right hamstring to join my calf. My body was trying to tell me something – any chance I would listen sometime?

I had a week off and then ran in the Victorian Veterans 10-mile Championships at Princes Park. I was running well but having a torrid battle to hold off Paul Twining when, 800 metres from home, I felt my right calf tear. I finished with a distinct limp but won the M50 narrowly (60 mins 36 mins) from Paul (60 mins 50 secs), and wouldn't you know it, Bronwen Cardy again (60 mins 57 secs) beating the remainder of the males.

I have this down pat by now – of course, a week off will fix it! Then after two weeks of training, I competed in the Veterans 25-kilometre Championship along the Maribyrnong River. A year prior, Colin Heywood had beaten me by seventeen seconds. This was another enthralling battle. I was pleased to cross the line first in 1 hr 37 mins 37 secs, a mere nine seconds clear of Colin and a couple of minutes back to Russell Johnson and Ernie Stewart.

By now, you know the story. My left calf, knee and hip were sore, so I had a week off and then tried to run the AV Burnley Half-Marathon. I didn't make it, as the left calf said, 'That's enough!'. After writing this, I find it ridiculous that I bothered to turn up for the World Masters Games a fortnight later, but that had been my aim all season. Yes, I had a week off, and our annual trip to visit Glyn and Rita Cox in Thornton, NSW. A week of training with Glyn and winning a low-key race at Maitland, and that was my preparation done.

The ten-kilometre road race was held on the streets around Albert Park in South Melbourne. It was a huge field as all ages were in together and you had no idea who your age competitors were. All you could do was run your best and find out after the finish where you were located in your age group.

World Masters Games M50 ten-kilometre result:

1: Klaus Goldammer (Germany), 33 mins 30 secs

2: Geoff Clarke (Australia), 34 mins 30 secs

3: Greg Wilson (Australia), 34 mins 58 secs.

This was an amazing result considering my lead-up. Geoff had beaten me by three minutes earlier in the season and now it was down to twenty-eight seconds. The next finishers behind me were David Standeven, a Sydney-to-Melbourne winner, and John Herridge. This was the first time I had competed against John, as we were in Townsville at different times, but he is the record holder for the King of the Castle footrace.

Two days later they held the eight-kilometre cross-country at Fairfield. This would be a real test as I seemed to have broken down after every race for at least a week over the past few years. This time, the field was limited to our age group and competitors would actually be able to see each other. The course was on undulating grass with four laps of two kilometres.

It made no difference at all to the result, which duplicated the ten-kilometre road race. I spent three laps grimly hanging on to Klaus and Geoff before giving a big 'Sydney or the Bush' kick up the hill the final time. I did it to find out if I could break them, but alas, they responded and then kicked clear to leave me with another bronze medal. I was third in the M50 at 29 mins 25 secs, a minute quicker than I had run at the World Masters Athletic Championship the previous year.

I suspected that my injury was an issue, but I turned up two days later for the five-kilometre track race. I had no hope from the start when I found that due to bureaucratic incompetence, I had been placed in the B field. No amount of argument from me or Klaus, who backed my stand, would make them alter their stupid decision. I ran a solo time trial out in front of the field; halfway through, my left calf strain caused me to step off the track.

Chapter 18 Paradise lost

Before leaving the event in disgust, I informed John Herridge of my injury and advised him to make sure he ran in the half-marathon. As he had a couple of fourth placings, I am sure he enjoyed the reward of a silver medal. I was really pleased that many years after my Townsville Road Runners days I had two TRR old boys in Joe Scott and John Herridge, join me with medals at a World Masters Games. Running-wise, that was pretty much the end of the road. I had a few pro runs in 2003, and when I complained about my ridiculous handicap as I had chronic injuries which were not going to improve, there was little sympathy. In a parting aside, the wife of the handicapper said I should just retire. I thought that if that was the attitude when I had been intermittently running with them for thirty years, I would!

*

One day in February 2003, Sandy returned from golf and said she had some diarrhoea issues that were not settling, and she would get it checked out at the doctors. The doctor booked her in for a colonoscopy, and the diagnosis was bowel cancer. A visit to oncology at Box Hill Hospital followed and the news was not good. At age fifty, Sandy had gone from fit and healthy, playing golf, to a fortnight later being given a death sentence. The specialist said he was amazed that she did not have more symptoms earlier. Her body was riddled with cancer which could not be eradicated, and she could expect only eighteen months more of life.

What followed was a roller-coaster of operations, chemotherapy and radiotherapy that went on for a long period. An initial major operation removed a large portion of Sandy's bowel and left her with a stoma to bypass the operation site. Recovery was slow and upon discharge, there were the difficulties of chemo and radiotherapy at regular periods. Quality of life after each of these was dubious to say the least, but it was life.

Kimberley was still causing disruptions to family life, and with her brother down in Melbourne, her angst was focused on Sandy. My half-sister, Donne, who had her own history of mental health issues, sent me a list of the signs and symptoms of borderline personality disorder. I ticked off eight of the ten factors as being exhibited by Kim and strongly suspected this was a likely diagnosis. However, nothing could be done if the sufferer was unwilling to admit they had a problem.

At one stage in the early days, we were both in separate hospitals, as I had surgery to repair an inguinal hernia. The biggest problem I had was being yelled at for trying to carry my own luggage at the time of discharge. Apparently, that could have undone all their good work, and I had an extended period of no heavy lifting.

Through it all, Sandy was optimistic and

non-complaining. When able, she got on with life as best she could and her boss-friend Michelle was a great support. Kimberley was living at home again for some of this period, and her behaviour had not improved. On one tragic evening, Sandy had cooked a meal and Kim came out and threw it over her mother. Without going into detail, Kim was removed from the house and placed short-term in a motel. Michelle arranged a bungalow in a suburban Kilsyth backyard where she could live without sharing with another, and we relocated her to this accommodation. This was not done lightly but in fairness to Sandy; she deserved the best quality of life available to her during her terminal illness.

In order to stay alive, Sandy needed to undergo further surgery, which she was willing to have to prolong her life. There was a serious problem in that she was so weak that she was unlikely to survive the operation, and so they kept feeding her through a PEG tube in order to build her up. At one stage, Sandy passed a record amount through her stoma (sixteen litres in twenty-four hours) but the nutrients were not being absorbed.

Eventually, the surgery was performed and after a long recovery, some vital time at home away from hospitals ensued. We even managed a trip to see Clitheroes at Burleigh Waters where Sandy got to do a whale-watching cruise on Moreton Bay. All the medical intervention was difficult, but it enabled Sandy to extend the eighteen months to three years.

John and Michelle were well along in construction of the Toolangi Tavern, but it was overdue and over budget. Rather than see them fall at the last hurdle, I contributed a loan and leaned on my boss to do likewise. Thankfully, this was able to get them through. When I visit and stand on the back deck looking out at the impressive mountain vista, I can brag that I stained this deck!

After one stay in hospital in 2005, Sandy was discharged to come home. When I noticed her condition, I kept saying, 'Surely you are not well enough to be at home.' I was too obtuse to realise that she had been sent home to spend her final days here instead of in hospital. On the way past Dixons Creek, we called in and collected a tiny Jack Russell-Maltese-Shih Tzu crossbred puppy to be her companion.

Not long after, Sandy suffered seizures and an ambulance was called for a final trip to hospital. After fighting it for a week, lapsing in and out of consciousness, Sandy passed away on 28 September 2005, aged fifty-two. What is the old saying? 'Only the good die young.'

CHAPTER 19
Back to Kyneton and family

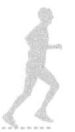

I don't think there is any rule book. I had long known what was coming and continued to work through so I would have employment. I just got on with life, except that employment was becoming an issue. I think the mantra in the timber industry was 'get big or get out'. Gary decided to close the Alex Demby Timber Company and merge it with a business partner's mill in Morwell. There would be a limited number of jobs in Morwell, so redundancies were offered to those who had that preference.

I settled for a redundancy, though I stayed around a while longer. After finishing up, I asked Gary what he was going to do with all the dry timber waiting to be processed. I arranged to stay on a temporary basis with a skeleton workforce to grade and process the stockpile. I also put my house on the market, as I had decided to move to somewhere larger, with a few more facilities.

My future home location was decided when I met

Frances online. She happened to reside in my old home town, and after a period, we decided that I would move over there. In due course, my house sold and thirty-eight years after leaving Kyneton, I completed the big circle by moving back. Sharing a holiday house converted from a machinery shed and helping Frances with work on her twenty-acre farm suited both of us. She was working full-time as a midwife at Kyneton District Health and I did some jobs around the place and most cooking until a job came along.

The initial job was courtesy of Frances. I was put on as leave relief at the supply department of Kyneton District Health. It was rather ironic that I had escaped computers arriving in the Army health system only to have to pick up that knowledge sixteen years later. The job continued when a new system called Oracle was adopted and I kept the supply department going while the regular storeman, Adam, went off to learn all about it. I then had to stay on to learn from him so I could do leave relief.

My only running was a low-key participation in the annual fun run that the hospital conducted. Since renewing acquaintances with Townsville Road Runners, I frequently went up there for a midwinter holiday. I stayed in either North Ward or over on Magnetic Island and occasionally went for a training run with the local runners. I was aware that they held an annual Townsville Running Festival but saw no need to coincide with that.

During this period, I went to see a top orthopaedic

surgeon for a diagnosis of my chronic left hip pain. Dr Peter Wilson happened to have also been the young doctor whom I assisted to perform wedge resections at 4 Camp Hospital in Townsville back in 1971. His advice was that I needed a hip replacement, but not urgently, as I would know when the time was right. I had seen TV footage of this operation and it was going to have to be incapacitating for me to undergo it.

As the years rolled by, we moved to an old house in Maxwell Street, Kyneton and spent some time renovating it. When the council wouldn't allow it to be subdivided, the decision was made to buy in the new estate across the Campaspe River and build a house there.

Sandy's little dog, Maggie, accompanied me and was soon best of friends with Fran's walk-in stray, Kev. Kev knew that Maggie was in charge, but she had more difficulty in persuading Frances of the pecking order. They enjoyed a walk along the river but as they grew older and wiser, they would just sit under the bridge and wait for us to put in the hard yards.

Frances retained her farm and a short trip across town ensured the goat herd were always happy. Maggie learned a lot up at the farm, like not to get between a goat kid and its protective mother. There was also the incident with the new pet doves. It seems they couldn't or wouldn't fly and so they were fair game; Maggie was only trying to return them to the stables but got excited. Newly born chicken culling was another specialty. One had a gammy leg and wasn't doing well; it was delicately lifted into Maggie's mouth and, err, culled!

I got a bit more early morning work in the 'box room' at the Kyneton Post Office, which fitted in fine, even when I was required at the hospital. As the local hospital work dried up, I applied for a similar position at Castlemaine Health. The supply manager gave the job to a friend he knew from Castlemaine, but his assistant Carolyn saw more in me and a few days later, I received a phone call. Peter, the supply manager, had been persuaded to hire me as well on a casual-temporary basis, particularly as I already knew the Chiron computer system.

I bounced around between the three jobs for a while and then chanced my arm at Castlemaine. With the new Oracle system coming in and my knowledge of it from Kyneton, I said I would give up my other jobs if Castlemaine were willing to put me on full-time. That is what transpired, and my new permanent job was half an hour north of Kyneton in a larger hospital.

A lot of my early work was in data entry for Oracle and in helping to set it up properly, I gained plenty of knowledge. All that was involved was ordering all the stores required to operate a medium-sized hospital and ensure they were delivered to the end user in a timely fashion. Castlemaine Health also had a fundraising fun run which I went in, and on my now annual trips to

Chapter 19 Back to Kyneton and family

Townsville, I would attend whatever club events were on.

*

Now it is time for an update of family. You will recall that my New Zealand maternal grandmother committed suicide at the time my father returned to Australia with young Gwen. Shortly after I was born, Gwen and my father separated and she moved to Woodend North with me and two siblings. My sister Lauren only lived for two years. When I was aged four, unbeknownst to me, my father was killed in a motor vehicle accident.

My mother married a widower, Don Wilson, and our blended family of five boys lived at the caretaker's house in the Woodend Cemetery. Later, Donne and Warrick were added to the large family. My brother Bryan had to change his name to Garth, as there was already an older Brian Wilson in the group. When I was aged ten, Gwen attempted suicide and very nearly succeeded. I imagine I was fortunate not to end up in care or be relocated with a foster family. The older stepbrothers have gone their separate ways and I have not kept up with their progress.

My brother Bryan married a Kyneton nurse, Pam Carne, and they had two children, Laurae and Daniel. When I was home on Christmas leave from Townsville in 1971, I had a hold of Laurae when she was very young. Her name is a combination of two people dear to them:

Lauren (deceased) and Pam's dad, Ray. I didn't see Laurae (Rae) again for many years.

After their divorce, Bryan moved back to New Zealand where he had been born and remarried. He and Helen had children Rachel and Matthew when living in Christchurch and then Geraldine elsewhere on the South Island. He ran a business called Bryan's Bargain Barn which sold pre-loved goods and ran a dry-cleaning service. I caught up with his new young family when I visited New Zealand for the Defence Marathon in 1984.

In the early 1990s, Bryan developed lung cancer, possibly due to a combination of many years of inhaling dry-cleaning chemicals and tobacco smoke. He did not have treatment except for pain relief and therefore his capitulation was more rapid than it needed to be. A few years later, his wife Helen also passed away and teenagers Rachel and Matthew were left parentless.

I caught up with my mother periodically as she bounced around between commission housing and periods of mental health hospitalisation. After Don Wilson's alcoholism got the better of him and he passed away with cirrhosis of the liver, the only one who was close to her was her only daughter, Donne. When I saw Gwen assaulting the only person who cared for her, that was the final straw for my (non-) relationship with my mother.

Donne grew to be a good and decent person who had her potential also affected by family history and genetics. She suffered from abuse in the family home, and this always affected her. As an adult, she married Adrian Roberts but unfortunately, he neglected to mention that he was homosexual. Then she had her own mental health issues and while an inpatient, she met another sufferer who managed to give her an STD. Donne then met a tall, dark and handsome stranger. In fact, Jean-Pierre Rausmakua was from Vanuatu and they may well have been in love, but it was very handy for him to have an Australian wife. For a while, they returned to remote Tanna Island in Vanuatu, where they lived a native existence. Perhaps this was a culture shock for Donne, and I am sure she resented being a possession in a male-dominated society. They soon returned to Australia. Keshet Lani was born and after some unfaithfulness by Jean-Pierre, the couple parted and their son Jourdain was born to a single mum. Mental health issues occurred after the birth of both children, but they got by. In a case of history repeating itself, Donne met and married a widower, David Morgan, who had a whole bunch of sons. The essential difference is that he was a nice, decent husband and father.

Years later, my sister Donne disappeared from the family home. The worst was feared and many months later, her body was found in a remote shed. The family genetics had taken another suicide victim. It is now left for her children Keshet and Jourdain to have a happy and long life.

I was never as close to her brother, Warrick, and had

little to do with him. He married Veronica and they had a couple of fine daughters before they also chose to live apart.

I have mentioned them at this stage because in 2012, Laurae (Rae) came back into my life and family life became even more interesting.

The phone rang at Fran's farm cottage; it was Rae, who arranged to visit for a catch-up. When I met her, she had certainly changed. She now had bright pink hair and was the manager of a well-known singing group called The Living End.

I should emphasise here that I knew absolutely nothing about my paternal line for most of my life up to this time. I had frequently questioned my mother, but all I received was a stony silence. On my birth certificate, there was no mention of a father, just mother, Gwendoline June Harvey. Many years later, I came into possession of a letter from 1957 from the Children's Welfare Department who had requested information about Bryan and me regarding compensation proceedings after the death of my father, Lloyd. I assume my mother just ignored the letter. Times were tough and I am sure we could have used some compensation!

Back in the 1990s, Donne passed a letter to me from a firm of solicitors located in Kyabram. It was dated 1971 and was regarding the death of a Della Tonks of Stanhope, back in 1965. After reading the letter, I realised that Della

Chapter 19 Back to Kyneton and family

was my paternal grandmother. The solicitors were trying to finalise the estate and were holding funds for the children of Lloyd Tonks, deceased. They had searched the Victorian Register of Births, Deaths and Marriages (BDM) but found no record.

Once more, if anything was done in response to this letter, my brother and I were never informed. It did, however, give me some useful information and I contacted the law firm to learn more. Their response was that, yes, there was information, but Gwen had left them instructions that no information was to be passed on during her lifetime. I now know why there was no information available from BDM. Bryan was born in New Zealand, I was born in NSW and my mother lied on Lauren's Victorian birth certificate. This dead end was not something I was going to mull over. I put the letter in the bottom drawer and got on with living.

Rae took this information and over the next weeks became an investigator *par excellence*. She learned of relatives and traced the Tonks family history right back to Richard Tonks' conviction for larceny in the 1800s and subsequent transportation to the penal colony of Tasmania.

A few weeks later we were in a lounge room in suburban Wantirna South, meeting my Uncle Dennis Tonks and Aunt Margaret. We were a little late in meeting Dennis as he was suffering Alzheimer's and was only partially aware of proceedings. Margaret, however, was a great help as she was able to fill gaps and personalise the bare facts that Rae had uncovered. Here, we also met for the first time my cousin Leighton.

I found it ironic that I had spent years visiting my half-sister Donne in Wantirna South and all that time my unknown relatives were living within a kilometre. Dennis was quite a bit younger than Lloyd and Geoffrey, but Margaret was able to tell of the hard life his older brothers had in assisting their father to share-farm in Kyabram. The older brothers were very close and often worked and played together as adults. I was further surprised to learn that I had followed in my father's footsteps by joining the military and working in the forestry industry.

My Aunt Phyllis had passed away, but I was amazed to learn that Uncle Geoffrey was still alive and well in his eighties. He was living under the name 'Jack Chivers' on a property he owned in the remote village of Mitta Mitta in north-eastern Victoria. The next trip was up there to meet him and get further insight into his adventures with my father in the pre- and postwar years.

It was amazing to find I had more family than I could have envisioned. While I got to meet some more cousins, I have not imposed myself on their lives. A lot of this is because I had spent a fairly solitary existence as far as family went, and I didn't really know how or how much

Chapter 19 Back to Kyneton and family

to interact. It is enough that we each know of our mutual existence and catch up when convenient.

When Don Wilson had passed away, he was buried in the Woodend Cemetery. The grave is located exactly where Gwen had tried to take her own life all those years ago. After many years of struggle, Gwen developed pancreatic cancer in her eighties and is now interred in the same grave site. She passed away, still refusing to discuss or acknowledge that I ever had a father.

In 2014, Dennis succumbed to Alzheimer's and a few years later, age caught up with Uncle 'Jack'. I got to meet Aunt Margaret's other children, Barry and Michelle, and their families. Jack also has several children from two marriages who are also my cousins. It was interesting to learn that in 2000 I had carried the Olympic Torch into the same town that my father and Winnie had been forced into marriage before I was born.

*

During my few years at Castlemaine Health, the supply manager retired due to ill health. Carolyn took over, which was fine by me until she decided to depart as well. I put my hand up for the position, which had been downgraded to supply coordinator, and was successful. In a few years, I had gone from temporary leave relief to being in charge, but all was not roses, as Carolyn had probably been aware. The plan was that I facilitate a change to Bendigo Health doing all the supply ordering and the local staff just delivering to the various users. Our jobs in supply would then be downgraded again. I thought this unethical, and as I had active service from my Vietnam days, I made my opposition clear by retiring in 2014.

I had served on in the Army upon my return from active service in South Vietnam and the unit I served in was disbanded at the end of Australia's participation. So, I just got on with my career, life, family and running. There was not much time or interest in becoming part of the ex-service social groups.

When I was working at Demby's Mill in Toolangi, I was lent a book called *Tiger Men: A Young Australian Soldier Among the Rhade Montagnard of Vietnam*, written by Captain Barry Petersen about his service in Vietnam. It was a thoroughly enthralling book about an amazing soldier. (Often, when I watch the movie *Apocalypse Now*, I wonder if Colonel Kurtz was modelled on Barry's service with the Montagnards in the mountains of central Vietnam.) It was then I realised that Petersen was a member of the Australian Army Training Team – Vietnam (AATTV), the very same unit that I had served in.

A bit more research saw me learn that the AATTV had served in Vietnam for ten years. Although only numbering about a thousand members in that period,

Chapter 19 Back to Kyneton and family

they were most highly decorated Australian Army unit that served in Vietnam. The only four awards of the Victoria Cross during the war went to members of the AATTV. Of these, two were posthumous to Major Peter Badcoe and WO2 Kevin Wheatley. WO2 Ray Simpson had since passed away and WO2 Keith Payne remains alive today. I was surprised to learn that in my Townsville days, when I had billeted Colin Payne, a young sprinter from Mackay, he was a son of Keith.

I have also learned that many of my fellow medics (RAAMC) with whom I had served were also members of the AATTV: people such as my first CSM Bob Allen, Peter Hulsing, Mick Dolensky and Ian Felton. In 2011, I travelled to Canberra for a reunion, the forty-fifth anniversary of the formation of 'The Team'. It was great to meet many of these legendary soldiers and renew acquaintances with some whom I had served with in 1972.

Part of the celebration was an afternoon tea at Government House, Yarralumla, where we were guests of the Governor-General. I met up with my fellow Long Hai advisors John Nolan, Bruno Carbone and Roy Chamberlain. I was also amazed to see that 'Captain Zero' Ed Nicholas from the Around Australia Relay was another former member of the AATTV. Keith Payne was also feted as, at the time, the only living winner of the Victoria Cross. I was also delighted to reacquaint with Don Targett with whom I had served at HQ AATTV in Ba Ria, as he was the only person there of a similar vintage to myself.

Five years later, the next reunion was held in Brisbane for the fiftieth anniversary. A highlight was a trip to the Land Warfare Centre at Canungra where a commemoration was held in The Grove. On the base where we trained before our AATTV service, a memorial grove has been planted. Every member of The Team has a tree and all too many have the ashes of a deceased member interred at their base. The Grove is a unique, sacred place and pays tribute to all who served and, in particular, those who failed to return home alive.

I remember Roy Chamberlain saying that if we hung around for a few years, we would be running the show as most of the members were ageing rapidly. This is because, particularly in the early 1960s, only officers and warrant officers with years of experience and service were considered for The Team. Ten years later, Don and I were able to be selected as young corporals, after passing a tough training period with limited experience. Hence, we are up to twenty years younger than many members of the AATTV.

We had left in a hurry in late 1972 when the Whitlam Government were elected. I spent my career with one medal for active service, as I had clocked up only four months before it all ended. Many years after my retirement from the Army, I read a book by Captain Terry

Smith, called *Training the Bodes: Australian Army Advisors training Cambodian infantry battalions - A postscript to the Vietnam War*. He had served down the road from Long Hai at our sister camp, Phouc Tuy. By reading it, I learned that I was entitled to wear two Meritorious Unit Commendation ribbons that we had been awarded for our service. All those years and nobody had seen fit to inform me! Even then, when I applied, the authorities rejected my application without giving a reason. I appealed the decision and common sense prevailed. It remains a privilege to have been able to serve with this elite unit of the Australian Army.

*

My story would not be complete without reference to my long-held passion for horse racing. This no doubt commenced on hearing Hi Jinx winning the Melbourne Cup over the loudspeakers at Woodend Primary. In those days, Don Wilson worked at Woodend's Shirley Park Stud which bred racehorses. There was also a local trotter named Delvin Dancer who won fifteen races in succession. For most of my life, this was generally the source of my Saturday entertainment if I had nothing else going on.

Later, when I had moved to Kyneton and had the freedom to direct my discretionary spending there, I went into horse ownership in a small way. It came about in 2011 when I won a small percentage of a Big 6 in a TAB wager. This was no ordinary win, as a little known former New Zealand trainer called Chris Waller trained two of the six winners. They were both imports and won at long odds; hence, the full prize dividend was more than a million dollars. My small share was an unexpected windfall and I decided to use it to buy a share of a racehorse.

I saw a handsome black colt sired by the champion Lonhro and bought into him. A factor in this choice is that the trainer was Chris Waller. I submitted my choice of a name and was delighted when Eight Straight received the most votes. I was even more delighted a year later when he ran second in metropolitan Sydney races at his first two starts, ridden by star jockey Hughie Bowman. At start three, in the last two-year-old event of the season on a bottomless Heavy 10 track and racing over 1600 metres, Eight Straight was victorious.

His future was rosy, and we knocked big offers from Hong Kong. He went for a spell and over the next two years, everything that could go wrong did. He never won another race and was retired injured as a mere four-year-old. My dine-out story from this is that I had a horse named Eight Straight with Waller and Bowman shortly before they became famous with Winx, who won about twenty-five straight. That's racing.

CHAPTER 20
Running as a Master

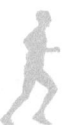

In 2015, aged in my early sixties, I adjusted my annual northern visit to coincide with the Townsville Running Festival. I entered the ten-kilometre event and ran along with the forty-minute pacemaker, having a chat to him. When I reached halfway, I was gasping for oxygen and couldn't hold the pace. I was disgusted to find my final time was forty-five minutes, a big personal worst even though I was first M60. After the guest runner had narrowly missed an attempt at breaking thirty minutes, it was recognised that the course was too long.

I gave little consideration to the fact that I hadn't competed for a dozen years or that I was getting old. I resolved that next year, I would train properly and return to do the marathon on the fortieth anniversary of my win in the Townsville Marathon, the only marathon I have won.

I commenced 2016 with a pipe-opener in January's

Victorian Masters ten-kilometre race at Braeside. I finished second as a M60 in a poor 44 mins 45 secs. Although it was agreed the course was 200 metres long, it was on a par with my Townsville effort and more training was required. In the first half of 2016, I managed to get some consistent training in without injuring myself.

In June, I had my first serious Victorian Masters competition since the World Masters Games in 2002. The question would be how much I had lost in the past fourteen years. I ran the Victorian Masters (VMA) Eight-kilometre Cross-country Championship at Yarra Bend. I placed third as a M60 in 34 mins 35 secs, well behind a bloke named Les Williams (32 mins 52 secs), whose name I remembered vaguely from my days as a professional track runner.

A month later was the VMA Eric Greaves Memorial ten-kilometre road race on the beautiful gravel paths of Braeside Park. In an earlier edition, I had copped a rubbishing from the club captain, Eric Greaves, when I took the incorrect path on the second lap. 'Wrong Way Wilson', he dubbed me, which was a bit rough as there was less of a crowd to follow on lap two. I always had good battles with Eric and on this occasion, I had thanked him for whistling me back by beating him.

In this edition of the M60 race, Les Williams (40 mins 3 secs) sped away from the start. Although he tired in the later stages, there was no pulling him back. I finished second (41 mins 32 secs) and a new runner, Yassine Belaabed, (41 mins 41 secs) was close behind. The M60 was turning out to be a very tough age group to be able to taste victory in. I did, however, get the feeling that if I could stay in touch with Les over a longer distance, I could wear him down. We all age-graded between 83 and 83.35 per cent, which is solid running and extremely close. A world best level performance is 100 per cent, and this was one of many days when Lavinia Petrie achieved just that with 101.12 per cent!

My previous marathon had been my over-ambitious debacle with an injury at the World Veteran Championship in 2001; that had put me off attempting a marathon for fifteen years. Now I was back in Townsville to see if I could still complete the distance. I hadn't done a Townsville Marathon for forty years, but of course I expected to win my M60 age group – based on nothing whatsoever!

I found the race difficult and there was some walking in the latter stages. My official time was 3 hrs 29 mins 28 secs (although I personally timed 3 hrs 27 mins), so it seems I had lost half an hour over my retirement period. Taking that into account, I was surprised when club president Brian Armit congratulated me on the excellent time. He also expressed surprise to see me running, as it seems I was (quite rightly) regarded as a former runner, only to be read about in old paper clippings.

I was a bit surprised, at the presentation, when a David Von Senden was announced as the first M60. It wasn't even close as he was about ten minutes clear of me. I had never heard of him, but then I hadn't followed athletics results for a long time. My bruised ego was soothed later when I discovered that David had won his age group in the Comrades Marathon for the past couple of years. This eighty-eight-kilometre event in South Africa is the world's most famous ultramarathon. What he was doing here in a Townsville Marathon I don't really know!

Once I had recovered, that should have been the end of my comeback. Townsville Marathon forty years on – tick, done! However, the VMA 10-Mile at Brimbank Park in September was an opportunity to see if Les Williams could be beaten. In his usual style, Les flew out, averaging under four minutes per kilometre, and it was difficult to stay in touch. I was fully aware that we were going way too hard. I must have learned something over the years. It took until a surge up the final hill, but I finally got past Les who appeared gone. The problem was that in doing so, I felt a strange tearing of tissue between my lower leg bone and my calf muscle. I still had 800 metres to endure and I knew Yassine would be coming hard. When I hit the line in 67 mins 22 secs, I had won my first M60 race since my comeback began and shown that Les was vulnerable when stretching out the distance. What about Yassine? Yes, there he was only four seconds behind me

Chapter 20 Running as a Master

again; he could really be a problem! Les was four years younger than us, and we had put a thirty-second gap up after catching him. I had an age grading of 83.08 per cent which is close to the best I am capable of.

Two post-race conversations remain in my memory. I had a good chat with Yassine and found out his background. He had not been in Australia long, after a journey from a childhood goatherd in Algeria to a long period in the US. The other was Lavinia Petrie who asked what the heck I was doing back running. She advised me not to think I was going to dominate my age group because there was a runner called John Shaw. My bemused reaction was that I had come back just to run the Townsville Marathon and had never dominated anything. I was hardly likely to at age sixty-four.

I had done a lot of training to get fit again and when I found that the World Masters Athletic Championship was returning to Australia, it seemed sensible to extend my comeback. There may have also been an element of unfinished business after what had eventuated in Brisbane in 2001. The only downside was that, once more, I was at the top end of my age group, which is quite a disadvantage.

In October, I flew to Perth, the venue for the championships. I had seen my AATTV mentor John Nolan at a reunion and now I had the pleasure of staying with him for the fortnight of the events. John lived in an outer suburb near Joondalup, well to the north, so I had a real tour of the city whenever I attended an event.

The eight-kilometre cross-country was at Perry Lakes, Floreat and consisted of four laps around a lake and parklands. I ran well and finished ninth of forty-seven starters in 33 mins 11 secs. An Australian, Alan Gower, won (30 mins 31 secs), a very close finish from Kiwi Tony Price who recorded the same time! A Tasmanian, Peter Lyden, was just six seconds in front of me, making me the third Australian. There was a team event, and I earned a silver medal as one of the three-member Australian team.

Melbourne Cup Day was on 1 November and there was a festive atmosphere at the Canning Park athletics track for the ten-kilometre track championship. The M60 event had a field of sixteen and was won by Dennis Wylie from New Zealand (39 mins 42 secs), with Ramez Riano (Columbia, 39 mins 44 secs) second and Samuel Koskei (Kenya, 39 mins 45 secs) third. That would have been a great race to watch, but I was still busy running on the far side of the track. I spent most of the race as first Australian, but Leon Brookes came home solidly to pip me by thirty seconds, with Peter Lyden a further thirty seconds back. I was the oldest runner in the field and was pleased with seventh place (40 mins 58 secs) and second Australian.

There were a couple of other highlights. When the Melbourne Cup was won by Mt Macedon local Almandin,

Chapter 20   Running as a Master

I heard someone shout that the winner came from his home area. I responded with, 'No, he comes from my home area!' That is how I got to meet fellow Woodend–Kyneton runner Gordon Muir. The other person I met for the first time was the meet celebrity. John Gilmour was competing and he had been a pioneer of Veteran competition in Australia and an international legend of the sport.

So far so good as far as backing up and not getting injured. The gap of five days between races no doubt assisted. My host John Nolan took me down to his son's property near Margaret River, where we enjoyed a couple of days of relaxation. As the marathon was down near Perth with an early start, I relocated to spend the last couple of days with my friend, Joyce, who lived at Ascot which was close to the event and Perth Airport.

The marathon course was a double out and back, starting near Crown Casino at Burswood and heading west along the Swan River. The only hill was The Causeway which took the field across the river. It was fairly chaotic at the registration area and they had to delay the start until they had everyone registered. I spotted only one person I recognised – Mick Francis from an earlier meeting in the Australian 100-kilometre championship twenty years previously.

With all age groups competing together as well as a concurrent half-marathon, there was no point in doing anything except running your own race. The first half was trouble free, but around the thirty-kilometre mark, I saw a toilet and thought I had better take advantage of it rather than have a problem later. This cost me a couple of minutes and then everything was a bit of a struggle. In the latter stages, I passed another Aussie and told him to keep going because he might be in the winning team. I had to do some intermittent walking in the final kilometres. Inspired by a different Australian coming past me and my proximity to the finish, I managed to run the final kilometres and be close behind him.

We were both so stuffed we just sat there on the lawn near the finish line. While recovering, we had a chat and I learned that his name was Peter Black and he was from Greenvale, a Melbourne suburb. After a while, Joyce and Chas located me and offered a lift back home to freshen up and recover. I was not going to pass that up. In farewelling Peter, I advised him to stay for the presentation as I reckoned he might be one of the first three Australians.

Much later that afternoon, I looked up the results and saw that the brilliant John Shaw (Australia, 2 hrs 55 mins 42 secs) had won from Alvaro Diez (Spain, 2 hrs 57 mins 20 secs). There were ten-minute gaps back to a Pole and a Brit and then there we were – Peter Black, fifth (3 hrs 24 mins 1 sec) and Greg Wilson, sixth (3 hrs 24 mins 17 secs).

At age sixty-three, John Shaw had come fifth in the

entire field and was a class act – Lavinia had not been exaggerating! Just as obvious was that Peter and I were the next best Australians and as such, we had won a team gold medal. What was just as certain was that I had been relaxing in the bath while I should have been at the presentation!

It was getting late on the final day of competition, and by the time we drove to the main athletics venue, they were packing up. Nevertheless, we found the responsible official and I was handed a medal. A very low-key celebration but totally my own fault. I was pleased with the five-minute improvement from my Townsville comeback. I had performed much better than my previous attempt at World Masters Championship level and seemed to have escaped injury. It seems I was a runner again, at least until my next retirement.

I commenced 2017 with my usual visit to Braeside for the Lindsay Thomas Memorial ten kilometres. My good efforts of last year carried over as I was second overall and first M60. In running 43 mins 13 secs, I was 1 min 30 secs faster than 2016. I followed up in April with the Victorian Masters three-kilometre championships and won the M60 in 11 mins 46 secs. Then in May in a real test against good runners, I came through with the Victorian Masters M60 ten-kilometre championship. The following result shows how close the top finishers were.

1: Greg Wilson, 41 mins 48 secs, 81.17 per cent

2: Ewan Wilson, 42 mins 13 secs, 80.37 per cent
3: Russell Johnson, 42 mins 32 secs, 79.77 per cent
4: Peter Black, 43 mins 16 secs, 77.02 per cent.

Finally, the age gods assisted me at a Masters meeting. Darwin was host for the first time of an Australian Masters Championship and due to the heat, they decided to stray from the Easter tradition and hold it in midwinter. As luck would have it, the first event was held on my sixty-fifth birthday.

The championships are held over four days and there is a race every day if you so desire. The problem is, of course, how will your ageing body cope?

Australian Masters M65 ten-kilometre championship result:

1: Greg Wilson, 42 mins 24 secs, 79.03 per cent
2: Ron Schwebel, 43 mins 21 secs
3: Ralph Henderson, 45 mins 53 secs.

I had won my first ever Australian Masters championships but didn't leave anything in the tank as I was keen to get home in front of M60 runner Peter Lyden. That was a mistake as I should have done what the runner-up did: coming off the podium, Ron said that he was saving himself.

On day two, I was stiff and sore from the ten-kilometre race and only decided to compete in the 1500 metres at the last moment. After a first slow lap, I threw caution to the wind and took off. Giovanni Puglisi was the only

Chapter 20 Running as a Master

one to follow and he kicked clear in the last lap.

Australian Masters M65 1500-metre championship result:

1: Giovanni Puglisi, 5 mins 26 secs
2: Greg Wilson, 5 mins 28 secs
3: Ron Schwebel, 5 mins 43.80 secs.

I was amazed that my age grading in this unsuitably short event was way better than my previous win at 83.25 per cent. Ron was again well back, and once more he said, 'I was saving myself'. By this time, I didn't know what to make of him, but he was running out of events if he didn't get fair dinkum soon!

Day 3 Australian Masters M65 5000-metre championship result:

1: Ron Schwebel, 20 mins 7 secs
2: Giovanni Puglisi, 20 mins 20 secs
3: Greg Wilson, 20 mins 55 secs.

I had started fast with a view to breaking twenty minutes, but in the second half I really struggled.

Day 4 Australian Masters M65 eight-kilometre cross-country championship result:

1: Ron Schwebel, 32 mins 56 secs
2: Giovanni Puglisi, 33 mins 37 secs
3: Greg Wilson, 34 mins 5 secs.

I lasted only three kilometres before becoming non-competitive and just plodding on to seal a minor placing. In the ten-kilometre, I had beaten Peter Lyden and now

I was two minutes behind him. However, four medals in four days was a great result and the lesson I learned from Ron Schwebel was even more valuable: pace yourself or suffer the consequences.

After Darwin, I struggled to run. I am not sure what the illness was, but nausea and dizziness persisted. I had a month in Townsville and couldn't run so I walked quite a bit. I had three lacklustre club races and a couple of three-hour runs for a poor marathon preparation. All things considered, I was happy to reach the finish in one piece, albeit with some walking in the last ten kilometres. I finished thirty-second in 3 hrs 47 mins, my slowest marathon and twenty minutes slower than last year, but I was first M65.

I didn't run another step until New Year's Day, 2018. Late in January, I ran in the Athletics Victoria ten-kilometre Country Championships at Ballarat. It was an extremely hot day, so the event was put off until 10 pm. I was the first M60 (43 mins) until the AV officials informed me that I wasn't eligible as I was a member of what they considered a metropolitan club. The club in question was Victorian Masters Athletics, which is an umbrella club for all Victorian Masters. After pointing out that I lived in a small town in central Victoria and very seldom visited Melbourne, I stormed off in disgust.

I hadn't met Yassine Belaabed in competition since those first few runs of my comeback in 2016. That was rectified at the Victorian Masters Championships in March.

1500 metres:

1: Yassine Belaabed, 5 mins 26 secs

2: John Cooper, 5 mins 28 secs

3: Greg Wilson 5 mins 36 secs.

5000 metres:

1: Yassine Belaabed, 19 mins 52 secs

2: Greg Wilson, 20 mins 45 secs

3: Greg Moore, 22 mins 13 secs.

My preparation was far from ideal, but it was apparent that Yassine had raised the bar and moved to another level. That 1500-metre victory was his first ever run at the distance! Not one to sulk, I was happy for Yassine and soon set off to Perth with him for the Australian Masters Championships. In fourteen years, I had been to only two and now it was in consecutive years.

You are never too old to learn, and I was now aware of two things. I was unlikely to beat Yassine again and I would need to spread the effort and leave something for later events. In the ten-kilometre, I advised Yassine to take it easy and save himself for other events, as demonstrated by Ron last year. However, Yassine does not really do slow. I was with him in the first half and then eased off to save myself.

10,000 metres:

1: Yassine Belaabed, 41 mins 39 secs

2: Greg Wilson, 42 mins 54 secs

3: Richard Pickup, 51 mins 12 secs.

The 1500 metres was a replay of the Victorian Championships, with one big exception. It was won by a South Australian star named Allan Mayfield.

1: Alan Mayfield, 5 mins 12 secs

2: Yassine Belaabed, 5 mins 24 secs

3: John Cooper, 5 mins 26 secs

4: Greg Wilson, 5 mins 54 secs.

I knew from Darwin that Giovanni Puglisi would be a tough opponent in the 5000 metres. Yassine conserved himself by sitting this one out. After a few laps, Giovanni had to stop for a shoelace malfunction. I took off, but to no avail – he was too fit and too good.

1: Giovanni Puglisi, 20 mins 48 secs

2: Greg Wilson, 21 mins 0 secs

3: Ron Schwebel, 22 mins 33 secs.

I was beginning to dislike these multi-day championships. Once again, in the eight-kilometre cross-country, I was flat, tired and sore for what should have been my best event. It would have been great to watch the fine bunch of placegetters, but I plugged around and it was well over by the time I arrived. Giovanni Puglisi won with Yassine Belaabed in second place and Alan Mayfield third. As for me, my buttocks felt like someone had been kicking them.

I needed recovery time, but my Townsville preparation

was now much too limited. The Townsville Marathon this time was 3 hrs 46 mins, just a one-minute improvement on last year. Something was not right, so what do I choose to do?

While up there, I got to meet fine local runners Gerry and Liz Maguire and renewed acquaintances with the man who told me to take up running. Bill Caulfield trained Liz, and although suffering cancer, was still lively and involved. He advised me that a second marathon in a year was always worse than the first. I had a different experience, but when I put it to the test, he was correct.

For some unknown reason, I decided to run the Melbourne Marathon in October, even though my previous experience there was not good. I missed my start group and spent fifteen kilometres dodging and weaving among slow and inexperienced runners. By the time I reached the 3 hr 40 mins pacer, I was already exhausted and it just got worse. It was hot and I spent most of the second half walking. The time was 4 hrs 15 mins, a personal worst by thirty minutes. It was enough for me to seriously consider going back into retirement.

CHAPTER 21
Trail to ultra

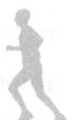

Being a late adopter of computers, smart phones, STRAVA (an app for recording running etc.) and social media, I had not been up with changes in running unless it was at the events I attended. I reluctantly got a mobile; it did phone calls, that's all! Finally, Telstra copped onto me and made G2 redundant. I was forced into owning something called a Smartphone and also had a Facebook page set up. Even so, I was not really in the new millennium.

All my training was done solo as there never seemed to be any other runners around Kyneton. Online, I discovered a Facebook group called Macedon Ranges Trail Runners and that got me thinking. Perhaps this was the place to meet some runners, but what was trail running? During my career, most of my good runs had been on rugged courses with steep hills, so it was worth a try. In November, I met Anna Jacometti at Woodend and went with her to join a group at the Macedon Scout Camp.

Chapter 21 Trail to ultra

There was a group of about ten, and off we went walking up a hill. I wondered what I had got into. Fifty minutes later when we summited Mt Macedon, I was grateful that we had walked. Then there was running, and it was nice, social exercise in invigorating bushland. I kept coming back for my weekly fix as well as doing my solo runs in Kyneton.

In December, Libby Nuttall organised a practice run for a nearby trail race called the Gold Rush Trail Run. I enjoyed the course along Sailors Creek and decided to join the group in my first trail race. I had noticed that once the course departed from the Hepburn Springs football field, the trail was very narrow, with passing an impossibility for a few kilometres.

On race day, I seemed to be one of very few warming up, as it doesn't seem a priority in a 24-kilometre trail race. It allowed me a fast start, so I would not be trapped behind slower runners in the early stages. The course took me 2 hrs 26 mins 19 secs and was much more fun than my Melbourne Marathon. I don't know where I finished but think I was the second over-50. I finished in front of our dozen runners, mainly because they all lost five to ten minutes behind a slow lady who was terrified of falling into Sailors Creek.

The start of 2019 was a complete rest, as I recovered from an injury to my left knee, sustained on a fall in the Wombat Forest. By mid-January, I had only five short runs and my long one was 1 hr 20 mins in the Cobaw Range. I was in Sorrento enjoying an annual holiday at the beach when Townsville ultra runner John Nuttall rang up. He was coming down to run in the Two Bays Trail Ultra and said I should run it also. As I was just down the road, I could not think of a reasonable excuse. In hindsight, perhaps I should have pleaded lack of fitness!

I felt I would be able to cope with the twenty-eight-kilometre course, because the Gold Rush Trail Run had been almost that far. The event was in a couple of days, but when I tried to enter, they informed me that it was sold out. The only other option was the fifty-six-kilometre race from Cape Schank to Dromana and then return. Gulp, I wonder why it wasn't sold out! Not for the first time in my life, I did something silly and ticked the box.

My first crossing of the Mornington Peninsula via Arthurs Seat was a comfortable and satisfying 2 hrs 54 mins, about the same pace as my Gold Rush run, except instead of getting into my car, I had to run all the way back. It was a hot, exhausting and painful 3 hrs 31 mins, but I completed the course. It took over thirty minutes before I could hobble from the recovery tent.

The result: one hundred and fourth (eighty-eighth male) of three hundred (forty-six who didn't make the finish), first M60 by forty-five minutes (6 hrs 20 mins 47 secs).

It seems that I was again an ultramarathoner after a retirement of twenty-one years. I was absolutely wrecked,

Chapter 21   Trail to ultra

but a week later I managed a 3 hr 30 mins training run on Mt Macedon. One of our runs took us on a climb directly up the steep face of Mt Macedon called The Beast. I use the term 'run' loosely, as it was definitely not runnable.

In February was the Roller Coaster Run of twenty-one kilometres at Mt Dandenong. Luke Berry said it would be fun, so four of us car-pooled to access a priority car park near the start. The course was well named as it was all up and down with a steep climb back up to the finish. Sarah Schroeder started really fast and Anna Jacometti was also in front of me to the halfway mark. Sarah was a very talented hill runner who had been well in front of me in the Melbourne Marathon. I was surprised when I picked her up on the awful climb to the finish. I ended up thirty-ninth of 183 and the first M60 at 2 hrs 17 mins 15 secs.

All my trail runs so far had been in shorts, singlet and road shoes because what else do you need? Up on Mt Macedon, I would just drink from the tank water at various toilet blocks. My companions were aghast when I disregarded the 'Do not drink' signs. They worked on me and eventually I became an 'equipped' trail runner. On the way to Warburton, I purchased my first pair of trail shoes.

In March was the Warburton TrailFest Lumberjack of fifty kilometres. Before my impulsive Two Bays race, I had entered this early to get the free T-shirt. The start was at remote Powelltown, where a lumberjack cut through a log to set us on our way. The first twelve kilometres was beautiful trail and then we hit the High Lead. The only thing that got me up this climb was my previous experience on The Beast. Above the climb was a plateau where the trail was a horror of tripping hazards on fallen and tangled stringybark. After the Ada Tree (2 hrs 30 secs), I had to walk all the way to Starling Gap (4 hrs). From there, the course was largely downhill and I was able to run, except for a dicey wade chest-deep across a frigid Yarra River. Two very talented females beat me home: Nicole Vaughan who prevented me taking a wrong turn (5 hrs 40 mins 26 secs) and Katherine Macmillan (5 hrs 50 mins 6 secs) who took that same wrong turn but still beat me. Result: twenty-second of ninety-six in 5 hrs 57 mins 54 secs.

I felt I was running well in these events, but I was never going to be up the front and there were no age divisions. The performance could not be measured as each event was so different. I became aware of a Trailsplus Mountain Trail Series fifty-kilometre which had an age graded section, so I decided to enter, to see how I measured up against all ages at sixty-six.

I had never run in our 'local derby', Run the Rock. It was a twenty-two-kilometre race that had some hills and dirt roads as it looped the local tourist attraction, Hanging Rock, and I decided to run it. For the first time,

Chapter 21 Trail to ultra

I was beaten by one of our trail running group, and another 'oldie' as well. I was with them until a shoelace came undone, a beginner's mistake that in the frosty morning took forever to re-lace. Result: sixty-seventh of 308, second M60 (1hr 48 mins 40 secs).

In April, my new sport of trail running came head-to-head with the more conventional type. The first leg of the Trailsplus Mountain Trail Series was up against the Australian Masters Championships in Melbourne. Never one to shirk an issue, I decided to emulate Ron Schwebel and attempt both, with the first one 'soft'. Yeah, right! A soft run at an Australian Championships can be done, but is there any point?

Mid-April was busy as I assisted Frances to clean up some of her best goats at the local dog wash. She then headed up north to attend the Royal Easter Show in Sydney and I headed off to Melbourne where I purchased all the essential items that a trail runner was supposed to need. The next day, we had a group training run in the Cobaw Ranges. The past few months of having a group to run with were so enjoyable compared to my mainly solo career since Townsville. On this occasion, it was mainly the Romsey–Lancefield runners with Luke up from Newtown. This was the first day I ran with Christy Lambert who was also in the early stages of a comeback. Sarah said that Christy was so good she would beat anything Sarah had done. Tall, slim and with an effortless running style, I could well believe it. We ran for more than two hours. The next day Matt Collins, Sarah Schroeder, Christy Lambert and I backed up by joining Mat Piper, Anna Jacometti and Ryan Hawson for another 2 hrs 30 mins on the steep slopes of Mt Macedon. We were backing up after a tough day and with the strongest group of local runners, so I was impressed when 'newbie' Christy was going as well as anyone.

On Saturday 26 April, Queenslander Ian Cameron was outstanding in the Australian Masters ten-kilometre championship and he lapped Yassine. I was a further lap back, cruising along, thinking I was third. Oops! Near the end, somebody I was unaware of lapped me and I was medal-less, exactly what I deserved (44 mins 55 secs). The highlight was catching up with Gerry Maguire and Bill Caulfield from Townsville. Bill had only one other in his 1500 metres, but it was David Carr, the best ninety-year-old in the world. Bill, as the only M85, won an Australian Masters Championship.

After my event, I rapidly changed back into trail runner mode and drove to my old stomping ground of Healesville for the Maroondah fifty-kilometre trail ultra. This event was the first leg of the Trailsplus Mountain Trail Series. Twenty-four years earlier, I had run in the event the first time it was staged. I competed three times for a win and two thirds, and they were my first trail runs, well before it became a popular sport.

Chapter 21 Trail to ultra

The course was now out and back, with an internal loop on the return journey. I was accompanied by Sarah and Luke as we set off from Maroondah Dam and did the steep ascent of Mt St Leonard. At the halfway point, I stopped for a toilet break and that was the last I saw of my companions. I probably ran a bit hard, attempting to reach them, and when I arrived at the internal loop, there was not enough oxygen in my brain. Instinct told me which direction to take to the finish and off I went. Eventually, Jon Lim caught me and I asked him if I should still have my bracelet. He said no and that I still had to complete the internal loop. The devastating news was that I had already run three kilometres further and had to retrace my steps or abandon! I persevered and eventually made the finish as twentieth male in 6 hrs 25 mins 26 secs, which is not bad for fifty-six kilometres! Waiting anxiously at the finish were Sarah, who had finished off strongly for first female (5 hrs 47 mins 10 secs) and Luke who was between us. It was a poor start to the Trailsplus Mountain Trail Series for me, and even had I stayed on course, it would have been difficult to stay with Sarah.

The following weekend, I did a bit of crewing and pacing for Mat Piper who was running in Australia's toughest trail race. The Down Under 135 is held in the rugged, isolated Lerderderg Gorge and is 135 miles up and down every hill possible. It takes a couple of days and rest is almost impossible as there are tough cut-offs, which if you fail to reach, you are out. Showing great endurance, Mat finished fourth and became the only person to have completed the course twice. It seems that most people only compete once. I wonder why?

In May, I competed in the Victorian Masters ten-kilometre championships and found Yassine untouchable. I was hanging grimly onto Ewan Wilson (former a 14-minutes five-kilometre runner) but with three to go, Yassine lapped us. I moved straight onto his back, and in doing so, finally managed to shake Ewan off.

Result:

1: Yassine Belaabed, 41 mins 27 secs, 83.7 per cent

2: Greg Wilson, 43 mins 10 secs, 80.1 per cent

3: Ewan Wilson, 43 mins 28 secs, 79.5 per cent.

The next leg of the Trailsplus Mountain Trail Series, the Mount Macedon 50 kilometres, was on our local training ground. All of us who trained on the mount knew how tough this event was. Most of the locals choose a shorter course and only Kate McMunn and Zoe Ravenscroft joined me in the 50 kilometres. This was the first time I had been afraid of competing in an event. I knew that when we ran through the finish line after thirty kilometres, it would be tempting to stop, so it was important not to go too hard early.

I was running near Kate and just behind the first female during the first half. By the time thirty kilometres was reached, I was so tired I dared not stop in case I stayed there. After a shorter loop around the mountain top, it was down the Chute Track, a mess of gluggy, red clay. The runners had thinned right out and for the next lonely hour looping around Middle Gully, I hardly saw a soul.

I was cold, wet and exhausted but the big challenge remained: a four-kilometre ascent of the Goat Track back to the peak of Mt Macedon. My back was aching badly and it was difficult to even maintain a walk up the steep, rough track. When I was 800 metres from the finish, I was finally able to run again, and just as well it turned out, as Kate was closing fast!

Result:

1: Ash Watson, 4 hrs 46 mins 47 secs
13: Lisa Wilkinson, 6 hrs 37 mins 14 secs (first female)
14: Greg Wilson, 6 hrs 40 mins 50 secs
16: Kate McMunn, 6 hrs 43 mins 9 secs (second female)
41: Zoe Ravenscroft, 8 hrs 10 mins 51 secs.

All of us locals managed to reach the finish. I was amazed at how close Kate and I were after fifty kilometres. In this second leg of the Trailsplus Mountain Trail Series, I was first age graded. An indication of the difficulty of this race is that I was twenty minutes slower than in the Two Bays race and I had run six kilometres shorter. This was just as tough as I feared, and I was proud of the result.

In mid-June, I helped crew for Mat Piper at another interesting local event, a 'last one standing' race called Mirrim Wurnit, held in a farmer's paddock at Deep Creek, east of Romsey. It was a Backyard Ultra where competitors had to do a rugged 6.7 kilometre-loop every hour. If you couldn't make the start line each hour, then you were out, until there was only one remaining.

While there, I heard that one of the competitors, Kevin Muller, was in the Army. Mat completed twenty-seven laps and finished sixth of thirty-five when an injury ended his race. Kevin had lasted almost as long and when helping them pack up, I learned a bit more about him. He turned out to be the Training Development Warrant Officer for the Army's Medical Corps, the same position I had filled thirty-four years earlier – small world!

A couple of weeks later, I thought my limited comeback, which had already been exceeded, was all over. The training run seemed simple enough, Romsey to Woodend, thirty kilometres. A group of five solid runners and – oh yes! – the course was a straight line over the top of Mt Macedon. It still shouldn't have been a problem, but my arthritic left big toe was very painful and I spent the latter part of 3 hrs 40 mins limping way out the back.

How do I fix running injuries? Ahh, I remember! A week off and then go again, which I did. Many of my cross-countries have been at the end of four days' competition and have been very poor. The Victorian

Chapter 21 Trail to ultra

Masters Eight-kilometre Cross-country Championship was a stand-alone event and I hoped for a better result. One of our trail running group, Ryan Hawson, had just turned forty and he had come along to test himself out in Masters competition. I felt we should both be suited by the undulating and technical course.

It was a very cold and frosty morning. Les Williams took off like he was in a hurry to get back to the clubrooms. Ryan sat with the leaders and by halfway assumed the lead, winning clearly (M40 31 mins 35 secs, 70.1 per cent). Meanwhile in the M65, something very strange was unfolding. I was sitting right with champion Yassine and could sense he was struggling. After halfway, I was enjoying the hills and sharp bends, and had cleared out from Yassine.

In the run to the line, I could sense runners closing on me and made sure I kept running hard, just in case they were from my age group. Unbelievably, they both were, and they weren't Yassine! Two former stars of the track, Ewan Wilson and Alan Hammond, were mowing me down with their superior speed, but the line came up just in time. As for Yassine whom I had not beaten since my comeback started in 2016, even a champion can have a bad day.

M65 Victorian Masters eight-kilometre Cross-country Championship result:

1:   Greg Wilson, 35 mins 47 secs, 77.7 per cent

2: Ewan Wilson, 35 mins 49 secs, 76.9 per cent
3: Alan Hammond, 35 mins 53 secs, 76 per cent
4: Yassine Belaabed, 37 mins 22 secs, 74.4 per cent.

This age group race had the most talented and deep field, and the closest finish that I have been in on road or trail. Nobody from any age grade managed 80 per cent, which demonstrates that the conditions were tough, and no doubt that suited both Ryan and me. It's a strange game when you can be contemplating retirement one week and beating Yassine the next!

My annual trip to Townsville commenced with a solid seventeen-kilometre training run with local stars Liz Maguire and Geoff Ford. On the return trip, they shook the cobwebs loose, while my toe was again sore, forcing me to limp. My run was completed in Bill Caulfield's car and I approached the marathon with little more training and low confidence.

In the end, my solid season of trail ultras stood me in good stead for my first marathon since the Melbourne disaster. I was much stronger in the concluding stages and improved by over seven minutes on last year. Result: thirty-ninth of 170 in 3 hrs 38 mins 58 secs, first M65.

A fortnight later, it was time for the Victorian Masters ten-mile Championships, which was held on a double out and back course on Knox bike paths. The course was flat and fast but it was blowing a gale. Top W35 female Kym Osmond set a good pace for Yassine and me early, but as soon as we got a tailwind, I lost contact. Once we turned and faced the headwind, I worked and worked and got back up with Yassine. Unfortunately, the final turn was in Yassine's favour and he floated away, propelled by the tailwind. Normal service resumed and Yassine was so hard to beat.

M65 Victorian Masters ten-mile Championship result:
1: Yassine Belaabed, 1 hr 11 mins 30 secs, 80.65 per cent
2: Greg Wilson, 1hr, 12 mins 30 secs, 79.54 per cent
3: Andrew Edwards, 1 hr, 19 mins 13 secs, 72.06 per cent.

While up north, I had missed the third leg of the Trailsplus Mountain Trail Series. The final event was the Wonderfalls Trail Run, fifty-two kilometres on the steep, forested hills near coastal Lorne. Just to get us awake, we had three crossings of the icy Kennett River in the first two kilometres and then a long steep climb on a single trail. As is usually the case, I found myself running with the first female for the first thirty kilometres. Whenever we hit downhills, Melissa Marshall would surge clear and then I would pull her back on the hills. There were five loops through a central aid station and they were all different, so it would be easy to get lost. There was a long downhill after the thirty-kilometre aid station and I never saw Melissa again after that. It was then a long solo grind to the finish which included a very steep climb and, of course, three river crossings. Melissa beat me in by ten minutes and won both Wonderfalls and the female Trailsplus Mountain Trail Series. I was ninth of fifty-five in 6 hrs 22 mins 3 secs.

As I had missed one race and got 'misplaced' in another, it was unlikely that I would feature in the men's event. I had beaten younger opponents by twenty-five minutes that day, so curiosity had me hang around. Sharyn Matthews was the other Macedon Ranges Trail Runner to compete and she had run in the marathon, finishing about when I did. She was about to depart after her debut trail marathon when I suggested she check in at the results tent before going. She was the first female in 5 hrs 57 mins 55 secs – some debut!

Male Trailsplus Mountain Trail Series result:

1: David Cripps
2: Greg Wilson
3: Michael Freiberg.

The Oceania Masters Championship were on in Mackay a week later and I read the results with interest. Townsville friends Geoff Ford and Gerry Maguire both won events, as of course did Yassine. I backed up in the Burnley Half Marathon as it included the final event of the Masters' Browne Shield competition. I ran most of the way with Eastern Masters teammate Nicky Hamilton-Morris, who was doing it as a last long run before the Gold Coast Marathon. My time of 1 hr 38 mins 12 secs was a narrow season PB (77.86 per cent). Knox (and

Lavinia) won the Browne Shield every year, but this time they got a fright when Eastern Masters were only nine points behind (1099.66 to 1090.18).

A busy year, but I decided to do the Run to the Maine Half Marathon because it was local and on dirt roads. I ran almost the same time as at Burnley, so in future I would stay away from half marathons and just write down 1 hr 38 mins 28 secs. The oldest age group they had was Over-40, so, at age sixty-seven, I was first M40! Sarah Schroeder (aged forty) took a nice scalp in the 10 kilometres when she defeated champion young ultra runner Nicole Vaughan (aged twenty-nine).

I had heard of a new phenomenon called parkrun, but I had never seen the need to do one. Then the locals decided to start a Campaspe parkrun and hold it in the park where I had my first primary school sprint race back in the early 1960s. The temptation was too great and, besides, I might go close in the age graded section. I spent an hour with Anna on a training run and we ran on to compete in parkrun. What I was unprepared for was the hundreds of runners who attended from all over, because it was the first one. I came twenty-first of 320 (21 mins 11 secs) and came second in the age grading with 80 per cent. The overall winner was young professional Michael Marantelli (15 mins 33 secs, 83 per cent).

I had never run in a Marysville Marathon, which was started as a bushfire recovery fundraiser by local doctor

Lachlan Fraser. I saw no reason to break that trend and so with Sarah and Daniel Van Boom, I challenged the 50 kilometres. The crew was all from Romsey-Lancefield except for me, and perhaps that indicated the start of a splintering of the Macedon Ranges Trail Runners group. We were well represented in the marathon by Matt Collins and Christy Lambert.

As it was held near the start of summer, hot conditions could be anticipated and that's probably why I had never run in a town I loved. It was therefore difficult to believe that it had snowed the previous day and that right up to the event start, rain was belting down. The three of us ran as a group for the first ten kilometres, which was a gradual uphill. Daniel had a toilet break and as he had not reached us by the base of a climb, we didn't see him again. Sarah and I are both fine hill runners and having us together up a steep hill meant trouble for any pursuers.

There was a drink station perched on the top and I had a brief chat with Robin Rishworth before continuing. Whoosh! Away went Sarah, really meaning business. There was a fairly flat out-and-back on a plateau, which was both slushy and interesting, because some of the previous day's snow was still settled. We slipped and slid all the way down Sund's Track and returned to the finish, with still twenty kilometres to cover.

I fluked passing through at the same time that Matt and Christy did on their marathon. A brief chat during

Chapter 21 Trail to ultra

which Christy expressed disapproval of my choice of white socks, then away they went. They were moving quicker than I was, but then veered off on a different path to mine, up Keppel Falls Lookout. I passed a couple on the steep climb and then after Steavenson Falls, it was all downhill to the finish, and away they went.

I was twentieth, seventeenth male and first M60 in 5 hrs 39 mins 11 secs, my fastest fifty-kilometre since the 1990s. Sarah Schroeder was second female (5 hrs 29 mins 6 secs) and Daniel Van Boom ran 6 hrs 15 mins in his first 50 kilometres. In the marathon, Matt Collins scored 4 hours 20 minutes and Christy was third female (4 hrs 21 mins).

I completed the circle of a very active year with a return to the Gold Rush Trail Run 24 kilometres. I advised Christy to warm up and start fast to avoid being stuck behind slow runners. She did exactly that and I still had her in sight throughout the first technical kilometres. Once we hit more open tracks, Christy just took off and the next time I saw her was at the presentation.

I was thirty-fourth and third over-56 (2 hrs 20 mins 37 secs). Christy ran a superb race in a quality field for nineteenth (third female, second 36-55 female, 2 hrs 13 mins 2 secs).

CHAPTER 22
Running through the Covid years

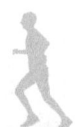

What a year of solid trail running! It was in 2019 that I had managed for the first time to compete well throughout a complete year. I was so pleased to have done it, as you just don't know what is around the corner. My thoughts on commencing 2020 were to increase my training and try to improve on the previous year's results. It started well.

In January, Sarah had booked accommodation for Two Bays Trail Run, and it was ideal as it almost backed on to the course. Less ideal was that Sarah couldn't make it and it was left to Matt Collins, Luke Beck and myself to compete. After last year, my plan was to go slower early and have a better second half, and I advised the others to do the same.

After a pre-start toilet visit, I lost track of the others among the large field. I just made my way further towards the front row due to the single track in the early stages. I ran comfortably and it wasn't until the turn around that I realised Matt and Luke were a little behind me and I became aware of my elapsed time. The halfway was reached in 2 hrs 41 mins, which was thirteen minutes faster than last year. I could be in real trouble in the second half. I did slow down (3 hrs 3 mins) but not as dramatically as last year, as I kept waiting for my teammates to come storming past.

Two Bays 56 kilometres result:

76: Greg Wilson, 5 hrs 43 mins 8 secs, second M60
122: Matt Collins, 6 hrs 1 mins 39 secs (his intended solid finish thwarted by injury)
167: Luke Beck, 6 hrs 55 mins 31 secs.

It is amazing what a difference being fit makes, as I improved my final time by 37 mins 40 secs on 2019 and was much healthier post-race. It took me only three days to recover and after that I even included some days of interval work to improve my speed.

In early February, we had a group run near Romsey to farewell Sarah who was moving to Ipswich in Queensland. Little did I know that that run was the beginning of the end of our wonderful group runs.

Since I had been travelling up to Townsville and running with John Nuttall, I became aware that he held some AURA Australian age group records for ultramarathons. It came to my attention that my oldest friend up there, Peter Lahiff, had set over a dozen of them! Peter was now living in care, as Parkinson's disease impeded his previous active lifestyle. The thought bubbled away that if they could, so could I, but it would mean making a comeback to 'real' ultramarathons.

By the end of February, I had a few track sessions under my belt and decided to have another crack at the age grade record at the Campaspe parkrun. I did the right thing and warmed up, but a toilet visit caused me to slightly miss the start and at the end, I missed the final turnoff.

After the event, I discovered the new record holder was my slightly younger and faster Masters nemesis, Les Williams. I had still taken thirty-seven seconds off my time (20 mins 34 sec, 83 per cent), so I would settle for being just off the top. Doing a fast five kilometres needed specific training and if I did a parkrun, I sacrificed my important long Sunday run.

There now seemed to be some anxiety around regarding a Chinese virus called Covid 19 and as a result, the Victorian and Australian Masters Championships were cancelled. That made my next run decision easy. I would return for another crack at the Warburton Trailfest Lumberjack 50 kilometres.

This event was unfinished business due to having to walk a lot because of the frustrating trip hazards on the middle section last year. I planned to go out slower and take it easy up High Lead, thus enabling my second half to be more pleasant. It went to plan, although I still passed nine runners up the High Lead, as some runners just do not like hills! Through to the Ada Tree and up to Starling Gap, I was able to maintain a good pace. My biggest issues were politely stepping off the track above a creek crossing, sliding down some metres and injuring a finger. I also repeatedly crashed my head into low overhead branches. On the lovely downhill from Starling Gap, I maintained a solid pace and avoided being washed away crossing the Yarra River. I maintained the pace all the way through, as I felt I may break 5 hrs 30 mins, and I was pleased to achieve that aim. My time was a satisfying 29 mins 15 secs faster than 2019. It seemed I had another top running season to look forward to.

I was eighteenth of ninety-eight (5 hrs 28 mins 39 secs), my best time during this comeback in what turned out to be my final trail event. David Bailey was first male (4 hrs 14 mins 12 secs) and Toni Garcia was first female (5 hrs 35 mins 45 secs).

Immediately afterwards, Melbourne began its long journey as the most locked-down capital city in the world. A few weeks later, the Victorian regional areas were included, as it seemed the city residents wouldn't stay home. My immediate running aim had been a trip to Canberra to attempt breaking John Nuttall's M65 AURA record for six hours. It was prior to lockdown, but the Australian Institute of Sport refused to allow use of their track, so the event was cancelled.

My training didn't change much, with a long trail run on a Sunday and very little during the week as I recovered. As there were no races, I invented a new challenge on Mt Macedon and called it 'Four Peaks in Four Hours'. It was a tough thirty kilometres with 1200 metres of climbing and took three hours and forty-seven minutes. It had climbs up Mt Towrong, Alton Rd, The Beast and the Camel's Hump and was a real challenge.

A few weeks later, the regional restrictions eased and so I repeated it with a strong group which included Matthew Collins, Christy Lambert and an extraordinary fifty-year-old 'mountain goat' called Steven Williams. Anna brought along a friend, Gemma, for this difficult introduction to trail running and they kept up well before wisely avoiding the final climb.

As there was no interstate travel, I arranged to complete a virtual Townsville Marathon on a two-lap course we designed near Woodend. I recruited a group of five and we stayed together during a comfortable first half of one hour and fifty-eight minutes. In the second half, all runners were free to go their own pace to the finish.

On lap two, Christy did an amazing twenty-one minutes negative split, for a PB of 3 hrs 35 mins. Phil Paton and I stayed together to record 3 hrs 43 mins 33 secs, which was his PB. Anna cruised through while pacing Gemma to her fine debut marathon of 3 hrs 51 mins. It was a memorable run by all – and just as well,

Chapter 22 Running through the Covid years

because we were then slammed back into lockdown.

At midnight on Tuesday following the marathon, we were to be shut down again with, would you believe, a night-time curfew. Matthew Collins decided to organise a group run at night to commemorate the occasion. Uninviting as it was at night in midwinter, a group of five hardy souls, which of course included Christy, set off along the technical single trail and 4WD tracks of the Cobaw Range.

We were cold but amused as it began snowing when we were halfway. Amusement turned to horror when I leaped onto the side of a deep, water-filled vehicle rut and my foot slipped in slowly but inevitably down into the puddle. The wet shoe was not a big deal, but down I continued as there seemed no bottom, until I was lying in a muddy, icy pond, thoroughly drenched. I was in grave danger of hypothermia, so the run was abandoned. Well sort of, as we still had to get back to our vehicles. What followed was a brisk forty minutes as I ran flat out to ensure I stayed warm. My hands, in particular, were freezing, even though Matt had given me his dry gloves. Oh yes! It was twenty-one kilometres in two hours and thirty-six minutes, and we all got home before we turned into pumpkins at midnight. A memorable way to get shoved back into lockdown again!

In August, only two people could exercise together, even in the middle of the night in the middle of nowhere.

Phil Paton wanted to attempt The Crossing to The Cross, a torture test that had been created by Mat Piper. One hundred kilometres from O'Briens Crossing through the Lerderderg Gorge, Pyrite Range, Wombat Forest, Middle Gully and twice up Mt Macedon – in the middle of winter. Christy decided it would be a good idea to accompany him in this real test of character and endurance. Some of us were spaced along the route to provide support and pacing.

I had the night shift to help them over the final cold, dark, foggy and slow nineteen kilometres. When I met them on Bawden Road for a climb up The Beast, it was getting dark and Phil was having some difficulties. They had already completed a tough eighty kilometres, so fair enough, but Christy seemed as fresh as a daisy. Off she went, setting a PB up The Beast and then sat at the top to wait for us. It was Phil's run and they stayed together all the way as we completed a loop of The Mount and then climbed back up through the fog to the Memorial Cross. The journey took them eighteen hours and fourteen minutes but on what I saw, Christy could have taken a couple of hours off that time. This run convinced me that Christy had outstanding endurance and great ultramarathon potential.

I had applied to be a member of the International Athletic Union (IAU) International Solidarity Virtual Six-Hour Run. The event was conducted to replace international events cancelled due to Covid 19. I won a spot on the AURA team to represent Australia, which was pretty cool as I had only done trail ultras during my comeback.

I selected the relatively flat Woodend Marathon course, as it gave me the best chance of seeing how close I could unofficially get to John Nuttall's M65 Australian record. I had a couple of handy pacers, although Christy slept in and I did the initial kilometres solo. Talent that she is, she jumped out of bed, drove over and was soon cruising easily beside me. We went through at my usual marathon pace (five minutes for each of twenty-five kilometres) and Anna joined me for the second half. I had a three-minute toilet break after forty-two kilometres and niggling leg cramps prevented a strong finish.

My STRAVA app recorded me at 65.591 kilometres in six hours, which would break the current record by a hundred metres. Later, I discovered the measurement of the track was inaccurate by up to two kilometres, but the performance showed that I was in the ballpark.

For the rest of the year, I continued to do long hilly runs on the Mount, mainly solo as Covid restrictions persisted. I pushed these out to forty kilometres, but it was to no avail as there were no events held. I had entered the Trailsplus Mountain Trail Series, but none of the events was held and I received no reimbursement. That was it for my trail running career, as I was not willing to be ripped off.

On Christmas Eve, I slipped on a wet tile at home and landed heavily on my right buttock. It was the worst fall I had experienced and it took months to recover. All that training for no return, and any training I did was with a pronounced limp.

In order to say something positive about 2021, I will include a horse story. I had bought into a few horses; most showed some promise and won a race or two. They were entertaining but not financially rewarding. In August 2020, I had taken up a five per cent share in a two-year-old chestnut filly with Sunshine Coast trainer Stuart Kendrick. By the end of the year for the second time, a name I had submitted was chosen for a racehorse. Funny Money was the filly's name, and with breeding of Capitalist out of Laughter, it had come to me in a flash. In February, the young filly won a 400-metre jump-out and followed up with an outstanding 850-metre jump-out win, where the jockey stopped riding halfway up the straight. In March, she debuted at the Sunshine Coast races where she led but was run down narrowly by a stablemate. It was a surprise to all. She was found to be shin sore and sent for a spell. Funny Money had only one speed and that was flat out until she got tired. On return from the spell, she was run down twice for close seconds and then held on for two narrow victories. Time for another well-earned spell, but if she never won again, that was a great start to her career.

Chapter 22   Running through the Covid years

I should have just left the running to Funny Money, as my year remained frustrating due to a mix of injury and Covid lockdowns. I did very little during the week and then tried to do a long run on Sundays. However I shouldn't have, as it was all done hobbling with what felt like a strained buttock from the fall. By May, I had gone to a physio and been given a set of strengthening exercises, which finally saw some improvement.

I went to the Victorian Masters ten-kilometre Championships, but only because I had convinced Christy and Ryan to compete. Yassine was in extraordinary form and ran 40 mins (age grade 88.7 per cent), which broke a long-standing Victorian M65 record. I was back in third more than four minutes behind (AG 79.8 per cent). My companions had more success, with Ryan still unbeaten, winning the M40 (36 mins 50 secs, 76.7 per cent). As for Christy, as expected (by me) in her debut ten-kilometre track race, she won W40 easily (39 mins 14 secs, 79.4 per cent).

Although Melbourne was still locked down, regional Victoria was given a reprieve and so I planned to fly to Sydney and be the only Victorian at the Southern Sydney six-hour event. With only two long runs under my belt, it was an ambitious undertaking, but I did want an official crack at John Nuttall's M65 record.

It did cross my mind that it was strange I could drive to Melbourne Airport and fly out, when no one from the city could. I stopped gloating about that, when at the last minute my flight was cancelled and no others were available. After a quick think, I threw my gear in the car and drove through the evening, heading north. I managed a few hours of sleep in the car and completed the journey on race morning. You would think with that sort of lead-up, I would be doomed to disappointment – and you would be correct!

I ran for six hours and was reasonably satisfied when I looked at STRAVA and it said 62.1 kilometres. It was a wake-up call when the official distance covered was 60.216 kilometres. With my preparation, I told myself that anything over sixty kilometres was a pass mark. Aged almost sixty-nine, I was well in front of the M70 record, but John Nuttall's M65 record of 65.491 kilometres seemed an impossibility. I should have been hunting it four years earlier, but I didn't know it existed, and running an ultramarathon of any kind had never entered my thoughts.

I had time to recover, but not to get fit, for my next event in July. It was the Victorian Masters eight-kilometre cross-country championship and when the 'Dream Team' were reunited on the M70 podium. Yassine dubbed us The Three Amigos. It's great to be a member of such esteemed company.

M70 results:

1:   Yassine Belaabed, 34 mins 26 secs

Chapter 22 Running through the Covid years

2: Les Williams, 36 mins 11 secs

3: Greg Wilson, 36 mins 21 secs.

My Macedon Ranges Trail Runners companions joined me in competing for Eastern Masters and had even more success. Christy Lambert was first W40 (34 mins 5 secs) and Ryan Hawson was first M40 (31 mins 49 secs), and both won very easily.

I had booked my flight to Townsville for the marathon long ago and then the Townsville Road Runners threw a spanner in the works. They advised that a celebration was planned to commemorate the fiftieth anniversary of the King of the Castle and it was only ten days before my flight up. I decided the easiest thing was to book a quick up-and-back trip and then return for the marathon.

It was great to catch up with my Townsville friends from the '70s. There was plenty of historic memorabilia on display, and three fossils lined up at the head of the field at start time. Bob Down, David Wharton and I had all run in the first King of the Castle, and we led for five metres before stepping aside. Well, the other two stepped aside, while I did the best I could to keep up. The course had been reduced by 500 metres and the climb was now a series of steps, but it was still a climb of 960 metres in a couple of kilometres. These days, it meant a walk-up and I clocked a sub-four-minutes per kilometre on the road down. Result: twenty-third in thirty-eight minutes and fifty-two seconds.

Had I a crystal ball, I would have remained in Townsville. I flew back to Melbourne and three days later, we were slammed back into lockdown. For the second year in a row, I did a virtual Townsville Marathon at Woodend. We couldn't have a group, but Gemma took the risk of catching Covid to accompany me through a 1 hr 55 mins first lap. A one-minute drink stop and a solo second half gave me a comfortable 3 hrs 51 mins 31 secs.

Towards the end of 2021, I returned to doing long Sunday runs with a couple of recovery runs mid-week. Covid had adversely affected my running and I am sure in the wider world it impacted people who already had issues and it contributed to fatal outcomes. My family's suicides had continued sadly. Bryan Harvey's son, Daniel, had been born in New Zealand, but then lived his life in Australia. He was in custody following incidents relating to drug use and was awaiting deportation to New Zealand. Rather than return to a country he did not know at all, he committed suicide in the cells. Donne Wilson's brother Warrick had, like her, a history of mental health problems and although separated, was sharing a house with his partner Terry in Far North Queensland. One day he disappeared into the bush where his body was later located.

Black humour, but it is nice to have discovered a whole paternal family who don't have this genetic problem. To the surviving descendants of the maternal line, have a good, long life and seek help if needed!

CHAPTER 23
On trail and track with Christy

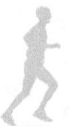

When you are in your high sixties and you lose two years of quality racing and training, it is difficult to get your running career back on track. I am sure that having Christy alongside for some of my training and races was invaluable in 2022, and we can both be proud of what was achieved. I will let that story unfold, but I'll begin with excerpts from a local newspaper article on Christy.

> For Christy Lambert every single run has a story and a proud moment. The 41-year-old Romsey mother-of-three made a triumphant return to the track after rediscovering her passion almost two decades on.
>
> Since 2019 Christy has made podium finishes at Gold Rush Trail Run, Two Bays Trail Run and Sri Chinmoy Marathon. She is also the Lancefield and Woodend Parkrun female record holder.

'Every single run has a story behind it that I am so proud of. It's a real journey to get to race day – a lot of blood, sweat and tears. I love pushing myself to the absolute limit. I seem to get emotional towards the end of a race, knowing that I have given everything that I have got and it's the end of all the weeks and months of training that have gotten me to this point.'

Christy grew up in Kyneton and began training through Little Athletics at age 14 before taking on senior athletics in South Bendigo. By the time she was 15, she wanted to improve her strength and began training under Olympian Pam Ryan. From a young age, she was competing in the 400 metres hurdles at state and national level.

'When I graduated from high school and started university I really struggled and lost my way. I dropped out of uni and started working in a horse racing stable. I took twelve months off from running and really missed the training and my coach.'

Christy returned to training for six months before learning she was pregnant with her son.

'I did try to go back to training, with the wonderful support of my family, friends and coach. I felt so guilty leaving my son with them so I could run, that I stopped.'

Chapter 23 On trail and track with Christy

Some years later Christy married Trevor, a passionate golfer and their family grew with two more children. Christy said she watched Trevor enjoy golf and craved hitting the track again.

'So one day I put my runners on and went for a run. I felt free and at peace with myself. When you love something so much you don't need much motivation.'

Christy's friend Erin Hansford introduced her to Macedon Ranges Running Club. She returned to competition with Run the Rock in 2019 where she finished second.

Now her training is up around 85 kilometres a week and includes MRRC runs, Tuesday Track Club and her own long trail runs. Christy said she feels so lucky to have her parents, husband and children cheering her on.

'I am truly grateful for all the people who have come into my life because of running and have even more gratitude and appreciation for the volunteers and marshals who make all the events possible.

'I joke around often with my running family, on how lucky we are to see, feel, hear and experience so many beautiful things. When we are all old and living in a nursing home, we will be able to look back and know that we have truly lived and didn't waste our lives.'

So, there we have a bit of background on a running friend I met in 2019 and who has, like me, made a comeback after many years of 'retirement'. It is a small world indeed when you learn that your training partner's mother attended Woodend Primary School just a year or two before you did. So, on with a year we will both remember with fondness.

After a lacklustre year, I decided to try for more training kilometres. Also, our interminable lockdowns seemed to have been lifted and there was more scope for events in which I could challenge some M70 ultra running age records.

It started with a blast on 2 January and my first training run with Christy for six months. On Mt Macedon, we stormed over thirty-seven kilometres, with almost 1000 metres of climbing, in 3 hrs 39 mins at an astonishing 5 mins 54 secs pace. Christy did some 'turn backs' so I could keep in touch, while collecting twenty-five STRAVA Segment awards!

I was impressed at Christy's fitness and during a post-run coffee, we discussed competing at Two Bays Trail Run. I didn't think I was ready for such a test but said, 'I will if you will.' This lady does not do half-measures. 'Let's do it!' said Christy. With only a debut marathon under her belt six months before, Christy was now challenging a strong and tough 56-kilometre trail race.

On the day, it was too hot and we both paid the price

Chapter 23 On trail and track with Christy

for starting too fast, but it felt like a good idea at the time. I was eighty-fourth (6 hrs 20 mins 35 secs) and Christy Lambert was third female (5 hrs 26 mins 30 secs), beaten by only two younger athletes of international standard. The event doubled as the AURA Australian Short Trail Championship, so Christy had placed third in that also in a sensational trail ultra debut. My time was similar to my debut, but I had been sensible and pulled up in much better condition. I spent several hours with Christy and family post-race, and I was the only one the next week who didn't have Covid.

I had entered the Sri Chinmoy Six-Hour at Canberra in late March. After looking at the M65 records, I changed my entry to forty-eight hours and decided to attempt one of the longest-standing records instead. Back in 1988, folk legend Cliff Young had run a hundred miles in 22 hrs 28 mins 5 secs, and it was still unbroken. It seemed an anomaly, as Cliff also had the twenty-four-hour record of 197.115 kilometres, a total which I hadn't achieved in my forties. Anyway, with no justification for thinking I could break it at age sixty-nine and three-quarters, I planned to do just that.

I set a schedule to surpass Cliffy's time and was well in front during the early stages. After fifteen hours I was tired, weaving a bit and my limbs were swelling with oedema. The same had happened in runs of this duration back in the 1990s and I was concerned that it was kidneys or heart. I stopped and lay awake in my tent until dawn and then went home.

Later on, I realised that although I had slowed down, I still had a buffer of one and a half hours before I dropped back to record pace. All I would have had to maintain was six kilometres per hour and the oldest record on the books would have been mine. At the time, I had no crew to advise me and thought I was behind the required pace. A further factor was that the longest I had run in 24 years was six hours, and I lacked faith that I could go for the required duration. Another thing I did was look into oedema in distance runners; it seems it is common and goes away a couple of days later. Hmm, the one that got away – I will never know! Result: 115 kilometres in fifteen hours.

Two weeks later, I had a 'Covid carry-over' entry for the 12-hour at Coburg. During a discussion with Christy about what was next, I mentioned it. When she asked what she should do, I replied that the main event was the 24-hour race, and that was where she belonged. Ever keen for a challenge, she agreed, although her longest race so far had been five hours and twenty minutes. I would only know if I had recovered from Canberra when I stepped onto the track.

For the Coburg 24-Hour Victorian Championship, the warm weather during the daytime detracted from overall distances completed. In a great exhibition of relaxed,

Chapter 23 On trail and track with Christy

solid running, Christy became leader of the women's field after three hours. By the time the event became difficult, she had a ten-kilometre lead over her nearest opponent. Walking became necessary and an ambitious 200-kilometre target was revised to surviving the night and achieving a 'miler', or 160.9 kilometres in twenty-four hours. During the second half of the event, Christy did more walking than running, but her opposition still couldn't make inroads on her huge lead. Time was lost off the track with 'stomach issues' due to an overcompensation for magnesium loss through sweating. The hundred miles was achieved after 21 hrs 23 mins 14 secs, and anything else was a bonus. In the final two and a half hours, Christy pushed her distance out to 175.340 kilometres, which was a mere 120 kilometres further than her previous longest race. In her debut at the distance, Christy had just won the Victorian 24-Hour Championship!

In the Coburg 12-hour, six hours after Christy started, I set off to see if I could run far enough to break my old Townsville friend Peter Lahiff's M70 record when I became old enough. I was relaxed and comfortable throughout the event until I realised that I was too relaxed and needed to lift the pace. An indication that I had not been working hard enough was that I could pick up after all that time. For the final couple of hours, I was one of the fastest runners out there as I strived to reach Peter's record mark. At one stage, chafing was an issue; John Vlahos stopped and organised some cream. Kindness is, of course, always rewarded and as the clock ticked over to twelve hours, I just managed to pass another runner; it was John. It turned out we were on the same lap. After twelve hours running, I had pipped my benefactor by a few centimetres!

I was pleased to achieve fourth place and 100.940 kilometres, which was a mere 304 metres further than the record and way off the M65 record for which I was eligible. John Nuttall was in the same event and flew out at the start with a view to breaking the M70 six-hour record. By midway, it was coming apart and he pulled out to fight another day. He suggested I needed to go out faster and while I agreed, I suggested he needed to go out slower!

During the period we were both out on the track, Christy had run four kilometres further than me in her second six hours. Then in the next six hours, I had run four kilometres further than her. Those figures make us look evenly matched, which I would take any day of the week. The huge difference is that Christy was out there for twice the time, and most of it was during the hot period.

Our local derby, the Run The Rock 22-kilometre race, was just three weeks later, which was a bit too soon after a 24-hour event. Taking that into consideration, three

Chapter 23   On trail and track with Christy

of us who train on nearby Mt Macedon took up the challenge. Outstanding fifty-year-old Steven Williams showed what he could do when he was third overall in 1 hr 25 mins. Christy also showed most of the younger runners up with second female in 1hr 42 mins 59 secs. I ran my quickest time for the undulating course, just four minutes further back in 1 hr 47 mins 18 secs. I really must race Christy more often just after she has completed a 24-hour, as I almost had her in sight.

A fortnight later, I made a last-minute decision to compete for Eastern Masters in the Victorian Masters 10-kilometre Track Championship. It was a good way to measure how I was going compared to previous years. My W35 teammate, Kym Osmond, was going quicker than I thought I could maintain, but I clung on during the first half. Gradually, I felt comfortable and with eight laps to go, took up the pacemaking. I did a negative split and made sure Kym was with me after all the work she had done.

I was first M65 with 42 mins 56 secs, equal to my Perth Australian Masters back in 2018. Putting my good performance into perspective was Yassine who was first M70 as he had suddenly become older. It hadn't slowed him down as he ran 40 mins 13 secs and broke a Victorian age record that had been set back in 1985!

At the end of May, I flew for a few days in Townsville, to attend the fiftieth anniversary of the formation of the

Townsville Road Runners. While I was absent, Steven and Christy again put in superb performances, this time in the very tough Mount Macedon 50-kilometre trail event. Steven ran this, his first ultra marathon at age fifty and came third overall in 5 hrs 7 mins. Unfortunately, it might also have been his last due to the recurrence of a chronic hip problem. I had run this event three years ago and regarded my 6 hrs 40 mins as one of my best trail performances. I was close to and between the first two females. Christy just came out and ran an hour faster and won first female in 5 hrs 41 mins – outstanding! I think I have left both Masters and the trails in good hands and can now just go and concentrate on the pursuit of M70 Australian age records.

Townsville was a busy running week and I returned with a quad muscle strain. After four days to recover, I flew to Sydney for a six-hour track race that didn't really matter as I was four days short of turning seventy. Overnight, before my flight, John Nuttall had a great run in the Southern Sydney 48-Hour. He set new marks for M70 at six hours, at 100 kilometres and twelve hours before retiring with his job well done.

I took on John's Coburg advice that I needed to go out faster and did just that. I completed the marathon distance in 3 hrs 44 mins and was still feeling fine. My new shoes gouged an agonising chafe across the top of my ankles and I had to change into the pair that had ruined my big toe a year earlier. It happened again and one and

Chapter 23 On trail and track with Christy

a half hours later, I had to stop and change again. I was off the track for six minutes which turned out to be crucial. My heart and lungs were fine right throughout, but niggling leg cramps prevented any heroics in the later stages. Result: fourth with 65.230 kilometres in six hours.

I missed John Nuttall's M65 record by a mere 261 metres, running five kilometres further than last year. Although I couldn't get the record, at age 69 years and 361 days, I had age-graded the best ever by an Australian M65. Performances are impossible to compare over fifty years, but this must be up among my best performances.

M65 six-hour Australian all-time list:
- 2022: Greg Wilson, 65.230 kilometres, age grade 87.171
- 2017: John Nuttall, 65.491 kilometres, age grade 84.027
- 1992: Randall Hughes, age grade, 83.791.

I now had a new bunch of John Nuttall M70 records to pursue, as he had overtaken the last of those held by my old Townsville mate, Peter Lahiff. The 'book end' records look just about impossible for me. They are held by two great runners with whom I competed back in the 1990s. Randall Hughes ran an amazing fifty kilometres in 4 hrs 7 mins, and my arithmetic tells me don't bother. Cliff Young covered 653.600 kilometres in the Colac Six-Day Race in the 1996 as an M70, and that would have won last year's Adelaide Six-Day!

CHAPTER 24
Chasing the records

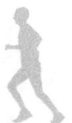

The Australian 24-Hour Track Invitational was the first suitable event for me to attempt a record after turning seventy. The event is held to enable elite ultra runners to achieve personal bests and set records in small fields and ideal conditions. For the first time, they were also holding an Open event on the outside lanes, suitable for the old, new or not so fast to compete in. This is the event Christy and I entered to pursue our respective goals. Christy was no doubt aiming at the tough benchmark of 200 kilometres, while I had a more modest 166.33 kilometres to achieve on legs still recovering from Sydney.

Christy's previous visit to the Australian Institute of Sport's (AIS) track in Canberra was about twenty-five years ago. The seventeen-year-old aspiring 400-metre hurdler completed her gruelling event and promptly bounded up into the stands to chat with her support team. Her coach (Olympian Pam Ryan) asked Christy to turn around and look down onto the track – her opponents were still sprawled on the track in varying stages of exhaustion. This learning experience may well have been to show Christy that she could have put more into the event, but much more likely it was to bring home the depth of her running endurance.

Fast forward to Saturday 2 July 2022 and Christy's second attempt at running for 24 hours a couple of months after debuting with victory in the Victorian 24-Hour Championship at Coburg (running 175 kilometres). With a sensible, conservative start, Christy was able to overcome the bitterly cold conditions and various health ailments to achieve first female (open event) with a personal best of 184.044 kilometres.

The last time I was at the AIS track was in February, when I failed in my belated attempt on Cliff Young's long-standing M65 record for one hundred miles. Moving to the present, in the same event as Christy, it was time for my first serious attempt at records in my new M70 age group. It must be said that if aiming to complete a 24-hour event, it is not a good race plan to attempt a series of records at intermediate distances. Going too hard early is a recipe for much discomfort later; however, if you doubt you can complete the long distance, it would be foolhardy to bypass records along the way. Hence, the plan was to aim for intermediate records, use up petrol in doing so, and whatever happened later was probably going to happen anyway.

Australian M70 age group records set on 2 July 2022:
- 6 hours: 61.777 kilometres, formerly 58.531 (John Nuttall, 2022)
- 50 miles: 8 hrs 32 mins 39 secs, formerly 8 hrs 38 mins 23 secs (Harry Davis, 2014)
- 100 kilometres: 11 hrs 18 mins 15 secs, formerly 11 hrs 42 mins 29 secs (John Nuttall, 2022)
- 12 hours: 105.590 kilometres, formerly 102 kilometres (John Nuttall, 2022).

A brief respite here, as this was really 'job done'. By the time I passed the first record, I was not feeling great and so had a break before resuming at a slower pace. That wasn't going to achieve the tough 50-mile record, so I lifted back to my earlier pace and nabbed it by six minutes. A few slow laps to recover, and then I picked up the pace for a period before taking a brief break. I then settled on three-lap runs and three-lap walks, calculating that this should be enough for me to attain the 100-kilometre and 12-hour records. This proved to be the case as I was able to shave twenty-seven minutes off the 100-kilometre mark and accrue an extra four kilometres for the 12-hour record.

All that effort, and I was still only halfway. It was 8 pm in frigid Canberra and the next record seemed mentally and physically impossible, needing a further ten hours of effort.

Chapter 24 Chasing the records

I walked until I was later informed that I would have to run to be in the ballpark of record times. So I tried running a few laps, but I couldn't go in a straight line and I knew from experience that this was not a good sign. I managed a good period of running three and walking three. The problem now was that both my running and walking pace had deteriorated badly and I needed a new plan. When I couldn't manage a straight line after 326 laps, I steered towards my collapsed tent, wrapped myself in a doona and just lay there.

I could hear crew member Frankie lying straight-faced to Matthew Eckford, the race director, saying, 'Don't worry, it's all part of the plan!' Christy was still out there gamely completing laps, while no doubt feeling as bad as I did. Crucially, the thought niggled away that this was exactly what happened at this stage when I was last in Canberra.

Though I had no plan, I eventually stumbled back out onto the track, having taken 47 mins 50 secs to complete lap 327. I have never spent a night as cold as that one and much of it was spent with many layers of clothing trying to stop the wind cutting through. I got walking, and then I was able to run again.

At Matthew's suggestion, I tried running the straights and walking the bends. I managed to cope with that but I cannot recall doing it for six hours. He asked me if I was aiming at one hundred miles and I replied, 'That is the aim.' The slight difference is that I was talking about a total for twenty-four hours and Matthew was talking about the 100-mile record.

When I had been out there persevering for almost twenty-two hours, I realised that I was going to finish this thing and that the 100-mile record was in reach, even after my break. I hadn't paid much attention to these final two records as they seemed most unlikely. With a few laps to go, it sunk in that I had already passed the 24-hour record mark, so I just walked, smiled, danced around Christy and did enough to ensure I totalled more than 170 kilometres.

Australian M70 age group records set on 3 July 2022:

- 100 miles: 22 hrs 32 mins 30 secs, formerly 22 hrs 39 mins 55 secs (Deryck Skinner, 2005)
- 24 hours: 170.395 kilometres, formerly 166.33 kilometres (Deryck Skinner, 2005).

This achievement would have been the ideal place to complete my running comeback, and this story, as it would be difficult to top. I did train and plan to attain all six records, but the fact that I managed to carry it out seems surreal. It almost came unstuck at record ratification time when a small clerical error was discovered, but I had surpassed the old marks by enough to retain the records. The one record it did cost me was the one I couldn't challenge because I was too old. I narrowly beat Cliff Young's M65 record that still stands from 1988, but the ratification process put me just behind it. Four months earlier, had I kept going ... !

While I was ecstatic at being able to complete a 24-hour run, the year was not over. I had a trip to Townsville for their fiftieth marathon and was not at all sure how it would be affected by my ultra a month earlier. I had three light weeks of training and then hoped for the best.

The marathon started early (4.45 am) to beat the heat, which was a good plan, as with cloud cover keeping the warmth in, it was a humid twenty degrees minimum. There were 160 starters but the conditions caused an abnormally high dropout rate. I set out faster than usual at around five minutes per kilometre and once we all settled in, I was not passed by anyone. In the later stages, I made my way through the field as others slowed due to heat or starting too fast.

I surprised a few, including myself, by finishing twenty-second of 121 finishers in a solid 3 hrs 43 mins 33 secs. I would like to think that if I concentrated on the marathon, was not post-ultra and the weather was kinder, I would give 3 hrs 30 mins a shake. In any case, at the time, my run was rated as the second best in Australia by an M70 for 2022, behind Bob Lane of Western Australia.

On the same October day that Wayne Thompson was bumping me down to third-best seventy-year-old marathoner, I was at Thorndon Park in Adelaide. With some misgivings, I had entered the second six-day race of my life. I took a campervan and enjoyed a stay with my lifetime friends, Ian and Marilyn Leet, pre- and post-race.

I felt a bit of an imposter among all these multi-day runners, as I had come with a much shorter goal. My plan was to attempt the M70 records for 200 kilometres and 48 hours, and anything else was a pipedream. I set up my tent and gratefully shared a gazebo, lent by eighty-year-old competitor, John Timms, who had shared my previous brief attempt at the Colac Six-Day many years earlier. It was interesting being there, absorbing the atmosphere and meeting a whole new bunch of athletes.

Thorndon Park is a lovely spot near the Adelaide Hills and the event is held on a 1.425-kilometre concrete path around a reservoir. It's scenic and traffic free, but pre-race I had misgivings with regards to running on a concrete surface, the weather and the distance. As the laps went by, I soon realised that it would be difficult to break records on this course due to having to ascend ten-metre high 'Thorndon Everest' each lap. Now I enjoy a hill more than most, but they do take energy and slow progress.

I survived through the first night and was in about sixth spot when I made the decision to save myself for another day. Of course, I was tired having been awake all night and running for twenty-two hours, but I had been conservative and could have continued. It is much easier to find a reason to withdraw than to keep going, and you don't know whether you just 'wimped' it!

Chapter 24 Chasing the records

Without bothering to stay and record a 24-hour distance, I retired with a grand total of 136.8 kilometres covered in 22.7 hours. By coincidence, the race leader, Annabel Hepworth, had retired with health problems some time earlier on exactly the same distance. So, if I never do another Six-Day, I can say I dead-heated for last with a champion Six-Day runner. It is still possible that I could have broken the records I was aiming at, but it was an unknown. I was unwilling to put myself through all that effort, perhaps miss the records and then not recover from what I had put my body through. Far better to stop while still in one piece and find a flat and fast track to give myself every chance of success next time. I don't pull out of an event lightly and I wouldn't know if my reasons were valid until I had another record attempt.

There is not a lot I feel the need to achieve, but folk legend Cliffy seemed to have a guardian angel on his records. If my body and fitness allowed it, there were a couple more records to chase before I would be satisfied. They might not be achievable, but at least I would know that I'd tried.

There are the two records that I am unlikely to attempt as they seem out of my reach: the M70 50 kilometres (4 hrs 7 mins, Randall Hughes, 1998) and the Six-Day (653.6 kilometres, Cliff Young, 1993). For the first, I would need to lower my time for the marathon to 3 hrs 30 mins and throw in a few five-minute kilometres, which takes a vivid imagination; one for John Shaw in his comeback, perhaps. The latter M70 record is fourteen kilometres further than the M65 record and would win a six-day race nowadays!

Logic tells me that I should be able to improve on my intermediate records if I raced at just that distance each time. So, there was a six-hour, 12-hour and 24-hour on the wish list. Another factor was that Cliffy had a 100-mile and 24-hour slightly better than my performances, but they were not ratified as records. It would be tough, but I might be able to go beyond them, particularly as I had brief rests, or walks, after achieving my records, when due to the clerical error I hadn't quite arrived!

It was an interesting end to the year, even without any competition runs. In October, a deluge of rain onto already sodden ground caused the nearby Campaspe River to rise rapidly. The river is usually a small sluggish stream at the base of tall banks and seldom breaks them. Within a day, it became a raging torrent and overnight, it almost cut the only access road to my neighbourhood. Some lower-lying sections of Kyneton were not so fortunate, and a week later, downstream towns like Rochester had terrible flooding.

At the start of December, I finally caught Covid and spent a couple of days feeling quite ill. At the same time, I noticed some vision issues that persisted even as my Covid symptoms abated. My GP had me attend

Chapter 24 Chasing the records

the Emergency Department at Bendigo Base Hospital to have the cause of my double vision assessed.

It was awful there as I waited many hours to be seen and a total of forty hours before getting a hospital bed. Then I was kept awake all night by loud and disturbed patients. After investigations, they decided to put me on medication to cure a very rare condition called myasthenia gravis. At the same time, I was prescribed Covid antiviral medication. After a day or two there on medication, I asked to go home where I could find some peace and quiet to recover. This was permitted and the double vision resolved. A week later, my GP informed me that blood tests for myasthenia gravis had come back negative and I ceased taking that medication.

Obviously, I had discovered a new side effect of Covid, and the antiviral medication was what cured my symptoms. After a further week, I eased back into training and was relieved to have no lingering Covid symptoms. All in all, it was a rare visit to our health system for me and a reminder of how quickly your life can change if you are unlucky. For instance, around this time, the Townsville Road Runners lost another club legend when Joe Scott passed away after a long battle with cancer. I was soon back to averaging seventy kilometres a week to be fit enough for my next competition.

In January 2023, I had contact from Barbara MacKay-Cruise who had dreamed up the Around Australia Relay back in 1986. She has written a book about the event and was requesting further input from team members, to give the story a bit more 'oomph'. I spent a few weeks re-typing the surviving copy of my 'book' written back then and forwarded it to her. Some sections may still find their way into print all these years later.

In March, the World Athletics Cross-Country Championships came to Australia for the first time and were conducted at Bathurst, NSW. I was tempted, as there were M70 Masters events as part of it; however, they were only four kilometres. I decided not to tempt fate and just keep training for ultras. Champions John Bermingham and Yassine Belaabed excelled as usual, while Ron Schwebel was very game in doing cross-country, Masters champs and the 48-hour! Using the same rationale, I didn't travel to Sydney for the Australian Masters Track Championships, as they were only two weeks before my first ultra record attempt for the year.

The Sri Chinmoy Australian 48-hour Championship meant another trip to Canberra. The records I had not yet challenged but felt might be achievable for me were the 200 kilometres (Deryck Skinner, 35 hrs 32 mins, 15 secs, 2006) and 48 hours (Cliff Young, 264.8 kilometres, 1993). I had broken Deryck Skinner's shorter records and so felt I could also surpass his 200-kilometre time. However, I had never run that far before and everything had to go right in training and on race day.

Cliffy's 48-hour was a whole different kettle of fish. The longer an event the more difficult it would be to challenge his records, as he had proven a superb multi-day athlete; there was a reason why this record was still standing thirty years after being set. I would need to be well inside Deryck's record to achieve this one. It was only my most recent 24-hour that I regarded as a success and the extra day was a total unknown. All I knew is that it would be difficult.

CHAPTER 25
Record-breaking ultramarathoner

In mid-March, I had a last, long run and then, deciding not to tempt fate, took it easy for a week. In Woodend, I had a coffee and interview chat with local journalist friend Phoebe Hartley as she gathered information for a story in her quarterly *Bush Journal*. The following week, I was still feeling flat and a minor injury was niggling, so I did no running and just hoped it would be okay on the day. A few days before the event was due, Nicole Vaughan put up a Facebook post declaring how lucky fellow Victorian ultra runners Rachel Sykes and Greg Wilson were, as they would be running with the world's best female ultra runner, Camille Herron. That was the first I knew of it.

I spread the drive to Canberra over two days to ensure I arrived fresh. Dinner was at one of Canberra's oldest buildings, The Old Canberra Inn, built in 1860. The next morning, I had a short drive across Bruce from my Airbnb to the AIS track. My new Canberra friends gave

Chapter 25 Record-breaking ultramarathoner

me a hand with my gear and then I registered, chatted a bit and had a relaxed wait for the start of the Sri Chinmoy 48-Hour Australian Championship at 10am. There was little time to get to know my shared crew, Justin Hiatt, who had been advised about me only on race morning! As he had last year's winner, Matthew Griggs, to prepare as well, I just showed him my schedule and another page with a list of instructions.

Camille was nearby and I considered a cheeky selfie with her, but everyone wanted a piece of her, so I left her in peace. Twenty-one of us toed the start line while Robert de Castella gave us some words of wisdom and then sent us off on our journey of discovery.

For the first ten hours, I just ran as I felt and put no pressure on myself. This was about eight to nine kilometres per hour. Meanwhile at the 'sharp end', Camille was consistently lapping in two minutes and building a huge lead on Matthew Griggs, who was also in splendid isolation in second.

Well aware of my vulnerability at fifteen hours, I pre-empted it and chose a brief rest at ten hours. On resumption, I reverted to what had worked last time, running the straights and walking the bends. This reduced my speed to around six kilometres per hour, but it was sustainable and better than walking. I was hugging the inside, as any wide running is not helpful in record attempts.

At some stage, there was a sustained downpour and the track flooded. The drainage couldn't cope and we spent many laps sloshing through inches-deep water, or running wide to find the shallow end. Eventually a sterling job with a squeegee and picking litter from the drain openings improved the situation.

After a period of we 'speed humps' causing problems for Camille and her world record attempt, we were told to move to lane two on the bends if walking. I was not pleased, but my brain must have been still getting enough oxygen. Instead of complying, I just changed to running the bends and walking the straights. Gotcha! I was fully aware of the importance of Camille receiving an unimpeded run, but what I was attempting was pretty important to me! Ironically, my running was not much faster than walking, so I probably remained an obstacle. Really, Camille was causing problems for herself. If she wasn't running so damn fast, she would not have to lap us so frequently. To her credit, she never complained and just kept pounding out two-minute laps.

There was a big change in the race at about eighteen hours. I heard Camille throwing up nearby and within a lap, Matthew Griggs suffered the same fate. Amazingly, Camille went back to her scheduled pace, but unfortunately Matthew had to call it a day a few hours later.

Through all of this, Justin and some relief crew had done a great job of keeping us both fuelled and out on the track, except for breaks of around twenty minutes when needed. At around twenty hours, I asked Justin whether I could break the 100-mile and 24-hour records if I picked up the pace. His response was no, I would need a couple of hours at eleven kilometres per hour. That's what I needed: clear-cut information, save the energy and focus on reaching 200 kilometres.

As I neared the 100-mile mark, I deviated from my sensible race plan. I was not near my record pace but decided I at least wanted to be in the same hour. For five laps, I ran flat out at about 5 mins 25 secs per kilometre and crossed the mark in 22 hours 59 mins 48 secs. I cut it very fine, but job done – now, settle down and get professional again!

I must have totalled about 165 kilometres by the time I reached the 24-hour mark, some five kilometres short of my record for the distance. Niggling in the back of my brain was the thought that it was frustrating to do all this work and not surpass my intermediate records. My focus, though, was firmly set on reaching 200 kilometres for the first time and they would have to wait for another day.

As I set off into the uncharted waters of a second day, the male field received a shake-up. Matthew Griggs had set up a huge lead but was forced to retire from the event. Clear second place James Quaife had battled injury for some hours and after much perseverance, he was also forced to the sidelines. I was having a quick break in the gazebo when Martin Fryer dropped by and informed me that I was the leading male. My immediate response was to compare myself to Steven Bradbury, the Olympian who won when the rest of the field fell over. It was ludicrous and beyond any ambition of mine that as a seventy-year-old, I would be leading in an Australian championship.

My co-inhabitant of the gazebo was a walker that I only knew as 'Joff'. All I knew of him was that he was out in front of David Billett and therefore he must be some sort of walker. As a 'thoroughbred runner', I had no idea of what to make of Joff with his thickset build, tie-dyed T-shirt, bushy beard and kilt, all topped off with a bushman's hat. A little later, Justin asked me what was most important, winning the championship or breaking the records. He stated that at my current pace, Joff was going to overtake me! My immediate answer was, 'The records', an instant clear-cut decision to ignore everyone else and just maintain a schedule that took no risks of injury or illness and achieve the records goal. In the back of my mind, I was wondering why I couldn't win the championship and get the records; common sense told me to listen to Justin and get on with it.

Justin alerted me that in five laps, I would reach 200 kilometres and gain my first record. Somehow, my brain informed me that if I ran absolutely flat out for

Chapter 25 Record-breaking ultramarathoner

five laps, I may be able to sneak the 200 kilometres in under twenty-nine hours. With no other reason except the desire to have a twenty-eight in front of the record time, I took off and managed to get down around five mins 25 secs per kilometre. When I crossed the line, I was overjoyed that the effort had not been wasted and a time of 28 hours 55 mins 32 secs was on the clock. My brain couldn't work it out after that effort, but I knew I had obliterated the Australian M70 record for 200 kilometres (formerly 35 hrs 32 mins 15 secs, Deryck Skinner, 2003).

Okay, refocus! There were still nineteen hours left to complete the event, so what was all that sprinting about? Justin informed me that even my walking pace would see me achieve the Holy Grail of Cliffy's 48-hour record. I found that difficult to believe, but Justin had not told me any fibs so far. I promptly took him at his word and settled into a long walk, during which I was lapped many times by a real walker in Joff.

It was mid-afternoon on my first experience of a Day 2. I still had a long night ahead, and although I felt fine, there was the expectation that my body would just reject what I was putting it through. Hence, the no-risk strategy to ensure I attained the record, even though perhaps I could have gone faster and stayed in one piece.

In all, I totalled one and a half to two hours off the track in lie-downs of under half an hour, and never slept. I trudged on through the long night and was pleased to see the dawn and to still be out there. Not long after, I walked down the back straight as rapturous applause was building for Camille who was following and approaching the line to break the current female world record for 48 hours.

I didn't get to see much as at the time, I was struggling out of my cold-weather walking gear before tottering back out onto the track. It was an instant decision for me to change so that I looked like a runner as I passed Cliff Young's M70 48-hour record. A similar but smaller crowd enthusiastically greeted my achievement, and it was a gratifying moment to achieve my long-strived-for goal.

Then something unplanned and unexpected occurred – I kept on running. I was aware that I still had two-and-three-quarter hours to go, but it felt comfortable. Suddenly I was running at close to Camille's pace. There were a few factors that contributed to my revival: the frustration of having to walk for such a long period, the pleasure of being able to almost match Camille's pace and pulling laps off Joff who had a long lead in the Australian 48-hour Championship. Mainly, though, it was sensational to be carried along by the crowd's enthusiasm and feel like I could finish really strongly and after forty-six hours of circulating, make a record I could be proud of achieving.

I kept it going all the way through to 10 am when a gun sounded and we all retired to strategically placed chairs while measurements were conducted.

Chapter 25 Record-breaking ultramarathoner

- New female world record: Camille Herron, 435.366 kilometres by 23.884 kilometres
- New Australian M70 48-hour record: Greg Wilson, 287.404 kilometres by 22.604 kilometres.

I had another record, Camille had many and Joffrid Mackett had some huge walking records. There were many other fine achievements; for example, Matthew Griggs placing second in the M50 section after pulling out at halfway. That was as crazy as a seventy-year-old finishing second to Joff in the Australian Championship.

Finally, my huge thanks for being an adopted Canberran for the duration. The support and friendship I received had a large influence on my result. Vital, however, was the job performed by crew Justin Hiatt. He took the thinking out of it. I just ran and walked while he kept me fed, watered and motivated. If I stopped, he was soon on my case to get back out there. The way we did it, I was never distressed and always confident of completing my first 48-hour event. Eternal thanks.

At the awards presentation, I had the honour of receiving my trophies from Martin Fryer, who until recently had been the only runner on the all-time top ten list for 48 hours other than Yiannis Kouros. Today, Martin was relegated to fourth all-time by Camille's extraordinary performance.

My Canberran friends assisted my packing up, then Matthew Griggs said, 'Come home and have a sleep.' This was an offer I could not refuse and the following day I was capable of the long drive back to Victoria. There were many facets of the last few days to absorb, but perhaps it is best summed up as: what an experience to be part of Camille's historic run, and to have vindicated my decision to DNF ('did not finish') in the Adelaide six-day, in such spectacular fashion!

Once back in Kyneton, it was straight back into my routine of feeding farm animals, eating, sleeping and waiting and wondering how long it would take for my body to recover. A couple of days later, I travelled to Melbourne to attend the book launch of the biography of running mate Les Williams. I was delighted that Yassine was also in attendance, making it a reunion of the Three Amigos.

My highlight reel was not quite complete yet, though. I was pleased that my 48-hour had been so successful that it might even match my run of records over 24 hours last July at the same track. I had thought it greedy and fanciful that I could reproduce what I had done then.

A few days into my recovery, I received an invitation to be the Australian M70 representative at the Abbott WMM WANDA World Marathon Age Group Championships. My time of 3 hrs 43 mins at the Townsville Marathon had been my only one for the year, and as I didn't have a second qualifier and there were a couple of faster Aussies, this was totally unexpected. Friends urged me to take this opportunity and so, after a few days, I entered the Chicago Marathon and cancelled my entry for the Australian six-day.

If this wasn't enough, a day later I was notified that I was one of five finalists in the Australian Ultra Runners Association (AURA) Ultra Performance of the Year for 2022. It seems my run last July at the Australian 24-hour Invitational was thought highly enough of to have me join four other outstanding performances to be voted on by AURA members.

The performances by Allicia Heron, Phil Gore, Stephen Redfern, Cassie Smith and me cannot be measured against each other in any meaningful way as they are so different. Whatever the final result, I am humbled to be mentioned in such company. It was a cold winter night in Canberra with a small elite field and a smaller group of us in the outside lanes. I was proud of achieving all six available M70 records but wasn't aware that any others had noticed. Many thanks to whoever nominated me and the AURA panel for including my performance.

A few light weeks of training followed, as I tried to balance recovery with being fit enough for my next challenge. The thought of having to complete three-hour-plus training runs was nauseating. Three weeks after the 48-hour, I managed a twenty-five-kilometre run and my feet felt strange. When I checked, there were large flaps of skin detaching from the ball off each foot. Residual damage!

A month post-race was our Run the Rock around

Hanging Rock. I was still warming up when the event started and so my 1 hr 48 mins 5 secs was satisfying, with just one fifty- and sixty-year-old in front at the finish. This year, Christy went in fresh and came away as first female in 1 hr 32 mins, a ten-minute improvement on last year.

While I wasn't awarded Performance of the Year for ultra running, it was an honour to receive the Cliff Young Award for the best single performance by a male over sixty. That was for the Australasian 24-hour Invitational (Open), but I am still not convinced it was my best performance for 2022.

The Southern Sydney Six-Hour was a month earlier. Aged almost seventy, I missed John Nuttall's M65 record by just 261 metres. During the event, I lost at least a kilometre due to having to change shoes twice. Age-graded, this is ranked at the top of the M65 all-time Australian ranking for six hours. The 65.230-kilometre distance that I achieved four days before turning seventy is longer than the best M70 distance recorded in the world.

Although a couple of running friends have mentioned world records to me since I turned seventy, I had never regarded myself near that level. It took me ten months to finally look up the M70 records just to satisfy my curiosity. It was as I thought. For example, I would have to shave 4 hrs 15 mins off my time for one hundred miles. In the 24-hour, my PB in my forties was 188.9

Chapter 25 Record-breaking ultramarathoner

kilometres and I would now, aged seventy, have to run 206 kilometres!

However, at the six-hour distance, there was a scarcely believable anomaly in that the IAU world record for M70 was held by Paul Aillery (France) at 60.994 kilometres. Not only was it a distance I felt I could achieve – I already had! During my 24-hour run, I had covered 61.777 kilometres in the first six hours and then kept going for another eighteen hours. I consulted AURA and they were happy to apply for the record on my behalf. There were superior performances on the German Ultra DUV Statistik site, but at this stage none had been ratified as world records. It would be interesting, and beyond all expectations, to see a positive outcome.

In one month at the Southern Sydney Six-Hour, I would attempt to improve on my Australian M70 record and if I could go close to last year's distance, it would be an undisputed M70 world record.

In mid-May, I made my annual trip to Clifton Hill for the Victorian Masters 10-kilometre Track Championship. I had done no speed work, which was normal for me at that time, but it would be a guide to my recovery and fitness. I was the slowest runner in the fastest of three heats and as such, I just had a twenty-five-lap time trial. In the later stages, Yassine lapped me and I managed to hold on until he kicked for the finish. I was surprised to average 4 mins 18 secs per kilometre, and I recorded my fastest time since winning the Australian Masters in Darwin on my sixty-fifth birthday. Pleased as I was with my effort, it paled into insignificance compared to Yassine's perennial excellence.

Victorian Masters M70 10-kilometre Track Championship result:

1: Yassine Belaabed, 40 mins 55 secs
2: Greg Wilson, 42 mins 39 secs
3: Greg Moore, unknown.

CHAPTER 26
My reasons for running

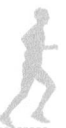

Leading into the Southern Sydney 6 Hour I should have been fighting fit, keen and enthusiastic, but I felt none of that. It often seemed the case that leading up to a big event my usual aches and pains seemed to worsen and I felt the event would be way beyond my capacity. Although I had been in similar form to last year, there was one ingredient missing: I had not been able to coax myself out for any long training runs since the 48-Hour. Camille Herron has a theory, based on her scientific knowledge, that those long runs are not necessary. I would soon find out if that applied to me also. In the meantime, I would just have an easy fortnight and hope that revived my interest in competing.

While I grapple with how much training I can tolerate, while freshening up enough to race well, it's reasonable to reflect on why I run at all. As a child of the 1950s and '60s, sport was one of the few avenues of recreation readily available. Those with the natural talent to gain a place on a sporting team were admired and the rest were left to find something else. Non-selection during my school years had me spending time reading, listening to music and making model aeroplanes.

At Kyneton High School, I ran the cross-country without any training, as all students were told to. Placing second and representing the school was my first experience of performing well in a sport. Kyneton had no athletics club, so during my mid-teens, I took up competitive cycling with some success. I found my weekends of striving for sporting success to be an enjoyable and memorable challenge.

Upon choosing running as my preferred sport, a rapid rise to local and Army sporting fame was achieved. Earning accolades for my sporting prowess was a whole new world for me and I no doubt lapped up the attention. My training increased with a focus on improving my times and results.

Achieving the balance between being as fit as possible and overtraining with resultant injury or illness is a challenge. This is particularly so for an older runner, with the realisation that you cannot achieve the training or results of your younger days. If motivation was all about trophies, personal bests and praise, then a running career would be completed by your mid to late thirties.

There is so much more to running, though, which

keeps me motivated to continue, perhaps for a lifetime. The general health benefits of being among the fittest of your age are considerable. The health issues I have detract from my running, but I am certain that running ensures they have less impact on my quality of life than if I were sedentary.

Then there are the people you meet at training and competition. It is such a pleasure to be mixing with runners who are generally cut from the same cloth. There are the champions who inspire with their natural ability and have the willpower, motivation and training to rise to the top. Many of us then think it worth taking up the challenge of making our own performances the very best they can be. I hope that I am counted in that latter group, as I enjoy doing the best I can, subject to the limitations of my body and mind.

Many friends are out there in training and competition for very different reasons that are just as valid. Those that are not blessed with an efficient 'running body' but overcome weight or health issues to become runners are to be admired. Others enjoy being out in the countryside, enjoying exercise and fresh air while taking in the scenery.

Much of my time in training has been solo for a variety of reasons, but there is much more enjoyment in being in a group with similar background and aspirations. The social aspects are invaluable, and the time spent training just flies by. Then there is a post-workout coffee and chat to be anticipated. I treasure the lifetime friendships formed with fellow runners, from as far back as fifty years ago in Townsville to my more recent Masters, trail and ultra running companions.

A running career and a healthy lifestyle seem to go hand in hand. One complements the other, and there is little room for unhealthy habits such as smoking and drugs. Given a choice, I will always gravitate towards people who share a similar lifestyle. It instils self-confidence and the discipline necessary to achieve optimum performance. There is a grey area we must all find between having confidence in ourselves and becoming an egotist.

Another enjoyable aspect of running is travelling to various events. I am sure I have travelled far less than most, but running has involved me in a few highlights. Having just sustained an injury, attempting two marathons in four days may not have been wise, but the New Zealand experience was well worth it. A trip around the world to orienteer in northern Norway is something I could never have imagined doing. The other trip of a lifetime was running around Australia in relay for three months.

I don't feel that running is an addiction for me, but then perhaps I am not the best judge. I often don't want to run due to illness, injury or being just plain flat from a long event or race. At those times, I generally listen to

Chapter 26   My reasons for running

my body and enjoy the break. However, niggling in the back of my mind is the thought that I shouldn't enjoy not going training in case that becomes habit-forming and I lose my fitness. If it is an addiction, then I had no problem with going 'cold turkey' for a dozen years at the start of the new millennium.

CHAPTER 27
Pie in the sky

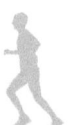

In 1992, I raced in my first ultra marathon that did not involve spending the final sixteen kilometres ascending Mt Buller in Victoria. It was an AURA six-hour track race at Burwood in suburban Melbourne. I won it, recording a touch less than eighty kilometres, with organisers Geoff Hook and Dot Browne announcing that I was now the Australian record holder. I thought that was pretty cool, and perhaps I would do some more of these events.

Within a month, Trevor Jacobs had brought his superior performance to their attention. Then Yiannis Kouros said his was better still and then he had kept going to complete twenty-four hours – couldn't argue with that. Thus ended my brief reign as king!

The next year, I was again victorious, but with just under seventy-five kilometres. I was not as fit and we had to endure a couple of hours of cyclonic conditions, causing most to retire to what tents were still standing

Chapter 27 Pie in the sky

to consume pancakes. That was it for my six-hour career of the last millennium. It was the only distance at which I remained undefeated.

Three years ago my track ultra career was belatedly resurrected in the Southern Sydney 6 Hour Ultra at Barden Ridge. I had come off the trails to attempt John Nuttall's Australian M65 six-hour record. Unfortunately, I had also come off my feet after slipping on a wet tile and spent months carrying an injury after a very heavy fall. Covid restrictions caused a last-minute flight cancellation and a rushed road trip. Alas, I lost my unbeaten record, which was entirely expected, but was disappointed to manage just more than sixty kilometres.

Fast forward a year and I returned by air with better preparation for a final record attempt at age 69.9. I had no expectations, but finished up running one of my best ultras, covering 65.230 kilometres but missing the record by a mere 261 metres. Bother!

So on to 2023 and some unfinished business at Southern Sydney Six-Hour, held this year at Leumeah. Three months earlier, I had completed my first 48-hour event and arrived hoping that I had recovered. I had set a schedule which gave me a chance of equalling last year if all went well. If not, then I would pay for my early heroics but not die wondering.

At the lower end, my ambition was to run further than my previous AURA Australian M70 age record of 61.777 kilometres. Seeing I had then run for another eighteen hours, this didn't seem overly ambitious. 'Pie in the sky' was to be able to exceed sixty-five kilometres, which would see me surpass some pesky non-record performances listed on the DUV Statistik. I had recently discovered the IAU M70 world best performance was 60.994 kilometres, held by Frenchman Paul Aillery.

At 10am, the field of twenty-nine were sent on our way and with a sub-five minutes first kilometre, I settled about sixth. My pace soon settled around 5 mins 20 secs per kilometre, which had me comfortably through the marathon distance in about 3 hrs 50 mins.

My legs then decided the marathon was over, so why was I still trying to run? It became a struggle to maintain the pace and I had to ease off to avoid cramps. It was only in the final half-hour, with the finish line in sight, that I was able to pick up the pace and finish in style. In the latter stages I had been informed by officials that I had surpassed the M70 world best performance. They probably wondered why I kept pushing with everything I had. It was those DUV characters and wanting to surpass as many as possible. In the end, there were two remaining with further distances, one of them only forty-seven metres! They were achieved in 2012 and 2019, so will not be claiming an IAU mark this far along. All in all, the 63.800 kilometres I achieved for a new IAU M70 world best performance was about where I had hoped

Chapter 27 Pie in the sky

to be distance-wise. It is an accomplishment I had never envisaged as the records at other distances vary from 'bloody difficult' to 'impossible'.

After a long drive home, my protesting legs were crying out for a long rest. A few days later, I could manage a walk, and after a week, running was slow and difficult. It was only a fortnight until I returned to Canberra for the Australian 24-hour Invitational (Open). The term 'going to the well once too often' sprang to mind. This, my final ultramarathon for 2023, was a return to the venue where I achieved my sweep of six M70 Australian age group records a year earlier. It was only three weeks since a flat-out six-hour at Southern Sydney and I was still not at all confident that my body had recovered from my exertions there. I had a long drive, followed by dinner with accommodation close to the track.

Race day dawned on a brisk Canberra morning, but this was a big improvement on last year, when rain bucketed down pre-event and then a strong wind blew in from the snowfields. An hour before the start, I caught up with Justin Hiatt who had kindly agreed to crew for me again. His assistance would be vital to a successful record attempt, as it had been during the Sri Chinmoy Australian 48-hour Championship a few months earlier.

I showed Justin the very optimistic schedule I had created to set me on a path to an M70 world best performance for twelve hours. It required me to average

9.5 kilometres per hour for twelve hours, and then I could stop and celebrate or continue at a slow pace for another twelve hours. Below it, I added a few goals that were more realistic and ended up being close to the mark.

The scheduled pace was fine throughout the marathon distance, as I felt relaxed and strong. Shortly after, I was working hard to maintain the pace and I knew a record 12-hour was not possible. Justin had an impeccable record as crew for outstanding performances and I had to find a way to keep that intact and ensure I didn't waste his valuable time. After hour five, I adjusted my goals with a view to improving my M70 Australian age group records for 100 miles and twenty-four hours. I settled into walking the straights and running the bends, which is what had worked last year. What I didn't know, and was about to discover, was whether I could maintain it for nineteen more hours. As race director Matt Ekford had said last year, 'If you want to break records, then walking will not achieve it.'

I had gone through six hours about nine kilometres behind my pace at Campbelltown three weeks earlier and my twelve hours (97.1 kilometres) was more than ten kilometres behind what I had aimed for. I then took a fifteen-minute break to avoid my fifteen-hour collapse of last year. We did the maths and I set off to attempt a better second half than last year. Simple really – all I had to do was continue my routine for another twelve hours

Chapter 27 Pie in the sky

and I would be in record territory in the final stages. Easily said, but it did entail hardly ever stopping and forcing my protesting legs into a run each time I came to a track bend. How long could I sustain it before settling into long periods of walking and resultant failure?

The hard part was from twelve to twenty hours as there was nothing to look forward to except many hours of cold, dark drudgery. If I got through that, I could then envisage attaining a new 100-mile record and two hours later the race finish.

If you don't keep putting fuel in, you grind to a halt – common sense, really. I tried to oblige whenever Justin offered me something; however, my brain and body were telling me that I was going to throw up if I had anything more. The signals were correct and now I had a problem, as there was no point in eating if it wasn't staying down there to get digested. In the final six hours, I cautiously resumed eating and drinking, just hoping that it would stay down. I had been 'banking' an extra kilometre every hour and when assured that I could walk for a bit and still reach my targets, I did so with much relief. Always niggling, though, was, 'Don't get too comfortable doing this, or it has all been for nothing!'

With my eyes on the 100-mile record, I was soon upping the pace again so I could ensure it was as decent a time as I could make it. How did I spend the final laps leading up to a new M70 Australian age group record?

Three laps of walking while nibbling a delicious hash brown I had been offered and then stopping to throw it all back up again. What a waste!

Back to it! Stuff the food and just run some laps to get to a hundred miles. I was pleased to improve my M70 age group record by 44 mins 8 secs by covering the distance in 21 hrs 47 mins 42 secs. It was only a day after the event that I realised I had also surpassed the longstanding M65 record held by Cliff Young. (Unfortunately, I didn't manage it a year earlier when I was in the appropriate age group.) That was better, as a goal had been achieved.

In an hour, the sun would be up for the final stages. Just keep doing more of the same and it might be possible to attain 175 kilometres. All the same, it was now an unusual experience to spend hours running on what almost resembled a skating rink: the track had become moist with dew and had now frozen solid. Wearing multiple layers, it was a constant challenge to stay warm enough while not sweating too much. Head coverings tended to become too warm and yet my ears had to be covered as they were freezing. My thick mittens had become moist with sweat and were now freezing up. *Super domestique* Justin found a heater and soon returned them to me warm and dry.

I continued with as much running as I could manage in the final hour, as the champions in lane one were all inspiring with their solid finishes. Out in lane six,

Chapter 27 Pie in the sky

the early leader, Ayden Boxsell, had been ten kilometres in front of me at the halfway mark. He had never run further than a marathon and now had a PB for 100 kilometres and 100 miles. Even though injured in the second half, he stayed out there at a walk and completed a courageous first 24-hour. Our sole female, Susan Marshall, was flying through the final stages, as she also attained the magical 'Miler' mark.

In my briefing notes to Justin, I noted my 12 Hour schedule was "Pie In The Sky", only be attained if everything went perfectly. I noted that otherwise I would be elated to achieve under twenty-two hours for 100 miles and 175 kilometres in 24 hours. I pushed the last few laps as much as I could, while having no idea of my actual distance, as it was approximately four to five kilometres less than my Garmin watch display. The gun sounded the completion of 24 hours and we rugged up on chairs while the distances were measured. Then it was off to the gazebo to lie down and keep warm until presentation time.

Some extraordinary performances were achieved by runners in the Invitational field. The depth was just what you would hope for in this type of elite event. For me, the superb running by Michael Hooker to attain 260.401 kilometres and a PB for Allicia Heron of 225.428 kilometres, including multiple W35 Australian age group records, were the highlights.

In the Open event, there was proof that the second half was as important as the first. As I remained uninjured and doggedly stayed the course, I won my first event against all ages this millennium. The distance achieved was 175.034 kilometres. With a sensible plan B and an invaluable crew in Justin Hiatt, I had improved my Australian M70 age group record by more than four kilometres. It was pleasing to finally get past Cliffy's non-record achievements after narrowly missing them the previous year.

We were just over halfway through 2023, but that just about wound up my ultra record hunt for another season. I had five weeks to allow my body to recover before my annual trip to Townsville for the marathon. During that period, I needed to decide between the Australian Six-Day in Adelaide and the World Age Group Marathon Championship in Chicago.

CHAPTER 28
A marathoner again

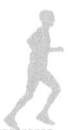

After a week of rest, I managed a couple of tentative weeks of fifty kilometres, culminating in a long run of twenty-five kilometres two weeks before the Townsville Marathon. A very unusual training preparation for my annual marathon, but I have had worse. Now for a couple of easy weeks so I could feel like racing. I had no idea what to expect, as it depended on whether all these ultras had made me fit or flattened me.

Townsville turned on its usual beautiful, dry season weather and I enjoyed catching up with old friends and revisiting some of my favourite spots. Early in the morning after arriving, I did an unplanned twenty kilometres with Gerry Maguire and Brendan Carter, followed up two days later with a brisk 8.8-kilometre Townsville Road Runners club race. A bit risky a week before a marathon, but I got through okay.

For race week, I moved from Ray Clitheroe's home in

suburban Annandale to Brendan's City Oasis Inn to be closer to the action. Townsville Road Runners had a low-key get-together where I joined Karin Thorburn as guest speaker. She was running her four-hundredth marathon! On race morning at 4.15am, I was appreciative of a lift from Brendan to the start area. I had about fifteen minutes spare to soak up the atmosphere, which I did by promptly removing myself for a necessary warm-up jog.

A brisk start had me settle in the top fifty runners, coincidentally feeling comfortable alongside Karin, for the first three loops along the beachfront of North Ward. About halfway, another 'mature' runner caught me and I clicked back up to five minutes per kilometre to keep in touch, in case he was in my age group.

On the long return trip out to Cape Pallarenda, I concentrated on picking off runners as they faded. For the first time in a number of years, I maintained a strong pace right through to the finish line. The ultra running must have been keeping me fit as the time I recorded was only bettered by my comeback run in 2016, 3 hrs 37 mins 16 secs, placing me twenty-eighth of 200 and behind only one runner aged over fifty. The six-minute improvement on last year was a qualifying time for next year's World Marathon Age Group Championships.

The last time I tried to follow up a Townsville Marathon with a big city marathon (in Melbourne in 2018), it was a personal worst time by half an hour. It was

Chapter 28 A marathoner again

a hot day, I was carrying injuries and I missed getting to my start group in time. It was with some trepidation that I signed up for Chicago Marathon. I would fly overseas for a run for the first time this millennium, in the hope that I could perform as well as I did in Townsville.

After recovering from Townsville, I had an injury-free solid month of training. Due to a head cold, I took a cautious approach with little training in the two weeks before my overseas trip, as I hoped to shake it for Chicago. I was off to a bad start when, after the long flight to Los Angeles, my luggage failed to make the connecting flight. There was nothing I could do as, after a swift inter-terminal run, I barely made it myself. In Chicago, I had to wait two hours for the suitcase with my running gear to catch up to me.

By then it was late. I headed directly to my Airbnb in suburban Wilmette. That evening, I met three Spanish guests who were over to watch the marathon. Injury prevented their participation but as they had spent the money, they came anyway. After meeting them, I arranged to share an Uber with them on race morning.

My intention to meet up with some of the other Australian competitors was often thwarted by my inability to communicate. On my only previous long overseas trip, smartphones had not yet been invented, so now I really struggled. I had purchased international roaming but they failed to inform me that it wouldn't work unless I purchased a US SIM card. Also, for some reason, my phone data would not work and it was only when I had wi-fi that I could communicate.

After no sleep on the eighteen-hour plane trip, I again spent a sleepless night due to jet lag and my body clock being out of sync. On Saturday morning, I walked and jogged for three miles to the Wilmette train station, using public transport to McCormick Place where I collected my race packet. The network was large, multi-faceted, confusing and frustrating for a first timer. Once in the city, I just followed a swarm of runners and after a long walk, arrived at the world's largest convention centre.

The Runners Expo was enormous and jam-packed with huge queues for every activity. I collected my race pack and my 'free' T-shirt, which I estimate had cost me near $5000. I decided to save all my remaining energy for race day and after some lunch, I endured the Chicago Transit Authority again. There were still no buses from the station, so it was more 'shank's pony' to get back to my accommodation.

That evening, I explained to my Spanish amigos that an Uber at 4.30 am would be necessary to ensure I was confident of not being late to the start line. I sensed a little hesitance but thankfully they were willing and organised the vehicle. Normally, I struggle to sleep before a race, and Chicago was no exception. I was concerned that three nights of very little sleep would adversely

Chapter 28   A marathoner again

affect my performance. At 3.30 am, I gave up and rose for breakfast and a leisurely preparation.

The Uber had us through the empty streets and into the city in plenty of time and I was deposited onto a footpath jam-packed with runners. I followed the crowd and after a couple of kilometres, located my entrance gate to Grant Park.

In a sea of humanity caused by 49,000 runners congregating in one park, our 2900 World Age Group Championship runners had a large, heated marquee in which to pass the early morning. As our event had stringent qualifying selection standards, it was crowded with fit and very talented athletes from most countries of the world. I relaxed, soaked up the atmosphere and procrastinated about how much clothing to wear.

An hour later, at 6.30, having added a long-sleeved top and gloves to my gear, it was off on a further kilometre walk to the start at corral five where a mass of runners waited. I worked my way towards a 3:40 pacer banner. Once there, I stood shivering in the cold as the clock ticked down, the US anthem was sung and, eventually at 7.30 am, the first corral of elite marathon runners were sent on their way.

Every ten minutes for several hours, another start corral was released. We were fifth in line and so another forty minutes passed until we shuffled around the corner and down to the huge start banner. When the clock counted down, we set off with a huge roar from the spectators. My Chicago Marathon adventure was under way.

With so many runners on the road, passing or being overtaken and frequent drink stations adding to the confusion, I spent my time running smoothly and avoiding accidents. Early on, I noticed a Brazilian lady, Gislene Calligaris, who stood out as efficiently and evenly running at an ideal pace for me. When she was still nearby at five kilometres, I had a few words and we spent the first thirty-five kilometres together. We keyed off each other and pushed each other along. Together, we overtook the 3 hrs 40 mins pacers and later the 3 hrs 35 mins pacers. This was now getting into seriously fast-time territory for the seventy-one-year-old version of me, but it still felt good.

At thirty-five kilometres, we were right on her aim of a Boston Marathon qualifier, and as she was going well, I suggested she kick for home. Soon after, she did so while I maintained the pace I had been on throughout, five minutes per kilometre. Everywhere along the course, there was loud encouragement from walls of supporters and it was great to hear shouts of encouragement for Aussies from them and other competitors.

Up to thirty-five kilometres, I had overtaken four M70 runners; from there on, I worked to maintain the solid pace and not let them come back. There was a long

Chapter 28 A marathoner again

haul up S Michigan Avenue and then a right turn, with the finish banner just a 300-metre climb on S Columbus Drive. I crossed the finish line in 3 hrs 32 mins 43 secs, which was a five-minute improvement on Townsville and a best time since my comeback year of 2016.

My feelings were mixed after the finish. On one hand, I was elated to have run such a strong and evenly paced race. There was also relief that, after all the effort and expense to run in Chicago, I had not wasted it by going too fast early and fading, or the other alternative of not being brave enough and running too slow to bypass problems when the going got tough in the latter stages.

Considering my training, which I considered to be light and lacking speedwork, I am satisfied that I ran the perfect race. When I later saw the results, that I was only 5 mins 26 secs behind the M70 winner, Tom Hutchison of Great Britain (3 hrs 27 mins 17 secs), I had misgivings. Had I concentrated, and survived, heavier and faster training, I may have gone very close. Only two minutes faster and I would have captured third placing. Perhaps, though, it was the ultra running that had me performing as well as I did.

I was placed eleventh M70 in the WANDA World Age Group Marathon Championship. Except for the first two, the remainder of my conquerors were within two minutes of my time. It was such a close and deep race. In the bigger picture, my Chicago Marathon placing was

11,363 in a field of about 49,000. Rough calculations had me coming home in front of 80 per cent of all competitors. On behalf of the top dozen M70 runners, I was very surprised that we were that far up the results.

It would be remiss of me not to mention a couple of unrelated performances that were outstanding. Apart from a world record, a couple of M75 runners broke age group records in brilliant fashion. They were W75 Jeannie Rice (3hr 34 min- World Age Group Record) and M75 Gene Dykes (3hrs 17 mins USA Age Group Record- while winning by about 45 mins!) The race winner, Kelvin Kiptum, also broke the world record with 2 hrs 38 secs. I can add this race to my March 48-hour in which Camille Herron also broke the world record.

After finishing, there was a long walk back to our marquee and there I encountered the only flaw in a superb organisation. The bag check system had been overcome by numbers and lack of volunteers. Hundreds of bags were strewn across the lawn in no particular order, and exhausted runners were getting cold and frustrated when told to search for their warm, dry clothes; I thought that a sit in the warmer marquee and a cup of hot tea would be time better spent. It was a good decision as I spotted my friend from Townsville, Liz Maguire. We enjoyed a chat, and when things died down a bit, located our gear and took off for a shower and change in her nearby hotel room. It is a remarkable coincidence that she also finished eleventh

Chapter 28 A marathoner again

in the W50 in 3 hrs 6 mins 22 secs. As she was aged among the oldest of her group, it was a top effort.

Later in the afternoon, another walk had us on a sightseeing river cruise, gazing at Chicago's architecture. We were joined by Melbourne runner Jane Webb and had such a good conversation going that we heard very little of what the cruise guide said. I then departed to again battle Chicago's public transport system and spend my final night in the city.

I said farewell to my Spanish friends, and my host Edward kindly dropped me at O'Hare Airport before noon, with quite a wait for my evening flight. Just when I was ready to depart, I discovered it was delayed until nearly 11 pm and I would miss the connection to the Melbourne flight. What ensued was a night in a nearby hotel and another long wait at the airport for an evening flight to San Francisco. I was starting to feel like I was in the Tom Hanks movie about a bloke stuck in an airline terminal! In fact, I had already starred beside him in *Castaway* – as a soccer ball!

There was a silver lining, though. As I wandered around the San Francisco terminal, I heard a shout; it was my Eastern Masters clubmate Brad Buyck and his family. Dinner and a chat saw the five-hour stopover pass pleasantly before we boarded for our long flight back home.

*

Upon hearing of the concrete paths and hot, humid weather, I originally decided to bypass the Australian 50-kilometre Championship in November, but a week after returning from a satisfying performance in Chicago, I decided to enter. My rationale was that there were very few races where I could test myself against Randall Hughes' long-standing Australian M70 50-kilometre record of 4 hrs and 7 mins. Logic told me that it was out of my reach, but is that a valid reason not to have a go?

A fortnight later, I was near Woodend attempting my first long training run since Chicago when a runner joined me for a few kilometres. His name was Mick Keating and he is father to Haley and Abby, a couple of ultra runners that I know. He seemed to run quite well and he mentioned that he was meeting his daughters at the Campaspe parkrun in a few weeks to celebrate turning seventy. I replied that it was a week before my Gold Coast run but I would join in the celebrations.

On the final weekend of October, I duly turned up for my third Campaspe parkrun, thinking I would probably run along with Mick. Nup! Whiteline fever struck and I was out there pursuing the leaders. After a solid run, I crossed the line in third place with a time of 21 mins 23 secs and age graded at a respectable 83.23 per cent. Had I managed that a few years ago, I would have set the inaugural age graded record. Unfortunately, over the years, the goal posts have moved and recently a

Chapter 28 A marathoner again

sixty-year-old Tony Kelly set a new mark of 85.87 per cent. My birthday present for Mick was that I prevented him from setting a venue M70 record!

A week later, I was up at the Gold Coast staying a couple of nights with an old ultra mate from the 1990s, Kelvin Marshall. Now, Kelvin loves a run so much he makes me seem like a 'weekender'. Though a dozen years younger than me, he is a legend at events as varied as the Melbourne Marathon, Six Foot Track Marathon (44.5 km trail), Gold Coast 50-kilometre, and until recently, he was the only runner to complete every Maroondah Dam 50-kilometre Trail Ultra. Glenn Lockwood joined us from Sydney so there were plenty of running anecdotes to share pre-race.

I have used the sayings 'let's not die wondering' and 'once too often to the well' before and they provide an apt summary of my final race of 2023. I knew it was warm and humid even this early, but my record pace was 4 mins 55 secs per kilometre. I thought, let's see what that feels like and hang back a little from the four-hour pacer, but keep him in sight. Wrong! He went out way too hard and I was ten seconds too fast through each early kilometre. I was through ten kilometres in 48 mins 17 secs and knew that my race was over in a competitive sense.

My pace eased back shortly after and my next ten kilometres was passed in 54 mins 43 secs. However, you can't turn time back, the damage was done and the sun was beating down and reflecting off the white concrete. I decided that it was a long way to come and pull out, so I switched to survival mode and spent the next twenty-five kilometres alternating walking and running. With five kilometres to go, I worked out that if I picked up the pace, I might finish in under five hours. My final two kilometres were back on record pace as I stormed up the finish chute to record 4 hrs 59 mins 35 secs and one-hundred-and-sixty-first position. Now, that's cutting it fine!

A post-race massage was welcome. By that time, Kelvin was back, having just beaten six hours for three-hundred-and-twenty-eighth in 5 hrs 55 mins 29 secs. Glenn was pretty much on schedule with his 6 hrs 20 mins 25 secs for three-hundred-and-fifty-ninth placing. As we made a weary journey to the car, I threw a casual 'I suppose I won my age group' to Kelvin and he consulted the phone. 'Not even close' was the stern reply.

Ron Peters had two things in his favour: he was an acclimatised Queenslander and he is a champion. Even his masterclass of seventy-third in 4 hrs 26 mins 20 secs couldn't get close to Randall Hughes' time of 4 hrs 7 mins from last millennium. The only other time I was in a race with Ron was the 2001 World Veterans Marathon Championship in Brisbane. While he was sublime winning the M45 World Championship (2 hrs 32 mins 58 secs), I went too hard early, was injured, unfit and

Chapter 28 A marathoner again

cramping almost half an hour behind. It seemed not a lot had changed!

It would be remiss of me not to record the first placegetters. Dean Edmonds won in 3 hrs 14 mins 7 secs, but the amazing performance was from second-placed Marnie Ponton. In the hot conditions, she managed to break the Australian female record with 3 hrs 15 mins 46 secs.

*

A day later after a badly needed sleep in my own bed at Kyneton, it is perhaps an appropriate time to finish this story with a final few words, and forward it to the publisher. That's not to say my running career is completed, nor my life story. I intend to live each day to the full, as none of us know how long we have. While I can set running goals and achieve them, I will pursue the challenge.

For next year, there are two that stand out. In April 2024, I'll return to Southern Sydney for my second 48-hour. I feel that 300 kilometres is possible for me and that would place me second-fastest behind the incomparable world best performance holder Radi Milev of Bulgaria (316 kilometres).

The other is the Australian Six-Day in Adelaide where I will see if at my third attempt, I can make it to day two and beyond. I have no idea how my body and mind will tolerate running for this period, but the challenge is there to be overcome. The prize at the end is the remaining record held by Cliff Young. At Colac, thirty-two years ago, the Aussie folk legend ran a total of 653.600 kilometres in six days and it has been unconquered in the intervening years. Then I could really retire, satisfied that all my running goals had been achieved.

But probably will not!

CHAPTER 29
Male Ultra Runner of the Year — 2023

Having an autobiography published is similar to an ultramarathon in that it takes quite a period of time to reach the finish line. Hence, we are still in the process and early in 2024, it is time for a further update on my running life.

I shall begin with an update on my sideline hobby as a very small time racehorse owner. Late in 2023, the bonny mare that I named Funny Money had recovered from a throat operation and I was anticipating a successful return to the racetrack for her. In a democracy, the majority rule and it was decided to put her in an online auction with a $20,000 reserve. The highest bid was less than a quarter of that and so her comeback trail continued.

I could see the writing on the wall, though, and I decided to take a share in a 'recycled' Sydney gelding called Seneschal. He was moved on as a last start winner from four outings, when considered not up to Sydney city class. Stuart Kendrick purchased him as an ideal horse for the more relaxed environment at the Sunshine Coast.

By February, Seneschal had two starts and looked promising at unsuitable short distances and Funny Money had trailed twice, the most recent being a dashing six-length win, while under no pressure. They were both due to race in Queensland mid-month and I considered attending until I priced the last minute airfares. Their respective fates just show the ups and downs of the racing industry.

Seneschal started long odds in a Brisbane 1600 metre event and, ridden perfectly, won clearly, to double his career prize money in one go. On the other hand, my favourite flying filly was found to be lame in her stall on race morning. A few days later, Funny Money was diagnosed with a fracture of her splint bone, causing her retirement to stud via the online auction.

Meanwhile, I had recovered from the Gold Coast race and resumed training with a view to running in the Australian 100 Kilometre Championship, scheduled for Canberra in mid-February. Within a couple of weeks, I developed some pain in my right knee. Having curtailed my prime of life running career with a similar problem, I was most wary of pushing on. I dramatically cut my training load with a view to making it to the start line, at the cost of being fully fit.

chapter 29   Male Ultra Runner of the Year — 2023

During this period, I saw a disturbing report on social media that was soon confirmed as fact. Kelvin Kiptum, who set a new World Record for the marathon in Chicago, had died in a motor vehicle accident. It does give one pause to be plodding around in your seventies and have the man who was to be the first under two hours for the marathon die so young. I reflected on what my non-running father could have achieved in life had he not died in a similar way at only thirty-two.

On the day I set off for Canberra, I noticed a phone text, requesting a call back. Thinking 'scam' I leisurely fed the boer goats at Fran's nearby farm, before noticing it was from an ultra event race director and friend, Matthew Ekford. With me thinking, 'I am sure I submitted the entry paperwork (belatedly) for his April 24 Hour,' I returned his call.

Matthew informed me that I had been chosen by the Australian Ultra Runners Association as the Male Runner of the Year — 2023. My reaction was to say that can't be correct as I wasn't even on the shortlist of five finalists. Once we established that panel was for a separate popular vote by AURA members, he said I had been chosen by the committee, due to my series of M70 Australian Age group Records and achieving a new World Best Performance at 6 Hours.

Somewhat in shock at being chosen by the AURA committee, I understood that the announcement would be made in coming days and I understood that I should 'keep it under my hat' until then. After thanking Matthew, I took a few moments of reflection to absorb the news. While on a personal level I was satisfied my M70 record chase had been very successful, that is very different to having those achievements weighed against many other younger and highly talented athletes.

No one can predict the future but it is highly unlikely that I will have another year of running up to the standard of the past two. It is realistic to acknowledge that age and injury will have an impact, while I continue to do the best I can with what I have on the day. News of this award and recognition by my peers as to the quality of my performances is most satisfying. I can only hope that as my time in the spotlight fades, it may inspire others to continue running into their twilight years.

The Sri Chinmoy 100 Km was timed to run overnight to escape potentially hot summer conditions, so I decided on a leisurely drive up the Hume Highway over two days. I had arrived in rural Tarcutta where I found a quiet spot to camp for the night. I parked on a dead-end road near the local rubbish tip and camped on a peaceful hilltop in nearby bush.

I seldom sleep well the night prior to a race and this evening proved no exception. Laying there awake, I could hear voices and see torchlight flickering through the trees. Reluctantly, I dressed and set off down the track to find

chapter 29   Male Ultra Runner of the Year — 2023

out what was going on. The first thing I heard was, 'At least we can let down all the tyres'. I soon pressed the unlock button on my keys and was rewarded with the sight of flashing lights and panicked feet running away from confrontation.

The rest of my night was spent driving my car to a safe area and then walking all the way back up to my camp site, before lying there mostly awake, my thoughts bouncing between annoyance that I had a further sleepless night ahead, to relief that I was not stuck in Tarcutta with four flat tyres. There followed an uneventful easy drive to Canberra for a race start near Lake Burley Griffin at 5 pm.

The weather gods had been kind and though the sun was warm, some lower cloud showed promise of heat not being an issue. Though I had given myself plenty of preparation time, I ran a bit short after assisting Annabel Hepworth in erecting her new tent, a process about which we both knew very little. There was just time for a warmup and toilet visit before the race briefing.

Well almost, as the crowd had gathered and I heard friend Yiannis advising me to get myself down there, as the announcer was calling for me. It seems Simone, the President of AURA, had a couple of delayed award presentations to make prior to the event starting. I was presented with the Cliff Young Award for 2022 'For the greatest single best ultra running achievement by a male over the age of 60'.

There followed presentation of International Association of Ultrarunners' certificates for my M70 World Best Performances over six hours in 2022 and 2023. Finally the event timer and former champion Martin Fryer was awarded a certificate for an Australian Age Group record from 2012, which had been set overseas and not previously awarded.

No pressure then to just come out and settle into a sensible race plan! There were relay runners all over the place setting off very rapidly and among them younger 100 kilometre stars out for the championship. Of course, I was sucked into starting too quickly, but I was aware of the danger and soon adjusted my pace to something more sensible. Well more sensible than at the Gold Coast, but then this was twice as far.

I flowed along at record-breaking pace, feeling great for around thirty-five kilometres, until just as suddenly I realised I would have to dramatically slow, or I was not going to complete the course. I hoped by doing this I would not have to walk before reaching the halfway mark, but that proved futile. Not even halfway and I was walking, nauseous and considering abandoning the race. At forty-five kilometres I crossed the timing mat and was then turning back to my tent when Martin said I couldn't as I would muck up the timing. So I was committed to another five-kilometre lap which would mean a fifty-kilometre time some forty minutes slower than I ran at the Gold Coast.

chapter 29 Male Ultra Runner of the Year — 2023

This time I veered off to my mattress as I approached the finish line ... I wasn't going to fall for that again! I spent fifteen minutes lying there and was just resuming with a grand total of six hours for my first fifty kilometres, when I heard the announcer Simone questioning where I had got to. I had also changed my shoes and shorts to relieve some pain issues.

I managed another twenty kilometres of running before I had to mix in some spells of walking, but at least now I was close enough to realise I could make the finish. There was nothing to prove so I could have just kept walking, but I really wanted to lie down and so I ran the final seven kilometres to hurry it along.

My final time for the hundred kilometres was just under thirteen hours and I should have been disappointed at being so far off record pace. However, all you can do is prepare the best you can and give it your best shot on the day. I did that and understand that the risk in running at record pace is spectacular failures when it doesn't come off. Having said that, I was the first Over70 competitor, in a field of ... err ... one!

Sometime during the night while I was busy, an amazing M50 athlete, Wayne Spies, was winning the event, defeating most of the relay teams and setting a new World Best performance for his age. Sorry I missed it.

My usual crewing mate Justin had been in a winning two-person mixed relay and then helped me pack. I managed the long drive home so I could have an undisturbed night of sleep. By the time I got back online, the 2023 AURA award winners had been announced and I was officially AURA Male Runner of the Year — 2023. Sore legs, tired, slow, but very satisfied with my running comeback, and especially in the last two years.

What follows will be the events I have earlier mentioned, hopefully performed at a sensible pace, if I am not in record hunting shape. To enjoy life in the company of friends, stay fit and healthy and if the occasional race achievements occur, then so much the better.

www.ingramcontent.com/pod-product-compliance
Lightning Source LLC
Chambersburg PA
CBHW030538080526
44585CB00012B/193